Quinones: A Privileged Moiety for Drug Discovery

Edited by

Ashutosh Kumar Dash

R & D, Drug Discovery Division
Macleods Pharmaceuticals, India

&

Deepak Kumar

Department of Pharmaceutical Chemistry, School of
Pharmaceutical Sciences, Shoolini University, Solan-173229,
Himachal Pradesh, India

Quinones: A Privileged Moiety for Drug Discovery

Editors: Ashutosh Kumar Dash & Deepak Kumar

ISBN (Online): 979-8-89881-027-6

ISBN (Print): 979-8-89881-028-3

ISBN (Paperback): 979-8-89881-029-0

Published by Bentham Science Publishers Pte. Ltd. Singapore, in collaboration with Eureka Conferences, USA. All Rights Reserved.

First published in 2025.

need for a court order if at any point you breach any terms of this License Agreement. In no event will any delay or failure by Bentham Science Publishers in enforcing your compliance with this License Agreement constitute a waiver of any of its rights.

3. You acknowledge that you have read this License Agreement, and agree to be bound by its terms and conditions. To the extent that any other terms and conditions presented on any website of Bentham Science Publishers conflict with, or are inconsistent with, the terms and conditions set out in this License Agreement, you acknowledge that the terms and conditions set out in this License Agreement shall prevail.

Bentham Science Publishers Pte. Ltd.
No. 9 Raffles Place
Office No. 26-01
Singapore 048619
Singapore
Email: subscriptions@benthamscience.net

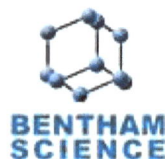

CONTENTS

Santosh Kumar Rath and *Ashutosh Kumar Dash*

PREFACE

Quinones constitute a major class of organic compounds that contain conjugated cyclic dione structures prevalent both in natural as well as synthetic organic chemistry. Naturally, quinones are rich in angiosperms, fungi (including lichens), bacteria, algae, ferns, conifers, sponges, *etc.*, and also in human beings. Hence, a lot of traditional Asian therapies include quinone as Ayurvedic medicine. These can be frequently accessed from reactive aromatic compounds, such as phenols or catechols, very easily. The topic "Quinone derivatives as drug candidates" is a vital point of discussion as they have a unique property to bind to multiple targets with excellent affinity. They are electrophilically reactive and covalently bind to nucleophilic sites within cells through the formation of oxidized cellular macromolecules, including lipids, proteins, and DNA. Hence, we can consider it as a privileged moiety for potential pharmacological activities. Due to its high redox ability, semiquinone radical can construct ROS (reactive oxygen species). Quinones are cast-off for electron and proton transport (Co-enzymes/ Cofactors) and are extremely tunable and versatile in function. With regard to biological activities, quinones and their derivatives have been proclaimed as antitumor, antibacterial, antifungal, antiviral, antimalarial, anti-AD, and anti-epileptic agents. They have various mechanisms of action for biological activities, including ROS, GSH, NADPH, P450s, (COX-2), glutathione S-transferase (GST), (NQO1), DNA, *etc.*, as receptors. If we collect quinone containing marketed drugs, we will get n-number. Some of them are Atovaquone, Flaviolin, buparvaquone, Seratrodast, doxorubicin, Emodin, mitomycins, Duroquinone, Mitoxantrone, Porfiromycin, Parvaquone, Valrubicin, *etc*. Quinones assist as indicators that transform in physical presence, hence used as dyes. The negative side of quinone is also an important point of discussion, such as toxicity profile (quinone toxicity can arise because of their use as well as by the metabolism of other drugs and various environmental toxins or dietary constituents). Quinones as drugs can also considered for organisms other than human beings, such as plants. Antifungal drugs include Chlonil, chlorothalonil, *etc*. Some napthoquinones (Duniones) have been marketed as insecticides, pesticides, *etc*. Some drug-like molecules containing quinones are under FDA approval, *viz* vatiquinone from PTC Therapeutics, which will be used against epilepsy. The modern trends of quinones are discussed as a concluding chapter of the book.

Ashutosh Kumar Dash
R & D, Drug Discovery Division
Macleods Pharmaceuticals, India

&

Deepak Kumar
Department of Pharmaceutical Chemistry
School of Pharmaceutical Sciences, Shoolini University
Solan-173229, Himachal Pradesh
India

List of Contributors

Adil Ali	Department of Biotechnology, Parul Institute of Applied Sciences and Research and Development Cell, Parul University, Vadodara 391760, Gujarat-India
Ankit Paul	Department of Biotechnology, Parul Institute of Applied Sciences and Research and Development Cell, Parul University, Vadodara 391760, Gujarat-India
Ashutosh Kumar Dash	Senior Research Scientist (R&D), Drug Discovery Division, Macleod Pharmaceuticals Ltd, Mumbai, India
Deepak Kumar	Department of Pharmaceutical Chemistry, School of Pharmaceutical Sciences, Shoolini University, Solan-173229, Himachal Pradesh, India
Divyani P. Patel	Department of Chemistry, Government College Daman (Affiliated to Veer Narmad South Gujarat University, Surat), Daman, U.T. of Dadra & Nagar Haveli and Daman & Diu, Gujarat 395007, India
Hiyashree Sharmah	Department of Pharmaceutical Chemistry, NETES Institute of Pharmaceutical Science (NIPS), Nemcare Group of Institution, Mirza, Kamrup Assam 781125, India
Lokman Ali Ahmed	Department of Pharmaceutical Chemistry, NETES Institute of Pharmaceutical Science (NIPS), Nemcare Group of Institution, Mirza, Kamrup Assam 781125, India
Mohd Hasan Mujahid	Department of Biotechnology, Parul Institute of Applied Sciences and Research and Development Cell, Parul University, Vadodara 391760, Gujarat-India
Priyanku Pradip Das	Department of Pharmaceutical Chemistry, School of Pharmaceutical Sciences, Shoolini University, Solan-173229, Himachal Pradesh, India
Ramesh Kumar	Department of Chemistry, Kurukshetra University Kurukshetra, Haryana 136119, India
Ram Sagar	Glycochemistry Laboratory, School of Physical Sciences, Jawaharlal Nehru University, New Delhi 110067, India
Rajendra Dighe	KBHSS Trust's, Institute of Pharmacy, Malegaon, Maharashtra, India
Ritu Gilhotra	Gyan Vihar School of Pharmacy, Suresh Gyan Vihar University, Jaipur, Rajasthan, India
Satish Kumar Singh	Department of Chemistry, Government College Daman (Affiliated to Veer Narmad South Gujarat University, Surat), Daman, U.T. of Dadra & Nagar Haveli and Daman & Diu, Gujarat 395007, India
Satyanarayana Battula	Department of Chemistry, Central University of Jammu, Jammu & Kashmir, 181143, India
Shashikant Bhandari	AISSMS College of Pharmacy, Pune, Maharashtra, India
Suryakant R. Rode	Jai Research Foundation Valvada, Valsad, Gujrat, India
Santosh Kumar Rath	School of Pharmaceuticals and Population Health Informatics, Faculty of Pharmacy, DIT University, Dehradun, Uttarakhand-248009, India

Sunil Sharma

Glycochemistry Laboratory, School of Physical Sciences, Jawaharlal Nehru University, New Delhi 110067, India

Tarun Kumar Upadhyay

Department of Biotechnology, Parul Institute of Applied Sciences and Research and Development Cell, Parul University, Vadodara 391760, Gujarat-India

Vivek Vivek

Amity Institute of Click Chemistry Research and Studies, Amity University Uttar Pradesh, Noida 201313, UP, India

Yogesh Yadav

Glycochemistry Laboratory, School of Physical Sciences, Jawaharlal Nehru University, New Delhi 110067, India

CHAPTER 1

Importance of Quinones in Drug Discovery

Priyanku Pradip Das[1], **Hiyashree Sharmah**[2], **Lokman Ali Ahmed**[2], **Ashutosh Kumar Dash**[3,*] and **Deepak Kumar**[1,*]

[1] *Department of Pharmaceutical Chemistry, School of Pharmaceutical Sciences, Shoolini University, Solan-173229, Himachal Pradesh, India*

[2] *Department of Pharmaceutical Chemistry, NETES Institute of Pharmaceutical Science (NIPS), Nemcare Group of Institution, Mirza, Kamrup Assam 781125, India*

[3] *Senior Research Scientist (R&D), Drug Discovery Division, Macleod Pharmaceuticals Ltd, Mumbai, India*

Abstract: Quinones, which are cyclic chemical molecules, have attracted considerable interest in the field of drug discovery because of their wide range of pharmacological effects and structural flexibility. This study examines the diverse functions of quinones in several therapeutic domains, encompassing their antioxidant, anti-diabetic, anti-inflammatory, anti-Alzheimer, and antibacterial properties. Having redox activity means that quinones can change important signalling pathways and create reactive oxygen species (ROS). This makes them effective against cancer cells and also protects against damage caused by oxidative stress. In preclinical studies, both natural and artificial quinone derivatives have publicised promising results. They act as antioxidants, getting rid of free radicals and stopping lipid peroxidation. Moreover, quinones have shown promise in the treatment of diabetes by blocking crucial enzymes and decreasing high blood sugar levels after meals. Quinones have anti-inflammatory properties because they are involved in the diminution of pro-inflammatory mediators and reduce oedema volume. Quinone derivatives have demonstrated reduction of β-amyloid aggregation, acetylcholinesterase activity, and monoamine oxidase in Alzheimer's disease research, suggesting them as possible multitarget-directed ligands for Alzheimer's disease treatment. Quinones also have antibacterial action against a variety of harmful microorganisms, indicating that they have the potential to tackle infectious disorders. Overall, quinones and their derivatives represent attractive possibilities for drug development across diverse therapeutic domains, emphasising their importance in advancing pharmaceutical research and solving unmet medical needs.

Keywords: Quinone, drug, drug discovery, disease.

* Corresponding author Ashutosh Kumar Dash and Deepak Kumar: Senior Research Scientist (R&D), Drug Discovery Division, Macleod Pharmaceuticals Ltd, India and Department of Pharmaceutical Chemistry, School of Pharmaceutical Sciences, Shoolini University, Solan-173229, Himachal Pradesh, India; E-mails: ashutosh.dash10@gmail.com and guptadeepak002@gmail.com

INTRODUCTION

The quest for novel therapeutic agents to address the myriads of human ailments necessitates exploration into diverse chemical classes. Quinones, owing to their unique structural attributes and pharmacological properties, have garnered considerable attention in drug discovery endeavours. Quinones exhibit a wide array of biological activities, making them versatile candidates for drug development [1, 2]. Quinones are capable of interacting with various cellular components, such as proteins and enzymes, due to their redox activity, thereby influencing essential signalling pathways. Furthermore, their ability to undergo redox cycling makes them effective generators of reactive oxygen species (ROS), which can induce cytotoxic effects in cancer cells. Additionally, quinones possess intrinsic antioxidant properties, enabling them to scavenge free radicals and alleviate oxidative stress-induced damage. This dual functionality of quinones, serving both as prooxidants and antioxidants, highlights their intricate role in cellular homeostasis and the pathogenesis of diseases [3]. It is well documented that quinone moiety in vitamins K_1 and K_2 is chiefly responsible for various biological activities [4]. Furthermore, quinones have been implicated in the inhibition of key enzymes involved in disease progression, such as topoisomerases and kinases, highlighting their potential as therapeutic agents. In addition to their direct pharmacological effects, quinones can also serve as versatile pharmacophores for drug discovery [5]. Quinones play multifaceted roles in cellular processes and pharmacology. Acting as electron carriers in cellular respiration and oxidative phosphorylation, they facilitate energy production. Additionally, quinones act as electrophiles, forming covalent bonds with nucleophilic residues in target proteins, a mechanism commonly exploited in designing enzyme inhibitors. Moreover, they participate in Michael addition reactions, enabling the conjugation of biologically active moieties to the quinone scaffold, thus imparting additional pharmacological properties. Beyond pharmacology, quinones are indispensable across scientific domains serving in electron transfer and photochemical processes with applications ranging from catalysts to energy storage [6]. Found abundantly in nature, sourced from plants, animals, bacteria, and fungi, they serve as building blocks for various technological advancements [7, 8]. In the pharmaceutical industry, quinone derivatives are crucial in drug development, offering promising pharmacological effects, including anticancer, antioxidant, antimicrobial, and anti-inflammatory activities. They form a major class of anticancer cytotoxins. One example is daunorubicin, which is antileukemic [9]. Additionally, in herbal medicine, quinone derivatives contribute to remedies for ailments, such as purgative (sennosides), antimicrobial and antiparasitic (rhein and saprorthoquinone, atovaquone), anti-tumor (emodin and juglone), and anti-cardiovascular disease (tanshinone), as well as in the inhibition of PGE2 biosynthesis (arnebinone and arnebifuranone). Furthermore, the natural world offers intriguing discoveries, such as *Malbranchea cinnamomea*, a thermophilic fungus capable of producing quinone antibiotics, highlighting the potential for novel pharmaceutical interventions derived from these compounds [10].

Quinones and their derivatives are essential and adaptable compounds that have far-reaching implications across scientific fields. Their multifaceted characteristics, spanning from fundamental chemical processes to advanced medical applications, underscore their enduring significance in advancing knowledge and meeting societal needs. In drug discovery, their wide-ranging biological activities, redox capabilities, structural flexibility, and potential as pharmacophores offer promise for creating innovative therapies for diverse diseases, including cancer, infectious diseases, and neurodegenerative disorders. Consequently, quinones remain pivotal in shaping and innovating various disciplines, showcasing their profound influence on both science and society.

CHEMISTRY OF QUINONE

Quinones constitute a group of cyclic organic compounds featuring a six-membered unsaturated ring where two oxygen atoms are bonded as carbonyl groups [11]. Quinone-based compounds exhibit thermal stability due to their aromatic ring structure, which enables them to maintain their integrity under heat. These compounds display reactivity because of the electron-rich regions present within their molecular structure. Additionally, the inclusion of oxygen atoms as heteroatoms enhances their reactivity against disease-causing microorganisms. Their ring structure being electron-rich allows them to undergo electrophilic substitution reactions, while the ketonic carbonyl carbon's electron deficiency adds to their versatility. This dual nature makes quinones highly active and promising candidates for fighting various disease conditions. Moreover, their propensity to undergo tautomerization, transitioning between quinone and hydroquinone forms, contributes to their variability in properties and reactivity [12]. When quinones are combined with heteroatoms like nitrogen, halogens, or sulphur to create medicinal compounds, they tend to exhibit enhanced bioactivity compared to standard molecules. The presence of these heteroatomic groups on the quinone structure introduces electron-donating or electron-withdrawing effects through resonance and inductive effects. This alters the reactivity of the compound, consequently influencing its pharmacokinetics and pharmacodynamics [13]. According to the Hammett equation concept, these effects lead to qualitative and quantitative changes in the activity of the compounds. Such changes in activity are attributed to variations in the sigma and rho values of the additional groups present in the compound, as well as their positioning and stereochemistry [14].

Among these, the quintessential representative is 1,4-benzoquinone, also known as p-benzoquinone, benzoquinone, or cyclohexadienedione, commonly referred to as "quinone", from which the class derives its name. Notable counterparts include 1,2-benzoquinone,   1,4-naphthoquinone,   and   9,10-anthraquinone.   1,4-Benzoquinone, with a melting point of 116°C, exhibits a yellow coloration and has a molecular formula of $C_6H_4O_2$ with a molecular weight of 108.09 g/mol. 1,2-Benzoquinone, also known as ortho-benzoquinone, is a red volatile solid with a melting point of 70°–80°C (with decomposition), and its molecular formula is $C_6H_4O_2$. 1,4-Naphthoquinone, with a melting point of 128.5°C, is yellow and has a molecular formula of $C_{10}H_6O_2$ with a molecular weight of 158.15 g/mol. Anthraquinone, having a molecular formula of $C_{14}H_8O_2$ and a molecular weight of 208.21 g/mol, displays a red coloration and a melting point of 286°C [15, 16].

PREVIOUS STUDIES ON QUINONES ANTIOXIDANT

Antioxidants are chemical substances that reduce the process of lipid oxidation reaction in food systems. Antioxidants are, by definition, compounds that prevent oxidation or inhibit processes that are facilitated by oxygen or peroxides. A large number of these molecules are used in diverse products as preservatives. According to biological definitions, antioxidants are artificial or natural materials added to goods to stop or slow down the degradation caused by airborne oxygen. As an illustration, consider enzymes or other organic materials like vitamin E or β-carotene. Antioxidants attach themselves to free oxygen radicals to stop them from harming healthy cells [17].

Muhammad *et al.* synthesised and demonstrated the antioxidant property of 2,6-di-tert-butyl-4-(4-methoxybenzylidene)cyclohexa-2,5-dien-1-one (**1**), as shown in Fig. (**1**). Compound **1** was tested *in vitro* and exhibited good antioxidant properties in DPPH, ABTS, and FRAP assay with percentage inhibition of 87.32 ± 0.17, 99.39 ± 0.44, and 0.731, respectively, at a concentration of 25 μg/ml [18]. Natural sources are prime sources of quinones, as demonstrated by Triveleka *et al.*, who isolated two quinone metabolites, namely 2-octaprenyl-1,4-hydroquinone (**2**) and 2-(24-hydroxy)-octaprenyl-1,4-hydroquinone (**3**), as shown in Fig. (**1**), from the sponge *Ircinia spinosula*, along with a series of synthetic derivates, and tested them for antioxidant activity. Metabolite **3** exhibited a strong effect against lipid peroxidation with an IC_{50} value of 220 μM [19]. Similarly, Cai *et al.* isolated five new quinone derivatives from *Chirita eburnean*, namely (R)-7-hydroxy-R-α-dunnione   (**4**),   (R)-8-hydroxy-R-α-dunnione   (**5**),   (R)-7,8-dihydroxy-R-α-dunnione (**6**), (R)-7-methoxy-6,8-dihydroxy-R-α-dunnione (**7**), and 1,7-dihydroxy-2-hydroxym-ethylanthraquinone (**8**), along with seven known compounds. Among these, compounds **6** and **7** exhibited DPPH radical scavenging ability, with IC_{50} of 124.82 ± 8.4 μM and 45.72 ± 3.6 μM, respectively, compared to 86.91 ± 6.8 µM for ascorbate [20]. Synthetic derivatives of quinones are very promising antioxidants, as demonstrated by Berghot *et al.*, who synthesised a series of novel naphthoquinone derivatives from 2,3-dihydro-2,3-epoxy-1,4-naphthoquionone. Among them, compound 2-(2--3-hydroxy-1,4-dioxo-1,4-dihydronaphthalen-2-yl)-1-(4-methoxyph-nyl)-3-oxo-3-phenylpropyl)malononitrile   (**9**)   and   compound,   (E)---(benzo[d]thiazol-2-yl)-1-(4-chlorophenyl)methanimine (**10**) demonstrated the highest antioxidant capability during the NBT assay with percentage inhibition of 82.8% and 80.5%, respectively, as compared to 71.3% of ascorbic acid [21].

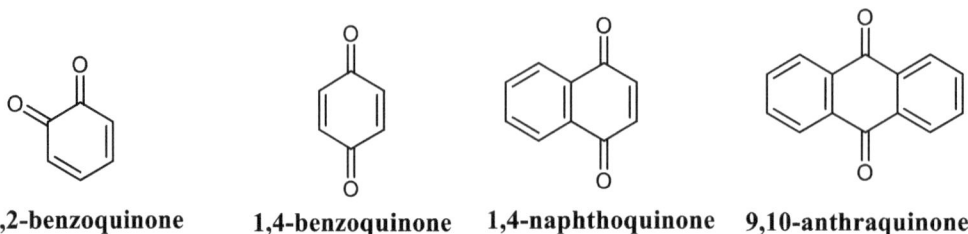

1,2-benzoquinone   **1,4-benzoquinone**   **1,4-naphthoquinone**   **9,10-anthraquinone**

Fig. (1). Structures of 1,2-benzoquinone, 1,4-benzoquinone, 1,4-naphthoquinone, & 9,10-anthraquinone.

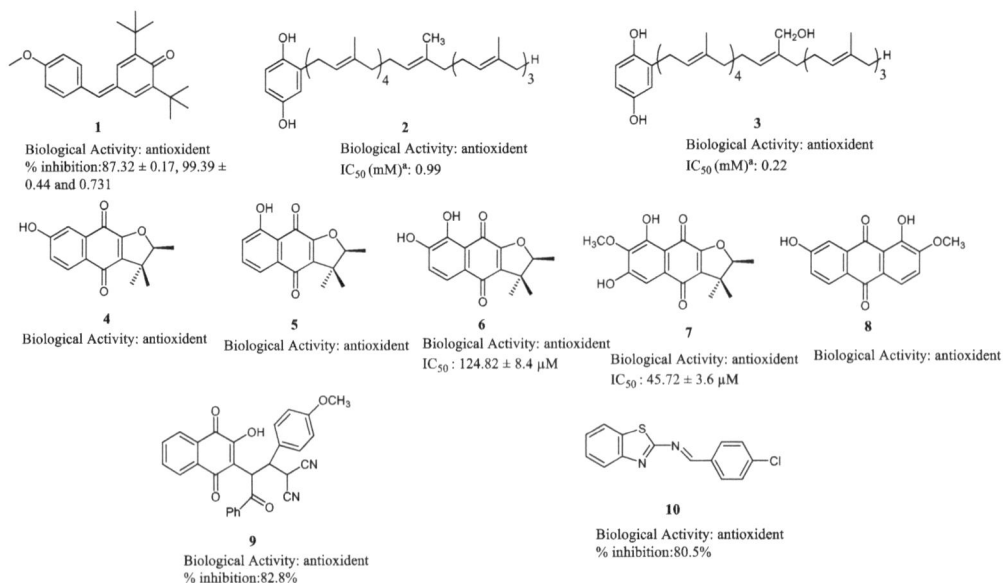

Fig. (2). Antioxidant quinone derivatives discovered or synthesised by researchers.

ANTI-DIABETIC

Diabetes is a long-term medical condition marked by high blood glucose levels and abnormal protein and fat metabolism. Because the pancreas is not producing enough insulin or the cells are not able to use the insulin that is being generated efficiently, blood glucose levels rise because the glucose cannot be metabolised in the cells [22].

Diabetes mellitus is classified into three categories: Type 1 diabetes mellitus, in which pancreatic β-cells are destroyed due to an autoimmune disorder leading to insulin deficiency. Type 2 diabetes is a metabolic disorder in which β-cells produce mutated insulin, leading to insulin resistance. Finally, gestational diabetes is defined as the presence of carbohydrate intolerance that first manifests during pregnancy, with the exception of women who most likely have overt pre-gestational diabetes. Pregnancy-related medical complications are widespread and are linked to a higher risk of unfavourable outcomes [23].

Demir *et al.* tested eight quinones against aldose reductase isolated from sheep kidney. All the tested quinones exhibited non-competitive inhibition against aldose reductase, with 9,10anthraquinone (11) exhibiting the best inhibitory action of aldose reductase with an IC_{50} value of 0.048 μM [24]. Synthetic quinone derivatives have high lead likeness for antidiabetic properties, as demonstrated by Zarren *et al.*, who employed a cupper-catalyzed one-pot relay synthesis to synthesise four anthraquinone-based pyrimidine derivatives and tested them against alpha-amylase for antidiabetic property where compound 1-((4-(5-(1-ethoxyvinyl)-6-methyl-2-oxo-1,2,3,4-tetrahydropyr-midin-4-yl)cyclohexyl)amino)anthracene-9,10-dione (12) exhibited significant antidiabetic property with an IC_{50} of 24.23 μM [25]. Nature is also a good source of quinones with antidiabetic activity, as demonstrated by Choi *et al.*, who performed the extraction off *Rheum undulatum* and isolated one stilbene and two anthraquinones, emodin (13) and chrysophanol (14), from the n-butanol fraction. These two quinones inhibited postprandial hyperglycaemia in ICR mice by 29.5 and 42.3%, respectively [26]. Similarly, Arvindekar *et al.* also performed tests on the *Rheum* genus, but they performed it on *Rheum emodi*, which yielded 1,8-dihydroxyanthraquinones (DHAQs), namely rhein (15), aloe emodin (16), emodin (13), chrysophanol (14) and physcion (17). During the oral glucose tolerance test, aloe compound 16 exhibited maximum lowering of blood glucose. However, on evaluation of alpha-glucosidase, compound 13 exhibited maximum intestinal alpha-glucosidase inhibition with IC_{50} of 30 μg/ml compared to 60 μg/ml of acarbose [27].

ANTI-INFLAMMATORY

The body tries to return the injured tissue to its preinjury condition through the intrinsic system of cellular and humoral responses known as the inflammatory response. These reactions can occur after exposure to heat or cold, ischemia/reperfusion, physical trauma, *etc* [28]. The reaction that is well described pertains to microbial infections, namely bacterial infections. In these cases, the innate immune system's receptors, such as Toll-like receptors (TLRs) and NOD-like receptors (NLRs)3, bind nucleotide-binding oligomerization-domain protein, triggering the response. Tissue-resident macrophages and mast cells are responsible for the first detection of infection, which triggers the release of many inflammatory mediators such as chemokines, cytokines, vasoactive amines, eicosanoids, and proteolytic cascade products [29].

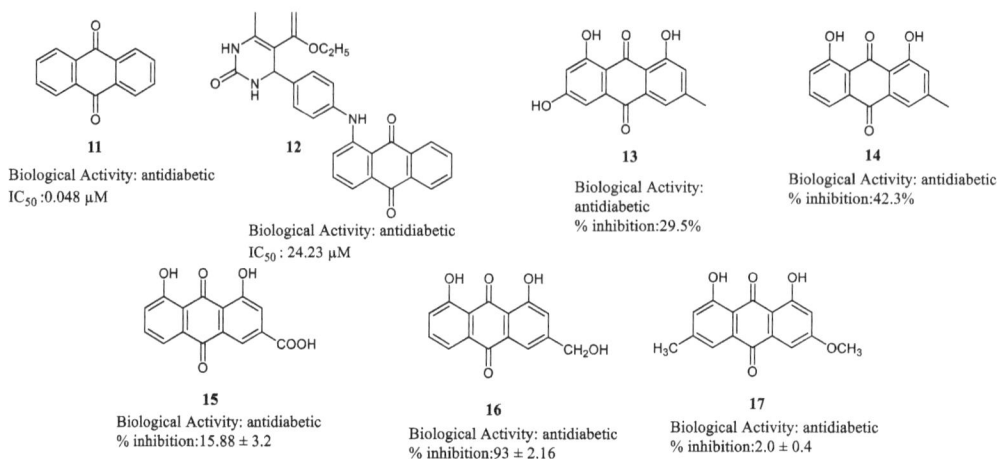

11
Biological Activity: antidiabetic
IC_{50} :0.048 μM

12
Biological Activity: antidiabetic
IC_{50} : 24.23 μM

13
Biological Activity:
antidiabetic
% inhibition:29.5%

14
Biological Activity: antidiabetic
% inhibition:42.3%

15
Biological Activity: antidiabetic
% inhibition:15.88 ± 3.2

16
Biological Activity: antidiabetic
% inhibition:93 ± 2.16

17
Biological Activity: antidiabetic
% inhibition:2.0 ± 0.4

Fig. (3). Anti-diabetic quinones isolated and synthesised by researchers.

Natural quinones can be modified to exhibit great anti-inflammatory properties, as demonstrated by Kshirsagar *et al.*, who performed synthesised 4,5-dihydrox--9,10-dioxo-9,10-dihydroanthracene-2 carboxylic acid **(18)** from aloe emodin **(16)**, a phytoconstituent of aloe vera. The researchers performed anti-inflammatory studies on compounds **16** and **18** *via* carrageenan-induced rat paw oedema. Both compounds **16** and **18** showed significant anti-inflammatory properties and had the ability to reduce oedema volume to 0.17 ± 0.0009 mL and 0.13 ± 0.009 mL, respectively, at 75 mg/kg compared to 0.08 ± 0.007 mL of diclofenac sodium at 10 mg/kg [30]. Similarly, demonstrating the potential of quinone as a nucleus for synthetic drug discovery, Petronzi *et al.* synthesized a series of derivatives of bolinaquinone, a hydroquinone marine metabolite known for its potent anti-inflammatory activity. Among this series of derivatives, 5-[(--Naphthyl)methyl]-2-hydroxy-2,5-cyclohexadiene-1,4- dionen **(19)** exhibited an IC_{50} of 4.0 ± 0.9 μM compared to 5.2 ± 0.5 μM of bolinaquinone on LPS-induced PGE2 production by LPS-stimulated RAW 264.7 cells [31]. Similarly, Liu *et al.* isolated twelve 1,4-napthoquinone derivatives from the endophytic fungus *Talaromyces* sp. SK-S009, namely Talanaphthoquionone A **(20)**, Talanapthoquinone B **(21)**, anhydrojavanicin **(22)**, 2,3-dihydro-5-hydroy-4-hydroxymethyl-8-methoxy-2-methylnaphtho[1,2-b]furan-6,9-dione   **(23)**, anhydrojavanicin **(24)**, anhydrofusarubin **(25)**, 2-acetonyl-3-methyl-5-hyd-oxy-7-methoxy-naphthazarin **(26)**, 6-ethyl-2,7-dimethoxyjuglone **(27)**, 6-[-(acetyloxy)ethyl]-5-hydroxy-2,7-dimethoxy-1,4-naphthalenedione   **(28)**,   5-hydroxy-6-(1-hydroxyethyl)-2,7-dimethoxy-1,4-naphthalenedione **(29)**, solaniol **(30)**, and javanicin **(31)**, among which compounds **21** and **22** are novel compounds identified. Compound **29** inhibited the LPS-induced inducible nitric oxide synthase (iNOS) and cyclooxygenase-2 (COX-2) mRNA expressions in RAW 264.7 macrophages with an IC_{50} of 1.7 ± 0.2 µM compared to 26.3 ± 0.6 µM of indomethacin. Compound **29** also reduced the mRNA level of pro-inflammatory factors like IL-6, IL1β and TNF-α [32]. Another natural source of quinones, the roots of *Juglans mandshurica,* was studied by Piao *et al..* The researchers isolated and identified two new quinones 4-(5-hydroxy-1,4-diox--1,4-dihydronaphthalen-3-ylamino)-butyric acid methyl ester **(32)** and 1,3-dimethoxycarbonyl-8-hydroxy-9,10-anthraquinone   **(33)**,   and   six   known compounds, namely juglanthraquinone **(34)**, 1-hydroxyanthraquinone **(35)**, galeon **(36)**, engelheptanoxide A **(37)**, sakuranetin **(38)**, and (-)-regiolone **(39)**. All the compounds isolated were evaluated for their ability to inhibit the production of NO and IL-6 by RAW 264.7 cell line after lipopolysaccharide stimulation *in vitro.* They observed that compounds **32-35** displayed potent anti-inflammatory effects, indicated by their ability to suppress NO and IL-6 production with IC_{50} of 27.03 ± 1.66, 20.9 ± 1.06, 24.18 ± 1.78, and 22.27 ± 1.26 µM for NO production inhibition and IC_{50} of 26.93 ± 1.24, 21.98 ± 2.91, 24.09 ± 1.21, and 27.63 ± 2.91 µM for inhibition of IL-6 production [33].

ANTI-ALZHEIMER

Alzheimer's disease, a progressive neurodegenerative condition affecting memory, cognitive function, and behaviour, has no cure at present [34]. However, ongoing research endeavours to develop medications and interventions to either prevent or slow its progression. Several approved medications aid in symptom management, improving the quality of life for those affected. Research into Alzheimer's aims to understand its causes, identify drug targets, and develop effective treatments, offering hope for future interventions by uncovering the disease's underlying mechanisms [35].

Natural and synthetic naphthoquinones have shown various biological activities. Therefore, Estolano-Cobián *et al.* synthesized amino alcohol derivatives from 1,4-naphthoquinone and evaluated their antioxidant potential using DPPH and ABTS·⁺ assays as well as their ability to inhibit acetylcholinesterase (AChE). Compound 2-((1,4-dioxo-1,4-dihydronaphthalen-2-yl)amino)butyl acetate **(40)** exhibited the highest antioxidant activity in the DPPH assay (51.52% at 1 mg/mL), while compound 2-((4-hydroxyphenethyl)amino)naphthalene-1,4-dione (**41**) displayed the highest antioxidant activity in the ABTS$\cdot^{+}$ assay (47.12%) and showed the most potent AChE inhibition, with an IC$_{50}$ of 0.0586 Mm [36]. Mezeiova *et al.* synthesized ten derivatives of 2-propargylamino-naphthoquinone and evaluated their biological properties, including inhibition of monoamine oxidase A/B, amyloid-beta aggregation, radical scavenging, and metal-chelating properties. Compounds 2-Chloro-3-[methyl(prop-2-yn-1-yl)amino]-1,4-dihydronaphthalene-1,4-dione (**42**) and 2-Chloro-3-[(prop-2-yn-1-yl)amino]-1,4-dihydronaphthalene-1,4-dione (**43**) showed high MAO-B inhibition, metal-chelating properties for Cu(II), and significant inhibition of Aβ aggregation. Compound 8-(Benzyloxy)-2-[(prop-2-yn-1-yl)amino]-1,4-dihydronaphthalene-1,4-dione (**44**) exhibited anti-inflammatory effects and strong radical scavenging activity [37]. Campora *et al.* synthesized two series of naphthoquinone and anthraquinone derivatives and evaluated them as potential multitarget-directed ligands for Alzheimer's disease. Among these derivatives, naphthoquinone derivative, namely 2-chloro-3-(phenethylamino)naphthalene-1,4-dione (**45**), demonstrated strong inhibitory activity against β-amyloid aggregation (IC$_{50}$ = 3.2 μM), PHF6 tau fragment (91% at 10 μM), acetylcholinesterase (AChE) enzyme (IC$_{50}$ = 9.2 μM), and monoamine oxidase B (MAO B) (IC$_{50}$ = 7.7 nM), making it a promising candidate for Alzheimer treatment [38].

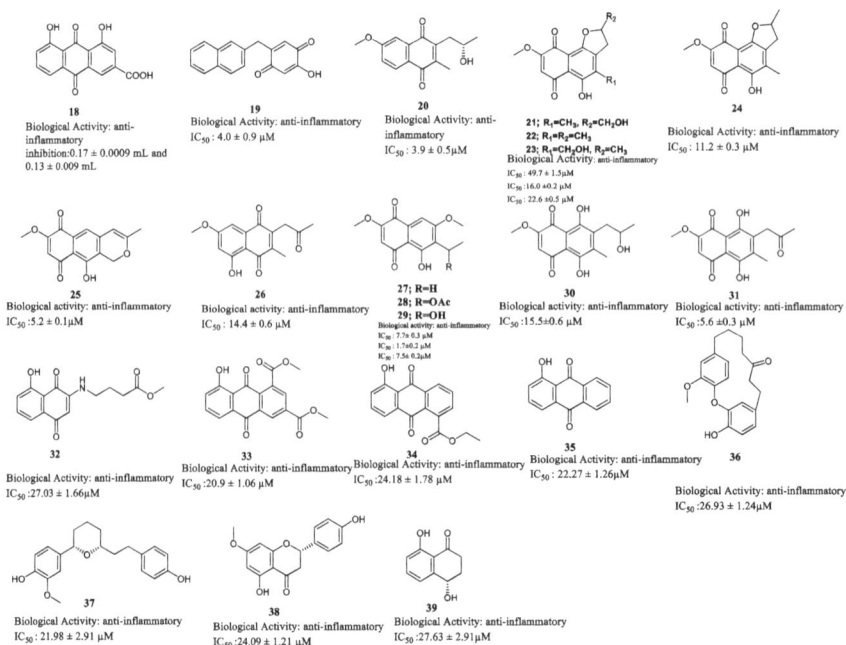

Fig. (4). Anti-inflammatory quinones synthesised or isolated by researchers mentioned in the section.

Similarly, Hosseini *et al.* synthesized derivatives of naphthoquinone conjugated with aryl triazole acetamide and assessed their anti-cholinesterase activities. Compound N-(2-chlorophenyl)-2-(4-(((1, 4-dioxo-1,4-dihydronaphthal-n2-yl)oxy)methyl)−1H-1,2,3-triazol-1-yl)acetamide (46) exhibited the highest inhibitory activity against both acetylcholinesterase and butyrylcholinesterase, with K_i values of 10.16 and 8.04 nM, respectively, surpassing Tacrine (used as a positive control), which showed K_i values of 70.61 and 64.18 nM, respectively [39]. Efeoglu *et al.* examined naphthoquinone thiazole hybrids as inhibitors of the cholinergic enzyme AChE. All the compounds studied demonstrated potent inhibition of AChE, with compound N-[3-(3-amino-1,4-dio-o-1,4-dihydronaphthalen-2-yl)-4-(4-bromophenyl)thiaz-l-2(3H)-ylidene]-2,6-difluorobenzamide (47) showing the most effective inhibition (K_i: 26.12±2.54 nM). In contrast, THA exhibited K_i values of 81.21 nM against AChE [40].

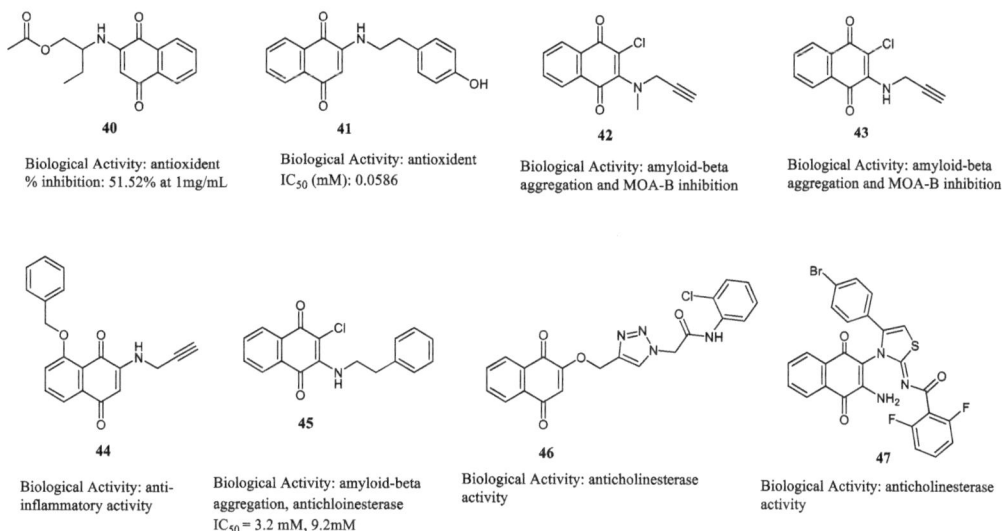

Fig. (5). Various quinone derivatives used for anti-Alzheimer studies.

ANTI-MICROBIAL

An antimicrobial is a substance that either kills microorganisms (microbicide) or inhibits their growth (bacteriostatic agent) [41]. These agents are classified based on the types of microorganisms they primarily target, such as antibiotics for bacteria and antifungals for fungi. They can also be classified according to their function. The use of antimicrobial medicines to treat infection is known as antimicrobial chemotherapy, while the use of antimicrobial medicines to prevent infection is known as antimicrobial prophylaxis [42]. While antimicrobials are vital in modern medicine for combating infectious diseases, the overuse and misuse of these agents have led to the emergence of antimicrobial resistance, posing a significant global health threat.

Molee *et al.* examined the antibacterial activity of a series of novel naphthoquinone derivatives against various gram-positive and gram-negative bacteria. Compound (R)-8,10-dihydroxy-3,5,7-trimethoxy-1-me-hyl-1H-benzo[g]isochromene-6,9-dione **(48)** demonstrated strong antibacterial activity with MIC values ranging from 200 to 400 µg/ml, while compound 2-hydroxy-7-methylanthracene-9,10-dione **(49)** showed moderate antibacterial activity with a MIC value of 25 µg/ml. However, the other derivatives did not show significant antibacterial activity [43]. Choudhari *et al.* discovered two new 1,4-naphthoquinone derivatives and assessed their effectiveness against various bacterial strains. Their research revealed that compound 2-chloro-3--(3-hydroxyphenyl)amino)naphthalene-1,4-dione **(50)** demonstrated strong antibacterial effects, specifically against *S. aureus* and *P. aeruginosa*. Conversely, compound 2-chloro-3-((4-hydroxyphenyl)amino)naphthalene-1,4-dione **(51)** exhibited superior antibacterial activity against all tested pathogens, with MIC values ranging from 32 to 512 µg/ml. Both derivatives demonstrated superior activity compared to the reference antibiotics, likely due to their distinct structural characteristics [44]. Rajasekar *et al.* studied the antibacterial properties of various quinone derivatives against different bacterial strains. They discovered that 3'-methyl-6-(methylthio)-[1,1'-biphenyl]-2,5-dione **(52)** exhibited potent antibacterial activity [45]. Yıldız *et al.* investigated the antibacterial activity of a series of new 1,4-benzoquinone derivatives against both gram-positive and gram-negative bacteria using the microbroth dilution method. They found that compounds 2-chloro-3-(4-isopropylpiperazin-1-yl)-5,6-dimethylcycl-hexa-2,5-diene-1,4-dione **(53)** and 2-chloro-3-(4-cyclohexylpiperazin-1--l)-5,6-dimethylcyclohexa-2,5-diene-1,4-dione **(54)** exhibited superior antibacterial activity against *S. epidermidis* and Amikacin, with MIC values of 4.88 µg/ml and 78.12 µg/ml, respectively, compared to the reference drug molecule Cefuroxime. However, the other derivatives showed no significant activity against the tested bacteria when compared to reference strains [46]. Andrades-Lagos *et al.* synthesized derivatives of 2,4-dimethylpyrimido[4,5-c]isoquinoli-e-1,3,7,10(2H,4H)-tetraone with antimicrobial properties. Nineteen compounds displayed antibacterial activity against Gram-positive bacteria with MIC values ranging from 0.5 to 64 µg/ml. Compound 8-((4-bromophenyl)amino)-6-ethy--2,4-dimethylpyrimido[4,5-c]isoquinoline-1,3,7,10(2H,4H)-tetraone **(55)** exhibited the most potent activity in the series, with MIC values of 0.5 µg/ml against both *Staphylococcus aureus* methicillin-susceptible strain and *Staphylococcus aureus* methicillin-resistant strain making it twice as potent as vancomycin [47].

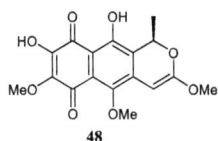
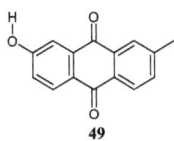
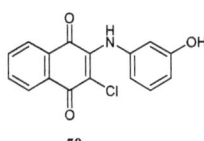
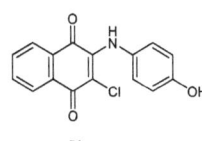

48

Biological Activity: antibacterial
activity
MIC value: 200 to 400 µg/ml

49

Biological Activity:
antibacterial activity
MIC value: 25 µg/ml

50

Biological Activity:
antibacterial activity

51

Biological Activity:
antibacterial activity
MIC value: 32 to 512 µg/ml

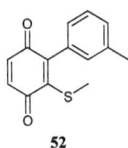
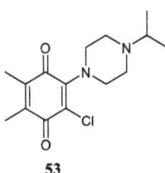
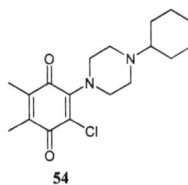
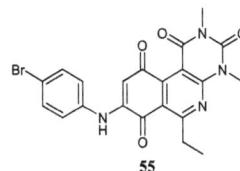

52

Biological Activity:
antibacterial activity

53

Biological Activity:
antibacterial activity
MIC value: 4.88 µg/ml

54

Biological Activity:
antibacterial activity
MIC value: 78.12 µg/ml

55

Biological Activity:
antibacterial activity
MIC value: 0.5 µg/ml

Fig. (6). Various quinone derivatives used for antimicrobial studies.

Table 1. Marketed drugs with quinone nucleus for various ailments.

Sl No.	Drug Name	Drug description	Reference
1.	Atovaquone	An antimicrobial drug recommended for the treatment and prevention of both *Plasmodium falciparum* malaria and *Pneumocystis jirovecii* pneumonia (PCP).	48,49
2.	Banoxantrone	A highly selective bioreductive medication called banoxantrone is preferentially harmful to hypoxic tumour cells and is activated in these cells. When combined with fractionated radiation, it has been demonstrated to effectively halt the development of tumours, outperforming the administration of either banoxantrone or radiation on its own. When paired with either cisplatin or chemoradiation, banoxantrone was also effective in tumour models.	50
3.	2-(4-tert-butylcyclohexyl)-3-hydroxy-1,4-naphthoquinone	2-(4-tert-butylcyclohexyl)-3-hydroxy-1,4-naphthoquinone is an experimental naphthoquinone antimalarial medication that, in human liver microsomes and in man *in vivo*, undergoes extensive alkyl hydroxylation to a single t-butylhydroxy metabolite. This process is primarily catalysed by a 54 kDa CYP2C9 form of cytochrome P450, P450hB20-27.	51
4.	Seratrodast	Seratrodast (INN) is a thromboxane receptor antagonist used primarily in the treatment of asthma.	52

Sl No.	Drug Name	Drug description	Reference
5.	Alvespimycin	Alvespimycin is an inhibitor of heat shock protein (HSP) 90 and a derivative of geldanamycin. As an anticancer agent, it has been utilised in studies investigating the treatment of solid tumours in different types of cancer. It demonstrates several pharmacologically favourable characteristics over the original HSP90 inhibitor, tanespimycin, including decreased metabolic liability, decreased plasma protein binding, greater water solubility, increased oral bioavailability, less hepatotoxicity, and superior anticancer efficacy.	53

CONCLUSION

Quinones, with their versatile structure and chemical properties, have emerged as a promising candidate in drug discovery and developed across various therapeutic fields. Their unique structural properties, redox capabilities, and pharmacophoric abilities provide them with invaluable usefulness in the fight against various ailments affecting humans, ranging from cancer and diabetes to inflammation, Alzheimer's disease, and microbial infections. This chapter summarises how researchers over the years have studied the quinone nucleus to understand and harness its therapeutic potential. Quinones are a rich source of molecules with a variety of biological functions, both natural and synthetic. Due to this, quinones are an excellent nucleus for the pharmaceutical field to study. There is still promise for developing the nucleus into clinically useful compounds *via* synthesis for drug discovery. Quinones are, therefore, long-lasting cornerstones for the creation of innovative therapeutic agents, offering promise for solving today's medical problems and achieving the best possible results for human health.

REFERENCES

[1]   Jiang JG, Huang XJ, Chen J, Lin QS. Comparison of the sedative and hypnotic effects of flavonoids, saponins, and polysaccharides extracted from Semen Ziziphus jujube. Nat Prod Res 2007; 21(4): 310-20.
       [http://dx.doi.org/10.1080/14786410701192827] [PMID: 17479419]

[2]   Jung HA, Ali MY, Jung HJ, Jeong HO, Chung HY, Choi JS. Inhibitory activities of major anthraquinones and other constituents from Cassia obtusifolia against β-secretase and cholinesterases. J Ethnopharmacol 2016; 191: 152-60.
       [http://dx.doi.org/10.1016/j.jep.2016.06.037] [PMID: 27321278]

[3]   Madeo J, Zubair A, Marianne F. A review on the role of quinones in renal disorders. Springerplus 2013; 2(1): 139.
       [http://dx.doi.org/10.1186/2193-1801-2-139] [PMID: 23577302]

[4]   Chadar D, Camilles M, Patil R, Khan A, Weyhermüller T, Salunke-Gawali S. Synthesis and characterization of n-alkylamino derivatives of vitamin K3: Molecular structure of 2-propylamino-3-methyl-1,4-naphthoquinone and antibacterial activities. J Mol Struct 2015; 1086: 179-89.
       [http://dx.doi.org/10.1016/j.molstruc.2015.01.029]

[5]   Zhang K, Chen D, Ma K, Wu X, Hao H, Jiang S. NAD (P) H: quinone oxidoreductase 1 (NQO1) as a therapeutic and diagnostic target in cancer. J Med Chem 2018; 61(16): 6983-7003.
       [http://dx.doi.org/10.1021/acs.jmedchem.8b00124] [PMID: 29712428]

[6] Jali BR, Barick AK, Mohapatra P, Sahoo SK. A comprehensive review on quinones based fluoride selective colorimetric and fluorescence chemosensors. J Fluor Chem 2021; 244: 109744.
[http://dx.doi.org/10.1016/j.jfluchem.2021.109744]

[7] Pereyra CE, Dantas RF, Ferreira SB, Gomes LP, Silva-Jr FP. The diverse mechanisms and anticancer potential of naphthoquinones. Cancer Cell Int 2019; 19(1): 207.
[http://dx.doi.org/10.1186/s12935-019-0925-8] [PMID: 31388334]

[8] Ma Q, Wei R, Sang Z. Structural characterization and hepatoprotective activity of naphthoquinone from Cucumis bisexualis. Natural Product Communications 2020; 1(15(1)): 1934578X20902898.
[http://dx.doi.org/10.1177/1934578X20902898]

[9] O'Brien PJ. Molecular mechanisms of quinone cytotoxicity. Chem Biol Interact 1991; 80(1): 1-41.
[http://dx.doi.org/10.1016/0009-2797(91)90029-7] [PMID: 1913977]

[10] Liu HW. Extraction and isolation of compounds from herbal medicines. Extraction and isolation of compounds from herbal medicines Traditional herbal medicine research methods: identification, analysis, bioassay, and pharmaceutical and clinical studies 2011; 10: 81-138.
[http://dx.doi.org/10.1002/9780470921340.ch3]

[11] Eyong KO, Kuete V, Efferth T. Quinones and benzophenones from the medicinal plants of Africa. InMedicinal Plant Research in Africa. Elsevier. 2013; pp. 351-91.
[http://dx.doi.org/10.1016/B978-0-12-405927-6.00010-2]

[12] Lapidot A, Silver BL, Samuel D. The tautomerism of quinones and the question of quinone methide intermediates in oxidative phosphorylation. J Biol Chem 1966; 241(23): 5537-41.
[http://dx.doi.org/10.1016/S0021-9258(18)96376-3] [PMID: 4288892]

[13] Badave P, Gaikwaid S, Jagtap SV. Versatile Remarkable Potent Bioactivity of Quinone based Compounds to Beat the Diseases. Eng Manag 2020; 83: 25605-8.

[14] Badave P, Gaikwaid S, Jagtap SV. Versatile Remarkable Potent Bioactivity of Quinone based Compounds to Beat the Diseases. Eng Manag 2020; 83: 25605-8.

[15] Dulo B, Phan K, Githaiga J, Raes K, De Meester S. Natural quinone dyes: A review on structure, extraction techniques, analysis and application potential. Waste Biomass Valoriz 2021; 12(12): 6339-74.
[http://dx.doi.org/10.1007/s12649-021-01443-9]

[16] Seigler DS, Seigler DS. Benzoquinones, naphthoquinones, and anthraquinones. Plant secondary metabolism 1998; 76-93.
[http://dx.doi.org/10.1007/978-1-4615-4913-0_6]

[17] Dontha S. A review on antioxidant methods. Asian J Pharm Clin Res 2016; 9(2): 14-32.

[18] Muhammad I, Pandian S, Hopper W. Antibacterial and antioxidant activity of p-quinone methide derivative synthesized from 2, 6-di-tert-butylphenol. Chem Int 2020; 6(4): 260-6.

[19] Tziveleka LA, Kourounakis AP, Kourounakis PN, Roussis V, Vagias C. Antioxidant potential of natural and synthesised polyprenylated hydroquinones. Bioorg Med Chem 2002; 10(4): 935-9.
[http://dx.doi.org/10.1016/S0968-0896(01)00346-7] [PMID: 11836101]

[20] Cai XH, Luo XD, Zhou J, Hao XJ. Quinones from *Chirita e burnea*. J Nat Prod 2005; 68(5): 797-9.
[http://dx.doi.org/10.1021/np049632f] [PMID: 15921435]

[21] Berghot MA, Kandeel EM, Abdel-Rahman AH, Abdel-Motaal M. Synthesis, antioxidant and cytotoxic activities of novel naphthoquinone derivatives from 2, 3-dihydro-2, 3-epoxy-1, 4-naphthoquinone. Med Chem 2014; 4(3): 381-8.

[22] Roglic G. WHO Global report on diabetes: A summary. Int J Noncommun Dis 2016; 1(1): 3-8.
[http://dx.doi.org/10.4103/2468-8827.184853]

[23] Egan AM, Dinneen SF. What is diabetes? Medicine (Abingdon) 2019; 47(1): 1-4.

[http://dx.doi.org/10.1016/j.mpmed.2018.10.002]

[24]   Demir Y, Özaslan MS, Duran HE, Küfrevioğlu Öİ, Beydemir Ş. Inhibition effects of quinones on aldose reductase: Antidiabetic properties. Environ Toxicol Pharmacol 2019; 70: 103195.
[http://dx.doi.org/10.1016/j.etap.2019.103195] [PMID: 31125830]

[25]   Zarren G, Shafiq N, Arshad U, Rafiq N, Parveen S, Ahmad Z. Copper-catalyzed one-pot relay synthesis of anthraquinone based pyrimidine derivative as a probe for antioxidant and antidiabetic activity. J Mol Struct 2021; 1227: 129668.
[http://dx.doi.org/10.1016/j.molstruc.2020.129668]

[26]   Choi SZ, Lee SO, Jang KU, *et al.* Antidiabetic stilbene and anthraquinone derivatives fromRheum undulatum. Arch Pharm Res 2005; 28(9): 1027-30.
[http://dx.doi.org/10.1007/BF02977396] [PMID: 16212232]

[27]   Arvindekar A, More T, Payghan PV, Laddha K, Ghoshal N, Arvindekar A. Evaluation of anti-diabetic and alpha glucosidase inhibitory action of anthraquinones from Rheum emodi. Food Funct 2015; 6(8): 2693-700.
[http://dx.doi.org/10.1039/C5FO00519A] [PMID: 26145710]

[28]   Serhan CN, Ward PA, Gilroy DW, Eds. Fundamentals of inflammation. Cambridge University Press 2010.
[http://dx.doi.org/10.1017/CBO9781139195737]

[29]   Medzhitov R. Origin and physiological roles of inflammation. Nature 2008; 454(7203): 428-35.
[http://dx.doi.org/10.1038/nature07201] [PMID: 18650913]

[30]   Kshirsagar AD, Panchal PV, Harle UN, Nanda RK, Shaikh HM. Anti-inflammatory and antiarthritic activity of anthraquinone derivatives in rodents. International Journal of Inflammation 2014; 2014.
[http://dx.doi.org/10.1155/2014/690596]

[31]   Petronzi C, Filosa R, Peduto A, *et al.* Structure-based design, synthesis and preliminary anti-inflammatory activity of bolinaquinone analogues. Eur J Med Chem 2011; 46(2): 488-96.
[http://dx.doi.org/10.1016/j.ejmech.2010.11.028] [PMID: 21163556]

[32]   Liu H, Yan C, Li C, You T, She Z. Naphthoquinone derivatives with anti-inflammatory activity from mangrove-derived endophytic fungus Talaromyces sp. SK-S009. Molecules 2020; 25(3): 576.
[http://dx.doi.org/10.3390/molecules25030576] [PMID: 32013142]

[33]   Piao S, Qi Y, Jin M, *et al.* Two new quinones and six additional metabolites with potential anti-inflammatory activities from the roots of *Juglans mandshurica.* Nat Prod Res 2022; 36(13): 3396-403.
[PMID: 33397154]

[34]   Srivastava S, Ahmad R, Khare SK. Alzheimer's disease and its treatment by different approaches: A review. Eur J Med Chem 2021; 216: 113320.
[http://dx.doi.org/10.1016/j.ejmech.2021.113320] [PMID: 33652356]

[35]   Atri A. Current and future treatments in Alzheimer's disease. InSeminars in neurology. Thieme Medical Publishers 2019; 39: pp. (02)227-40.
[http://dx.doi.org/10.1055/s-0039-1678581]

[36]   Estolano-Cobián A, Noriega-Iribe E, Díaz-Rubio L, *et al.* Antioxidant, antiproliferative, and acetylcholinesterase inhibition activity of amino alcohol derivatives from 1,4-naphthoquinone. Med Chem Res 2020; 29(11): 1986-99.
[http://dx.doi.org/10.1007/s00044-020-02617-1]

[37]   Mezeiova E, Janockova J, Andrys R, *et al.* 2-Propargylamino-naphthoquinone derivatives as multipotent agents for the treatment of Alzheimer's disease. Eur J Med Chem 2021; 211: 113112.
[http://dx.doi.org/10.1016/j.ejmech.2020.113112] [PMID: 33360800]

[38]   Campora M, Canale C, Gatta E, *et al.* Multitarget biological profiling of new naphthoquinone and anthraquinone-based derivatives for the treatment of Alzheimer's disease. ACS Chem Neurosci 2021; 12(3): 447-61.

[http://dx.doi.org/10.1021/acschemneuro.0c00624] [PMID: 33428389]

[39] Hosseini S, Pourmousavi SA, Mahdavi M, Taslimi P. Synthesis, and *in vitro* biological evaluations of novel naphthoquinone conjugated to aryl triazole acetamide derivatives as potential anti-Alzheimer agents. J Mol Struct 2022; 1255: 132229.
[http://dx.doi.org/10.1016/j.molstruc.2021.132229]

[40] Efeoglu C, Selcuk O, Demir B, *et al.* New naphthoquinone thiazole hybrids as carbonic anhydrase and cholinesterase inhibitors: Synthesis, crystal structure, molecular docking, and acid dissociation constant. J Mol Struct 2024; 1301: 137365.
[http://dx.doi.org/10.1016/j.molstruc.2023.137365]

[41] Webster M. Merriam webster online. Merriam-Webster Incorporated 2014.

[42] Leekha S, Terrell CL, Edson RS. General principles of antimicrobial therapy. InMayo Clinic Proceedings. Elsevier. 2011; 86: pp. (2)156-67.
[http://dx.doi.org/10.4065/mcp.2010.0639]

[43] Molee W, Phanumartwiwath A, Kesornpun C, *et al.* Naphthalene derivatives and quinones from Ventilago denticulata and their nitric oxide radical scavenging, antioxidant, cytotoxic, antibacterial, and phosphodiesterase inhibitory activities. Chem Biodivers 2018; 15(3): 1700537.
[http://dx.doi.org/10.1002/cbdv.201700537] [PMID: 29325221]

[44] Choudhari D, Lande DN, Chakravarty D, *et al.* Reactions of 2,3-dichloro-1,4-naphthoquinone with aminophenols: evidence for hydroxy benzophenoxazine intermediate and antibacterial activity. J Mol Struct 2019; 1176: 194-206.
[http://dx.doi.org/10.1016/j.molstruc.2018.08.066]

[45] Rajasekar S, Krishna TPA, Tharmalingam N, Andivelu I, Mylonakis E. Metal☐Free C☐H Thiomethylation of Quinones Using Iodine and DMSO and Study of Antibacterial Activity. ChemistrySelect 2019; 4(8): 2281-7.
[http://dx.doi.org/10.1002/slct.201803816]

[46] Yıldız M. Design, synthesis, characterization, and antimicrobial activity of novel piperazine substituted 1,4-benzoquinones. J Mol Struct 2020; 1203: 127422.
[http://dx.doi.org/10.1016/j.molstruc.2019.127422]

[47] Andrades-Lagos J, Campanini-Salinas J, Pedreros-Riquelme A, *et al.* Design, Synthesis, and Structure–Activity Relationship Studies of New Quinone Derivatives as Antibacterial Agents. Antibiotics (Basel) 2023; 12(6): 1065.
[http://dx.doi.org/10.3390/antibiotics12061065] [PMID: 37370384]

[48] Blanshard A, Hine P. Atovaquone☐proguanil for treating uncomplicated Plasmodium falciparum malaria. Cochrane Database of Systematic Reviews 2021; (1).

[49] Robin C, Lê MP, Melica G, *et al.* Plasma concentrations of atovaquone given to immunocompromised patients to prevent Pneumocystis jirovecii. J Antimicrob Chemother 2017; 72(9): 2602-6.
[http://dx.doi.org/10.1093/jac/dkx198] [PMID: 28651341]

[50] Patterson LH, McKeown SR, Ruparelia K, *et al.* Enhancement of chemotherapy and radiotherapy of murine tumours by AQ4N, a bioreductively activated anti-tumour agent. Br J Cancer 2000; 82(12): 1984-90.
[PMID: 10864207]

[51] Patil PC, Akamanchi KG. Simple and effective route for synthesis of parvaquone, an antiprotozoal drug. RSC Advances 2014; 4(102): 58214-6.
[http://dx.doi.org/10.1039/C4RA09934F]

[52] Terao S, Shiraishi M, Matsumoto T, Ashida Y. [Thromboxane A2 antagonist--discovery of seratrodast]. Yakugaku Zasshi 1999; 119(5): 377-90.
[http://dx.doi.org/10.1248/yakushi1947.119.5_377] [PMID: 10375998]

[53] Pacey S, Wilson RH, Walton M, *et al.* A phase I study of the heat shock protein 90 inhibitor

[53]   Pacey S, Wilson RH, Walton M, *et al.* A phase I study of the heat shock protein 90 inhibitor alvespimycin (17-DMAG) given intravenously to patients with advanced solid tumors. Clin Cancer Res 2011; 17(6): 1561-70.
[http://dx.doi.org/10.1158/1078-0432.CCR-10-1927] [PMID: 21278242]

CHAPTER 2

Chemistry and Synthesis of Quinones and their Derivatives

Divyani P. Patel[1], **Satish Kumar Singh**[1,*] and **Vivek Mishra**[2,*]

[1] Department of Chemistry, Government College Daman (Affiliated to Veer Narmad South Gujarat University, Surat), Daman, U.T. of Dadra & Nagar Haveli and Daman & Diu, Gujarat 395007, India

[2] Amity Institute of Click Chemistry Research and Studies, Amity University Uttar Pradesh, Noida 201313, UP, India

Abstract: Quinones are a group of organic compounds that have a wide range of chemical properties and applications in various fields, such as pharmaceuticals, materials science, and organic synthesis. They are highly versatile and can be modified to produce derivatives with unique properties. This chapter presents a comprehensive and current overview of the chemistry and synthesis of quinones and their derivatives. It serves as an invaluable resource for chemists, researchers, and scientists who are interested in exploring the diverse aspects of this significant class of organic compounds.

Keywords: Derivatives of quinone, Synthesis of quinone, Quinone.

INTRODUCTION

Quinones are fascinating chemical structures composed of a nonaromatic ring and two carbonyl functional groups positioned at either the 1 & 2 or 1 & 4 relative to one another [1 - 4]. Quinones have garnered significant scientific attention since their fundamental structure was revealed in 1838 [5, 6].

Quinones have a crucial function in photosynthesis by carrying electrons. They are a type of molecule that works as vitamins and can help prevent and treat various illnesses, such as cardiovascular diseases and osteoporosis. Quinones can also enhance overall health conditions due to their antioxidant properties [7]. Several cancer-fighting drugs that have either been clinically approved or are

* **Corresponding authors Satish Kumar Singh & Vivek Mishra:** Department of Chemistry, Government College Daman (Affiliated to Veer Narmad South Gujarat University, Surat), Daman, U.T. of Dadra & Nagar Haveli and Daman & Diu, India; Amity Institute of Click Chemistry Research and Studies, Amity University Uttar Pradesh, Noida 201313, UP, India E-mail: vmishra@amity.edu; drsatish.singh@ddd.gov.in

Ashutosh Kumar Dash & Deepak Kumar (Eds.)

currently in clinical trials are made up of quinone-related compounds. Quinones, which can be produced from air pollutants, also have toxicological effects.

Quinones can activate rapid redox cycles, which enables them to form bonds with hydroxyl, thiol, and amine groups [8]. Furthermore, several quinones have anti-inflammatory [9, 10], anti-osteoarthritis [11], antibiotic [12], antimicrobial [13], antioxidant [14], and anticancer potential (Fig. **1**) [14-16]. While the exact mechanism by which they operate remains incompletely elucidated, speculation suggests that DNA is their primary target. Some proteins participate in alkylation or intercalation with DNA, while others catalyze double-strand DNA breaks and also serve in DNA cleavage through the actions of both DNA topoisomerase I and II [17].

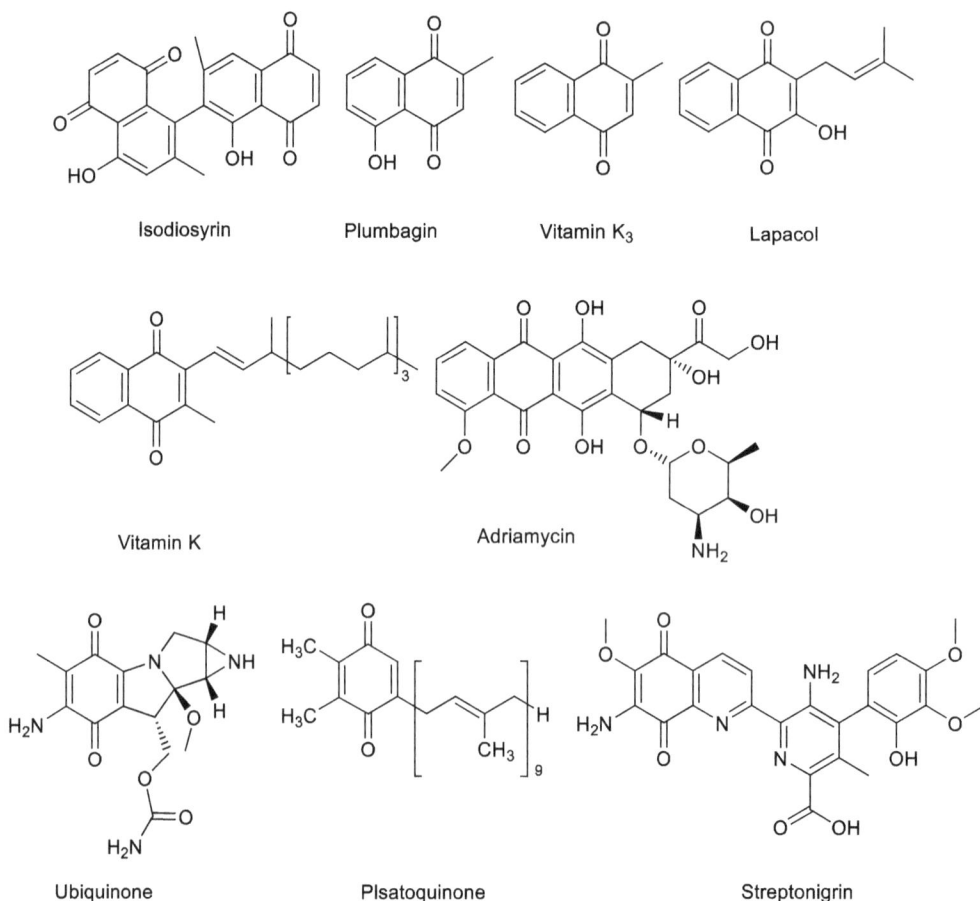

Fig. (1). Some naturally occurring quinone derivatives [25 - 27].

Quinones and their derivatives are essential in chemical, environmental, and pharmaceutical applications because of their distinct physical and chemical characteristics [18]. Quinones and their derivatives possess unique physical and chemical properties that make them essential for chemical, environmental, and pharmaceutical applications [19 - 21].

Furthermore, quinones serve as key components in the synthesis of functional materials, such as conducting polymers, organic dyes, and photoactive molecules, enabling applications in optoelectronics, photovoltaics, and sensor technologies [22]. Their redox chemistry has also been harnessed for energy storage devices, electrochemical sensors, and catalytic transformations, underscoring the multifaceted nature of quinone reactivity and its relevance to modern technological challenges [23, 24].

In this chapter, we explore the chemistry of quinones and their derivatives, underlying their reactivity, synthetic strategies for their preparation, and the myriad applications that exploit their unique properties. Through a comprehensive examination of quinone chemistry, we aim to illuminate the diverse facets of this fascinating class of compounds and highlight their enduring impact on science and technology.

Structure and Chemistry of Quinone

Quinones are colored compounds with a basic benzoquinone chromophore structure consisting of two carbonyl functional groups associated with two C=C bonds. Anthraquinones, benzoquinones, and naphthoquinones are the three primary classes of quinones, distinguished by their respective one, two, and three-ring structures. Benzoquinone is an essential component of quinones; specifically, 1,4-benzoquinone (4-benzoquinone) is a non-aromatic substance that may be readily reduced to produce hydroquinone [28]. Benzoquinone units play a crucial role as fundamental units in both the biosynthesis of biologically active chemicals and quinone synthesis. Anthraquinones are compounds characterized by the attachment of 1,4-benzoquinones to one or more C_6H_6 rings on a 2,3-carbon position. Two carbonyl groups are located at a single benzene ring in the naphthoquinone structure, usually in the ortho or para position [29, 30]. Naphthoquinones hold α- and β-unsaturated carbonyl functional groups. The electron delocalization facilitated by the presence of carbonyl groups and double bonds results in strong coloring in the visible spectrum. Anthraquinones, which belong to the third family of quinones, are molecules that consist of the anthracene nucleus and two carbonyl groups, often located on the B-ring. Due to the ability of quinone structures to accommodate various substitution patterns, there are several derivatives found in nature, particularly for anthraquinones.

Hydroxyanthraquinoids possess the ability to absorb visible light, resulting in their characteristic coloration [31]. The color of a quinone molecule is determined by the position, kind, and amount of -OH group and electron-donating or accepting components, referred to as auxochromes, on the different rings. These components influence the creation of intra-molecular H-bonding and steric effects [32].

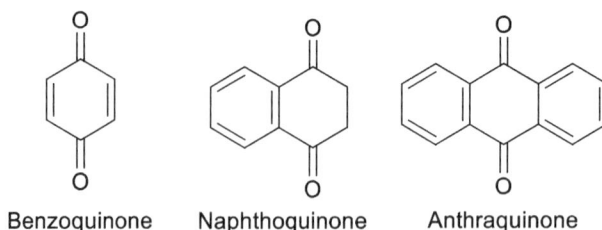

Benzoquinone   Naphthoquinone   Anthraquinone

Fig. (2). Structures of Quinone.

Quinones emerge as a category of chemical compounds obtained from the oxidative transformation of dihydroxyarenes. The fundamental quinones are generated from benzenediols, specifically 1,2-dihydroxybenzene and 1,4-dihydroxybenzene (Figs. **3** & **4**).

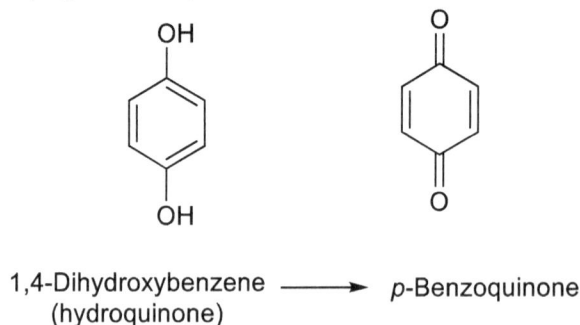

1,4-Dihydroxybenzene ⟶ *p*-Benzoquinone
(hydroquinone)

Fig. (3). Synthesis of *p*-Benzoquinone from 1,4-Dihydrobenzene.

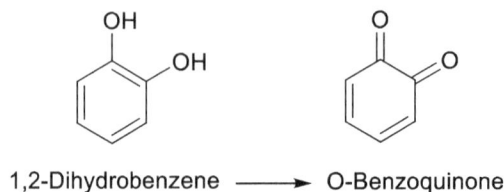

1,2-Dihydrobenzene ⟶ O-Benzoquinone

Fig. (4). Synthesis of O-Benzoquinone from 1,2-Dihydrobenzene.

Additionally, condensation of arenes may produce quinones, such as naphthoquinones (Fig. **5**).

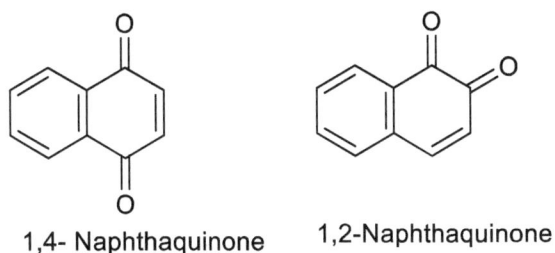

1,4- Naphthaquinone   1,2-Naphthaquinone

Fig. (5). Structures of 1,2-Naphthaquinone and 1,4-Naphthaquinone.

The oxidation of dihydroxyarenes to quinones is a reversible process that involves the transfer of two electrons. This process also involves the synthesis of the radical form of semiquinones as an intermediate step (Fig. **6**).

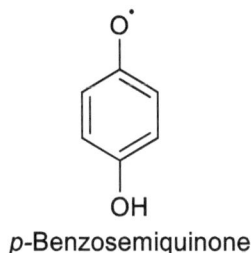

p-Benzosemiquinone

Fig. (6). Structure of p-Benzo semiquinone.

The quinone/diphenol (or quinol) redox systems are commonly seen in nature. Another example of a charge-transfer complex is quinhydrone, where diphenol acts as the electron donor and quinone acts as the electron acceptor (Fig. **7**).

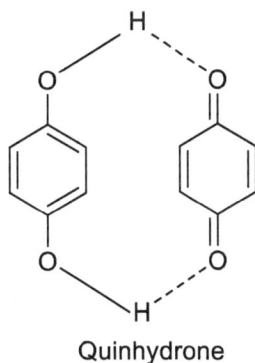

Quinhydrone

Fig. (7). Quinhydrone showing quinone/diphenol (or quinol) redox systems.

SYNTHESIS OF BENZOQUINONES

benzo-1,2-quinones

BAHA, known as Weitz's aminium salt (tris(4-bromophenyl)aminium hexachloroantimonate), can be utilized to facilitate the reaction between phenols and ethers, resulting in the formation of quinone derivatives. These derivatives can be used as valuable building blocks for obtaining quassinoids, which are the bitter compounds found in Simaroubaceous plants. Takeya and his colleagues have elucidated the procedure for synthesizing benzo-1,2-quinones, which primarily entails the oxidation of benzenes that have been dihydroxylated at positions 1 and 2. Benzo-1,2-quinones can be synthesized with a 70% efficiency by oxidizing 1-hydroxy or 1-*tert*-butyl dimethyl silyloxy-2-methoxybenzene using BAHA in tetrahydrofuran Scheme (**1**) [33].

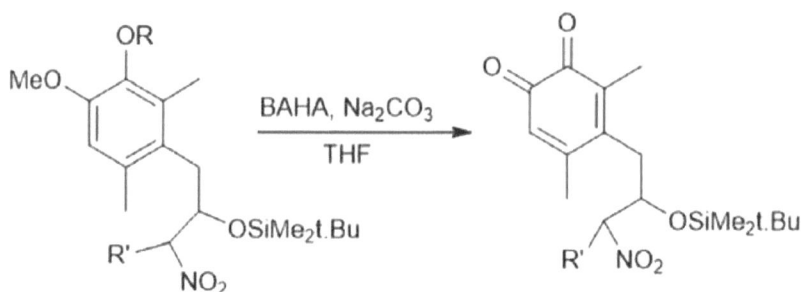

Scheme (1).   Synthesis of Benzo-1,2-quinones from 1-hydroxy or 1-tert-butyl dimethyl silyloxy--methoxybenzene using BAHA in tetrahydrofuran[33].

The process of galloyl monoethers oxidation using orthochloranil produces orthoquinones in high yield. These reactive electrophiles take part in various nucleophilic additions with carbanionic and heteroatomic partners. Furthermore, the use of Lewis acids to facilitate the combination of orthoquinones offers a highly efficient method for generating dehydrodigalloyl-type diaryl ether units. These units are known to be characteristic features of several ellagitannin natural products. Using o-chloranil to oxidize monoprotected gallates, benzo-1,-quinones may be produced in high yield Scheme (**2**) [34].

benzo-1,4-quinones

A wide range of methods have been developed to convert phenols into benzoquinones, with most of these approaches focusing on 1,4-benzoquinones. Phenols that have a substituent at the 4-position undergo oxidation when reacted with *t*-BuOH in EtOAc or C_6H_6. Afterward, when treated with $TiCl_4$, a substantial quantity (70-80%) of 1,4-benzoquinones with a substituent at the 2-position is formed. The substituent derived from the phenol group is relocated to the ortho-position of the 1,4-benzoquinones Scheme (**3**) [35].

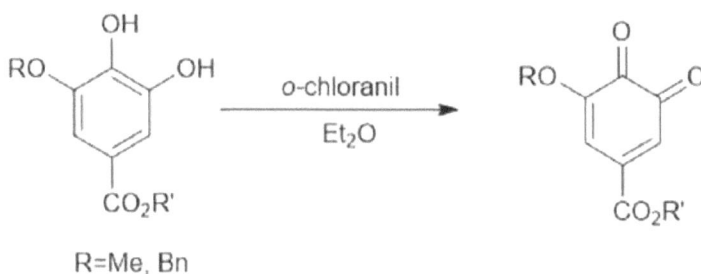

R=Me, Bn

Scheme (2). Synthesis of orthoquinones by Galloyl monoethers oxidation using *o*- chloranil[34].

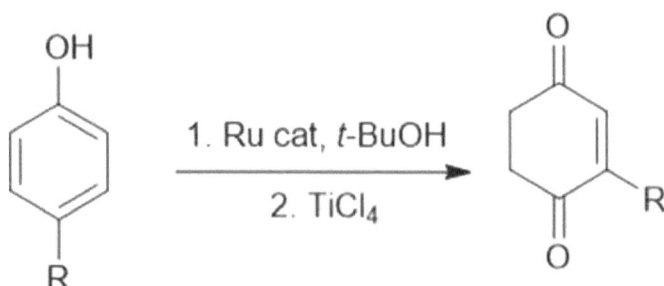

Scheme (3). Synthesis of benzoquinones from phenols[35].

Recent investigations have demonstrated that vanadium complexes supported on polymer materials exhibit remarkable catalytic activity in the phenols to 1,4-benzoquinones oxidation with high yield using *t*-BuOH as an oxidizing agent [36]. A recent investigation demonstrated that catalysts composed of Co and Mg-salts of silica gel-supported p-aminobenzoic acid exhibit exceptional efficacy in the oxidation of phenols to 1,4-benzoquinones with excellent product yields [37]. This conversion was achieved through p-sulfinylation followed by a Pummerer rearrangement utilizing TFAA $(C_4F_6O_3)$. The overall yield of this process is moderate [38]. Frémy's salt was used to oxidize the aromatic ring of 1-demethylthiocolchicine to form 1,4-benzoquinones Scheme (**4**) [39].

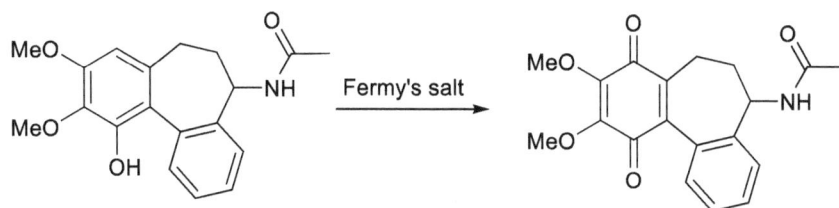

Scheme (4). Formation of 1,4-benzoquinones by utilizing Frémy's salt to oxidize the aromatic ring of 1-demethylthiocolchicine.[39]

Using acetonitrile-water as a solvent, CAN (ceric ammonium nitrate) oxidized 1,3-dimethoxy-5-alkyl-4-chlorobenzenes, resulting in the formation of 3-methoxy-5-alkyl-6-chlorobenzo-1,4-quinones. The quinones can then be hydrolyzed into 3-methoxy-5-alkyl-6-hydroxybenzo-1,4-quinones Scheme (**5**) [40, 41].

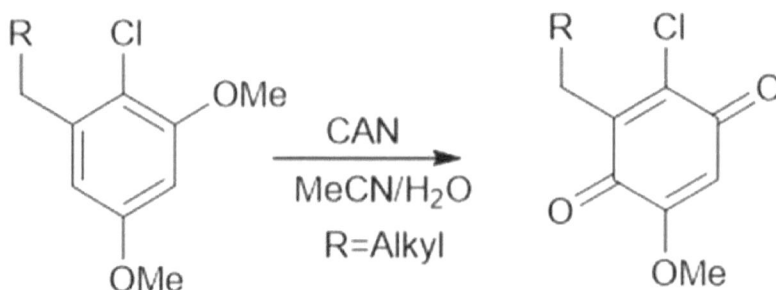

Scheme (5). Formation of 3-methoxy-5-alkyl-6-hydroxybenzo-1,4-quinones using CAN as an oxidizing agent from 3-methoxy-5-alkyl-6-chlorobenzo-1,4-quinones in acetonitrile-water solvent [40,41].

Through oxidation and chlorination, 2,3-dichloro-5,6-dimethyl-1,4-benzoquinone was generated from commercial 2,3-dimethylhydroquinone. The synthesis of novel 2,3-dimethyl-1,4-benzoquinone molecules was achieved by reacting the chemical with various piperazines, both chlorinated and substituted with piperazine, in water at moderate temperatures Scheme (**6**) [27, 42].

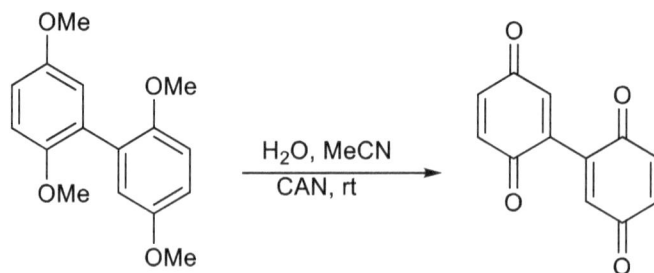

Scheme (6). Synthesis of [1,1'-bi(cyclohexane)]-3,3',6,6'-tetraene-2,2',5,5'-tetraone [27, 42].

To investigate the impact of the chlorine atom on the activity, researchers produced unchlorinated and piperazine-linked new 2,3-dimethyl-1-4-benzoquinone molecules using a one-step technique. This was achieved by utilizing commercially available 2,3-dimethylhydroquinone and various piperazines in the presence of $NaIO_3$ Scheme (**7**) [43].

SYNTHESIS OF NAPHTHOQUINONES

Naphtho-1,2-quinones were produced by oxidizing 1-tetralones with SeO_2 in AcOH with moderate yields. 2-Hydroxynaphtho-1,4-quinones have been synthesized with high efficiency (95-98%) through oxidation using potassium superoxide in dichloromethane Scheme (**8**) [44]. Naphtho-1,2-quinones have been produced from 1-tetralones through oxidation using SeO_2 and AcOH with high yields. Excellent yields of 2-hydroxynaphtho-1,4-quinones have been achieved by further oxidation with potassium superoxide in dichloromethane Scheme (**9**) [45].

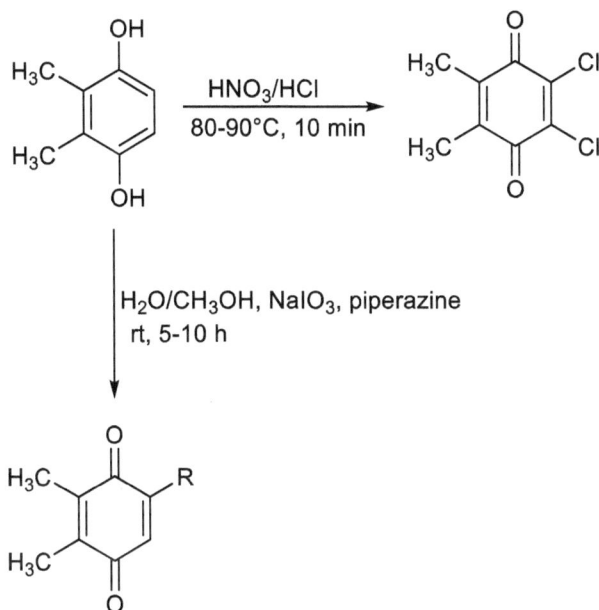

Scheme (7). Unchlorinated and piperazine-linked new 2,3-dimethyl-1,4-benzoquinone.

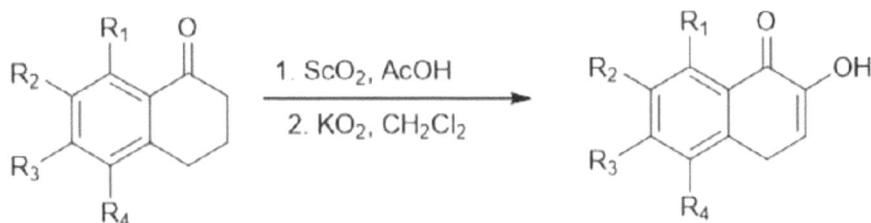

Scheme (8). Development of 2-Hydroxynaphtho-1,4-quinones.

Naphthoquinones and Benzoquinones Substitution

The cycloaddition reaction of styrenes with quinones (a class of organic compounds) has been observed to take place with the support of Lewis acid catalysts (like $MeAlCl_2$, $TiCl_4$, $SnCl_4$, or $BF_3.OEt_2$). This results in the formation of cyclobutanes, which can then be rearranged into dihydrobenzofurans upon treatment with protic acid Scheme (**10**) [46, 47].

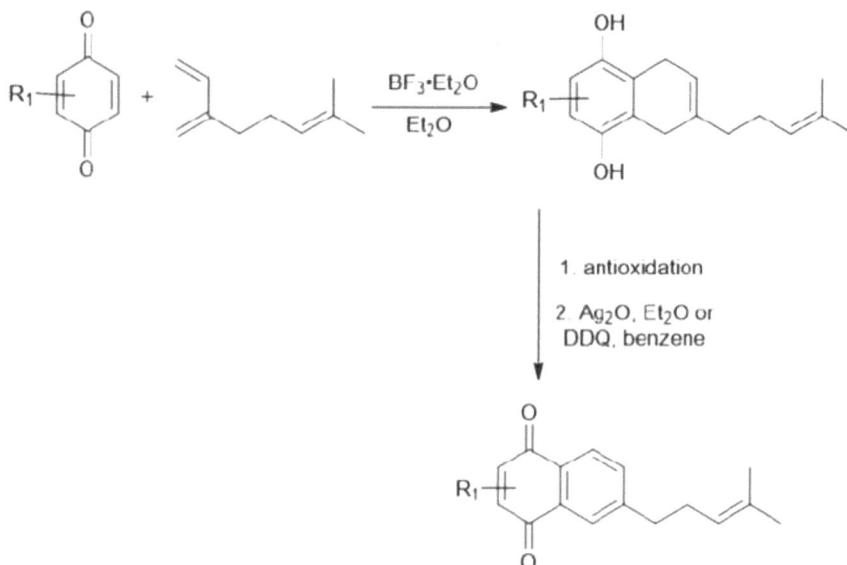

Scheme (9). Development of Naphtho-1,2-quinones.

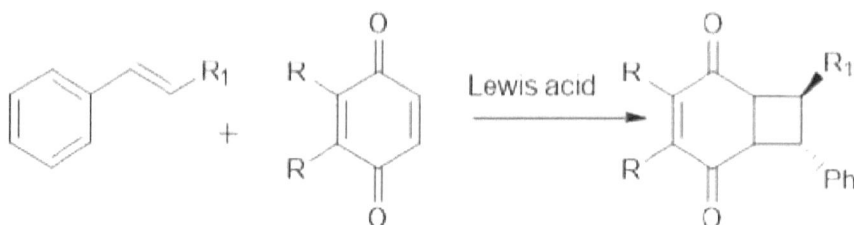

Scheme (10). Development of cyclobutanes *via* cycloaddition reaction of styrenes with quinones.

In the presence of catalytic concentrations of iodine, naphthoquinones have been successfully chlorinated using acetic acid and either $CuCl_2$ or $HgCl_2$ [48]. $CuCl_2$ or $HgCl_2$, along with catalytic amounts of iodine, have proven to be effective in chlorinating naphthoquinones in acetic acid. Additionally, it has been observed that benzoquinones can also be halogenated using these methods [49]. Innovative methods for introducing halogen atoms to quinones have been developed [50, 51]. Additionally, novel methods for the addition of halogens to quinones have been developed [52]. Furthermore, the combination of 2-bromonaphthoquinones with aryl stannanes, facilitated by Pd and Cu catalysts, led to the production of 2-aryl naphthoquinones with high yields. The compounds followed further reactions with *t*-BuOOH and Triton B, resulting in the formation of 2-aryl-3-hydroxyquinone (**Scheme 11**) [53, 54].

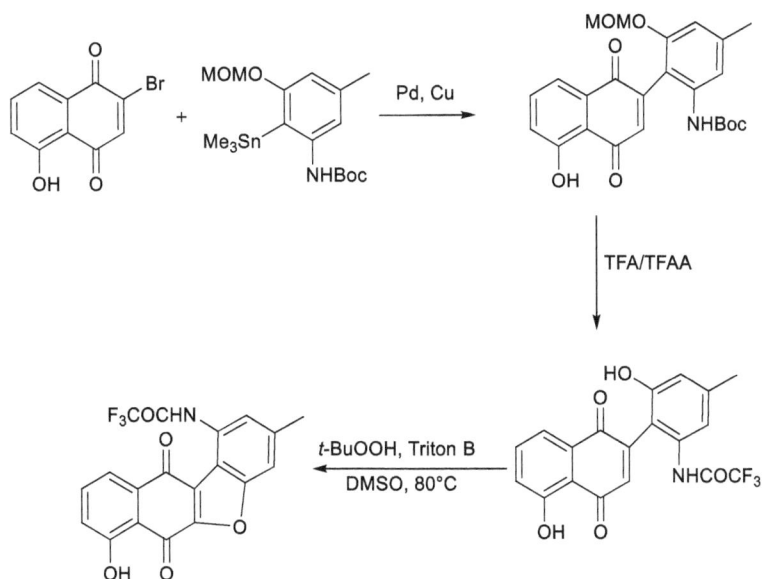

Scheme (11). Development of 2-aryl-3-hydroxyquinone.

Two synthetic versions of the antibacterial substance Juglomycin A have been identified. The first was asymmetric and demanded four stages from 5-methox--1-naphthol, whereas the second was a racemic mixture and required six steps from juglone Scheme (**12**) [55, 56].

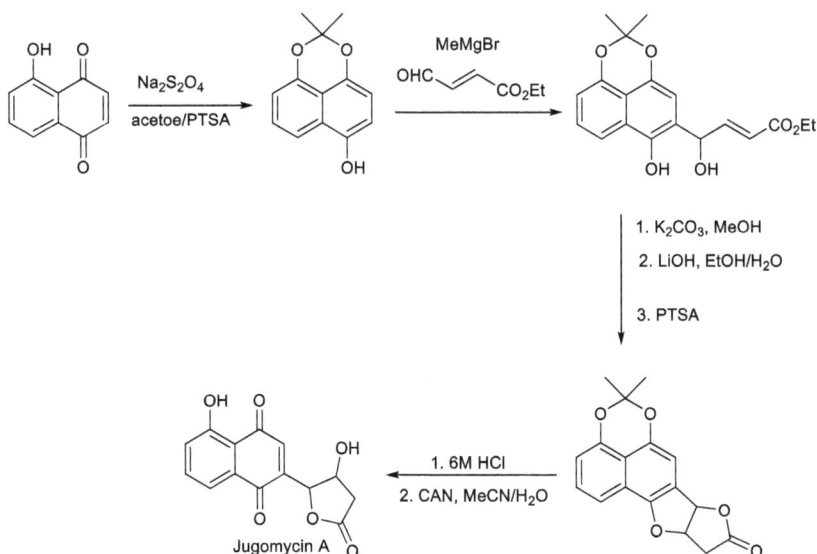

Scheme (12). Development of Juglomycin A.

SYNTHESIS OF HETEROCYCLIC QUINONES

Five-membered Heteroaromatic Quinones

Several publications have been made in the field of research on the synthesis of fused five-membered heterocyclic quinones, which has been extremely significant. However, the synthesis of heterocyclic quinones containing oxygen has not been explored much. One promising approach involves adding 2-lithiofurans to *tert*-butylcyclobutenediones, which is then quenched with methyl trifluoromethanesulfonate, and thermolysis is carried out with $(CH_3CO)_2O$. This leads to the production of 4-acetoxy-7-methoxybenzofurans, which can be further oxidized with CAN yield benzo [*b*] furandione with excellent yields after deprotection Scheme (**13**) [57]. Functionalized cyclobutenediones and 2-lithiofuran are employed as initial substances in the production of phenanthrafuranoquinones. A functionalized benzo[*b*]naphtho[2,3-*d*]furan was synthesized through the cyclization of a 2-aryl-3-hydroxyquinone [58].

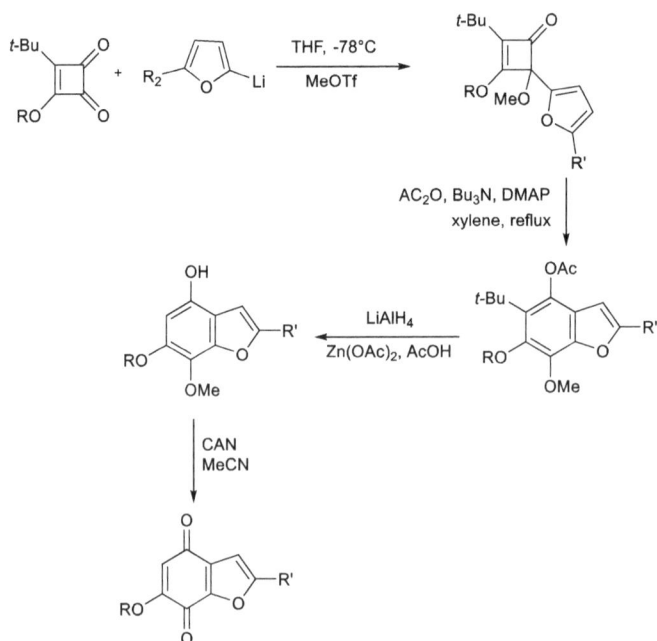

Scheme (13). Development of benzo[b]furandione.

Six-membered Heteroaromatic Quinones

Most research on quinones with six-membered heteroaromatic rings has been focused on heterocycles containing nitrogen. Synthesis of 8-hydroxy-2-methylquinoline yielded 7-*N*-substituted quinoline-5,8-dione derivatives. This was done as part of the overall process of creating the anticancer medication Lavendamycin. A crucial step involved the conversion of the amide of 5,7-bis(acylamino)-8-hydroxyquinoline into its oxidized form using $K_2Cr_2O_7$ in an aqueous CH_3COOH solution. This reaction yielded acylaminoquinolinediones with good yield Scheme (**14**) [59 - 61].

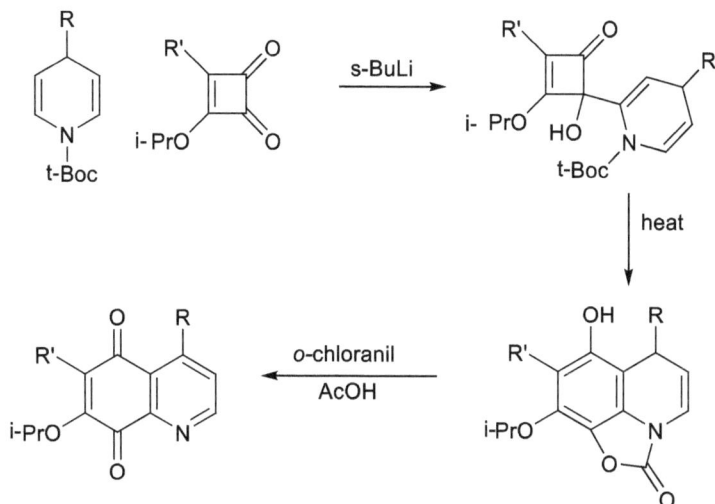

Scheme (14).   Formation of acylaminoquinolinediones.

Moreover, there have been reports on the chemical properties of these quinones. 4,6-Substituted-7-isopropoxyquinoline-5,8-dione derivatives were synthesized by reacting lithiated cyclobutenediones. Additionally, a sequence of azabenzisochromanequinones was developed using the condensation of Meldrum's acid (2,2-dimethyl-1,3-dioxane-4,6-dione) and trimethyl orthoformate, followed by a cyclization process. The quinones were synthesized as analogs of the benzisochromanequinone antibiotics, using a 6 or 7-aminochromane as the initial compound. Ultimately, the marine alkaloid Renierol was synthesized by producing 5,8-dihydro-7-methoxy-1,6-dimethylisoquinoline-5,8-dione using the isomeric 7,8-dione Scheme (**15**) [62, 63].

Saturated Heterocyclic Quinones

Depending on the phenolic substituent, spiro-fused piperidinonaphthoquinones or tetrahydronaphtho[*a*] [3] benzazepinediones can be produced *via* the ortho-position hypervalent iodine oxidation of phenol derivatives with aminoquinones. Azepinediones are synthesized from meta-substituted phenols Scheme (**16**) [64, 65].

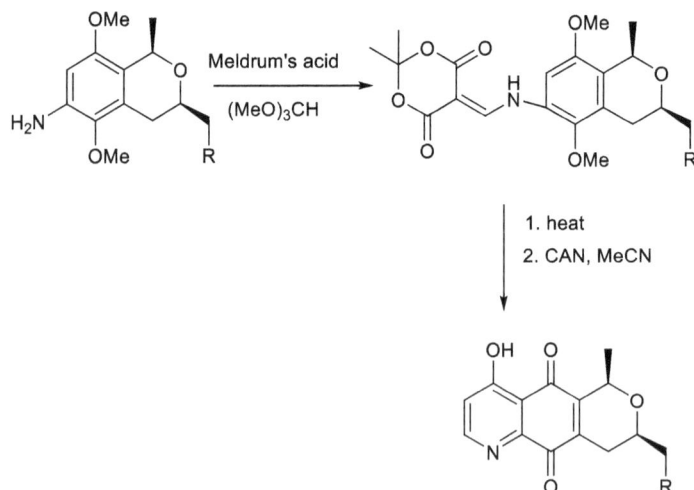

Scheme (15). Development of 5,8-dihydro-7-methoxy-1,6-dimethylisoquinoline-5,8-dione.

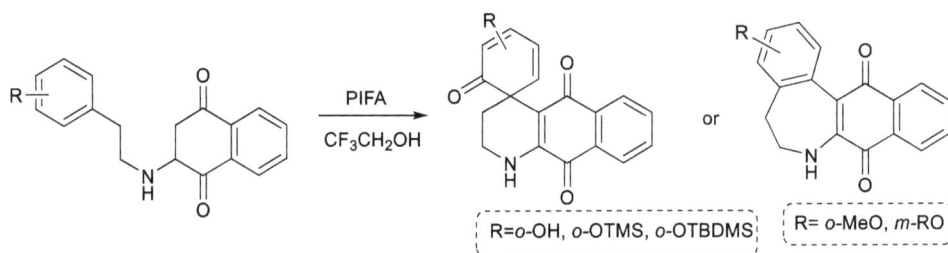

Scheme (16). Formation of spiro-fused piperidinonaphthoquinones or tetrahydronaphtho[a] [3] benzazepinediones and Azepinediones.

Using $BF_3.Et_2O$ to rearrange the phenols of spirodienone to form the azepinedione yields a naphtho[2,3-*f*]quinoxaline-7,12-dione with potential antileukemic effects. Piperidinoquinones are synthesized through the thermolysis of 4-hydroxy-4-[-za-1,6-dinyl]cyclobutenols, which are produced through the reaction of lithium salts of 4-aza-1,6-diynes with cyclobutene diones Scheme (**17**) [66, 67]. Several studies have extensively described the synthesis of benzo[*c*]pyran and/or naphtho[*c*]pyran ring structures including an oxygen atom at the fourth position. This oxygen substituent has been found to be essential for the observed biological effects. Benzopyran quinones can be produced through the mercury-mediated oxidative ring closure of 2-hydroxymethyl-3,6-dimethoxystyrenes, resulting in the formation of dimethoxybenzo[*c*]pyran, which is then oxidized using silver oxide. Naphthoquinonepyrans can be produced through the [4+2] cycloaddition reaction of benzopyran quinones, which are formed from isochromanes with 1-acetoxybuta-1,3-diene. Subsequently, these resulting compounds undergo oxidation in the presence of a base catalyst to form dehydroherbarin Scheme (**18**)

[35]. In natural naphthopyran derivatives, the synthesis of kalafungin and Hongconin has been achieved through diverse methodologies, all of which entail the generation or possible generation of naphthopyran quinones. Additionally, naphthoquinonepyrans have been synthesized by photoannulating 2-aryl-3-alkoxy naphtho-1,4-quinones under DDQ conditions. Excellent substrates for the reaction are benzyl or isopropyl ethers [68 - 72].

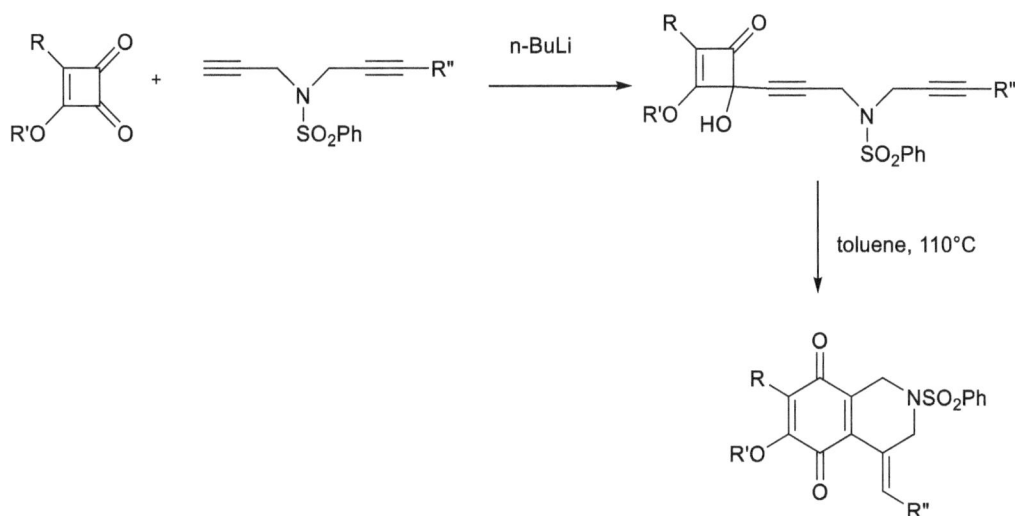

Scheme (17). Development of 4-hydroxy-4-[aza-1,6-dinyl] cyclobutenols.

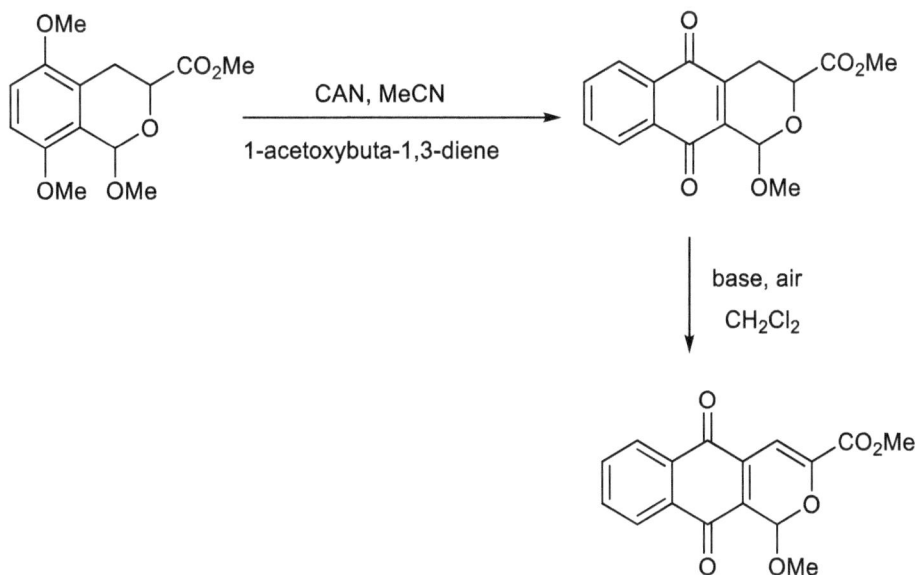

Scheme (18). Development of dehydroherbarin.

SYNTHESIS OF ANTHRAQUINONES

Anthraquinones are attractive for synthesis because of their diverse biological actions, which include anticancer, antibacterial, and antifungal properties. There are two easy techniques for synthesizing anthraquinones by oxidation. Phenanthrene-9,10-quinone was produced with a yield of 66% by oxidizing phenanthrene with dihydroxy phenylselenonium benzenesulfonate in refluxing dioxane-water. Anthra-1,2,5,6-quinones are synthesized *via* the process of oxidizing 2,6-dihydroxyanthracenes. Various oxidants, such as phenylseleninic anhydride, $K_2NO_7S_2$, and *tert*-butyl hydroperoxide, were examined. However, only phenylseleninic anhydride produced the expected products with high yields [73, 74].

Anthraquinones can also be synthesized using Diels-Alder methods. The synthesis of a silylketene acetal was followed by a reaction with 2,6-dichlorobenzo-1-4-quinone, which produced a chloro-substituted benzoquinone. The Diels-Alder reaction was performed using 1-methoxy-1,3-bis[(trimethylsilyl)oxy]buta-1,3-diene as the reactant, resulting in the production of benzo[*a*]naphthacenequinone G-2N with a yield of 83% Scheme (**19**) [75]. The synthesis of thiazolo anthraquinones involves the reaction of 4-methylene-5-(bromomethylene)-4,5 dihydrothiazole with naphthoquinones. Polyfunctional silylketene acetals can be used to generate derivatives of kermesic acid. Moreover, 2-(*p*-tolylsulfinyl)-benzo-1,4-quinone has been known as a highly responsive dienophile for cycloaddition reactions. It can react with styrenes to form phenanthrene-1,4-quinones, with vinyl naphthalenes to produce benzo[*c*]- and benzo[*a*]phenanthrene-1,4-quinones, and with two equivalents of 1-methoxycyclohexa-1,3-diene to produce tetrahydronaphthacenequinones. In addition, the researchers developed a different approach for producing 2,3-dimethoxy-6-methylanthra-9,10-quinone by a Diels-Alder process [76 - 83]. 7-Aryl-7-deoxyanthra cyclinones, which are derivatives of anthracycline, have been synthesized. The crucial intermediate tetracyclic ketone is synthesized using the Diels-Alder reaction between 1-aryl-3-trimethylsiloxybuta-1,3-diene followed by ethynylation, hydration, and oxidation. The ketone yields a final product with a 32% production rate. Angucyclines are a class of antibiotics that have a broad range of pharmacological actions, including anticancer, enzyme inhibitory, antiviral, and antifungal properties. Angucyclines were produced using a process including two subsequent aldol cyclizations and aromatization with *N*-methylmorpholine-*N*-oxide. This process facilitated the addition of the necessary phenolic hydroxy group. The starting material for this synthesis was 2-bromo-3-(bromomethyl)juglone Scheme (**20**) [84]. A study was conducted to synthesize highly substituted anthraquinones with a high yield. This was achieved using the base-induced anionic cyclization of a naphthoquinone generated from 2-bromo-

3-(bromomethyl)juglone Scheme (**21**) [85]. A simple yet versatile method for synthesizing anthraquinones from *o*-bromodiphenylmethanes has been reported, achieving high yields Scheme (**22**) [86].

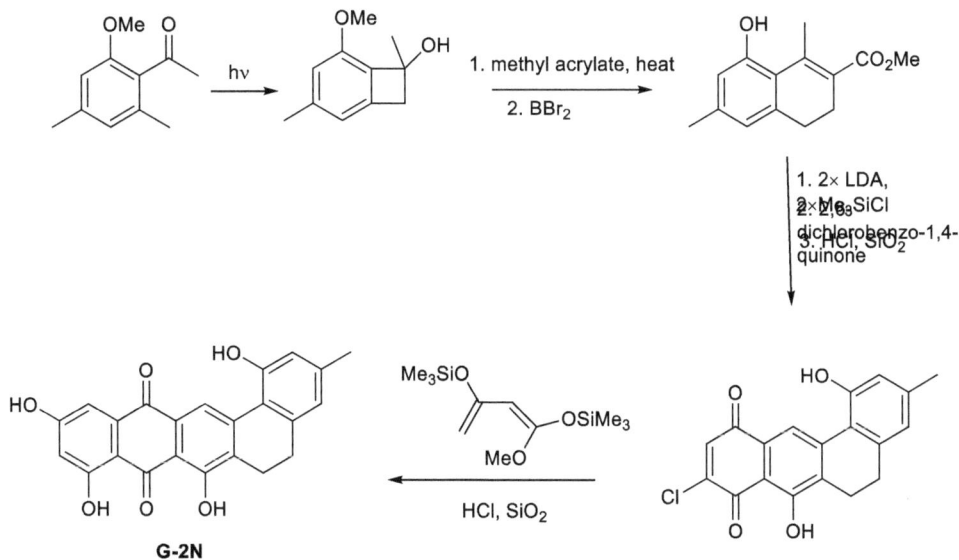

Scheme (19). Development of benzo[a]naphthacenequinone (G-2N).

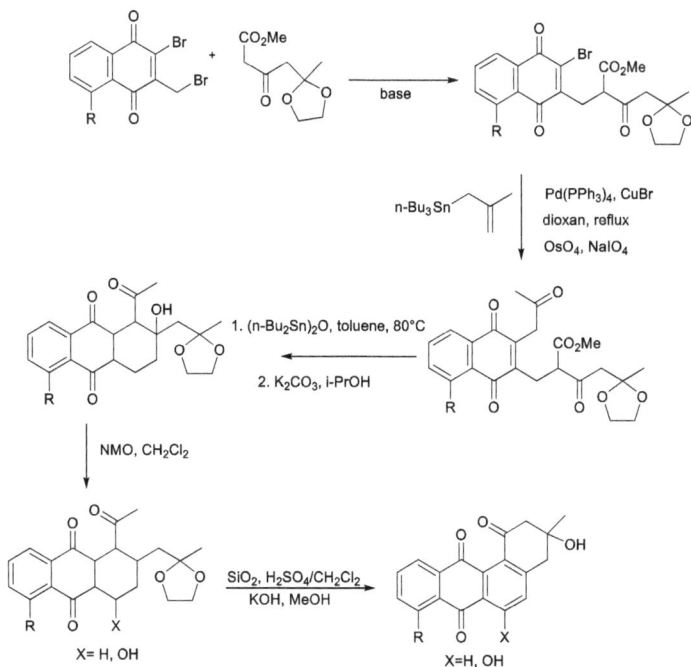

Scheme (20). Development of angucyclines.

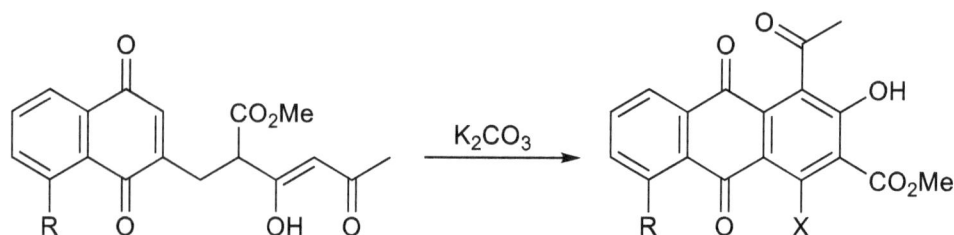

Scheme (21). Development of base-induced anionic cyclization of naphthoquinone.

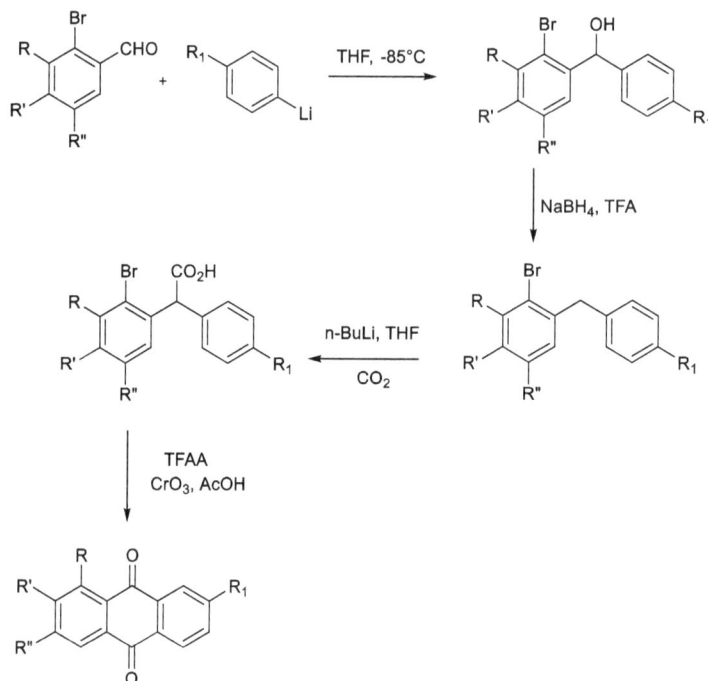

Scheme (22). Synthesis of anthraquinones from o-bromodiphenylmethanes.

QUINONE DERIVATIVES

Because of their distinct physical and chemical characteristics, quinones and their derivatives are important in chemical, environmental, and medicinal uses. Quinones and their derivatives are physiologically active chemicals that play a significant role in electron transport and photochemical reactions [87]. They are also used in the synthesis of drugs for treating conditions such as cancer, malaria, and bacterial infections. Quinone derivatives show a wide range of applications, including MOFs, chemosensors, batteries, polymorphs, catalysts, ROS, dyes, energy storage, and electron transfer [88]. In addition, both natural and synthesized quinone derivatives play a crucial role as essential constituents of effective or potential therapeutic molecules in pharmaceutical sectors [89].

Quinone Tethered Amino Derivatives

Several different metal salts, including those from alkali metal and alkaline earth metal, d-block metals, and lanthanides, can be effectively detected using amino quinones as molecular sensors. The predominant reason for this is the existence of -NH groups along with many binding units [90]. Kumar and his group have recently published a report on the production of amino anthraquinone derivatives from 1-(2-aminoethylamino)-anthracene-9,10-dione [91]. When these derivatives are mixed with salicylaldehyde in ethanol, a diamine-salicylaldehyde-based Schiff base chemosensor **2** is formed. This Schiff base demonstrates diverse optical responses in chromogenic sensors, which can be induced by adding Cu^{2+} (red to blue) and Ni^{2+} (red to green), allowing simultaneous estimation of Cu^{2+} and Ni^{2+}. In 2012, a group of researchers synthesized anthracene derivatives by reaction of 1-(2-aminoethylamino)-anthracene-9,10-dione with various aromatic aldehydes in ethanol. As a result, they obtained azo-methine derivatives (chemosensor **3-5**) in the form of dark red solids (**Scheme 23**).

Moreover, when they stirred 1,8-di-(2-aminoehylamino)anthracene-9,10-dione with 2-hydroxybenzaldehyde in ethanol, chemosensor **6 was produced**[92]. The excellent UV-visible absorption properties of the 1-aminoanthraquinone chromophore enabled efficient visual identification and measurement of Cu^{2+} and Ni^{2+} in buffered aqueous solutions Scheme **24**).

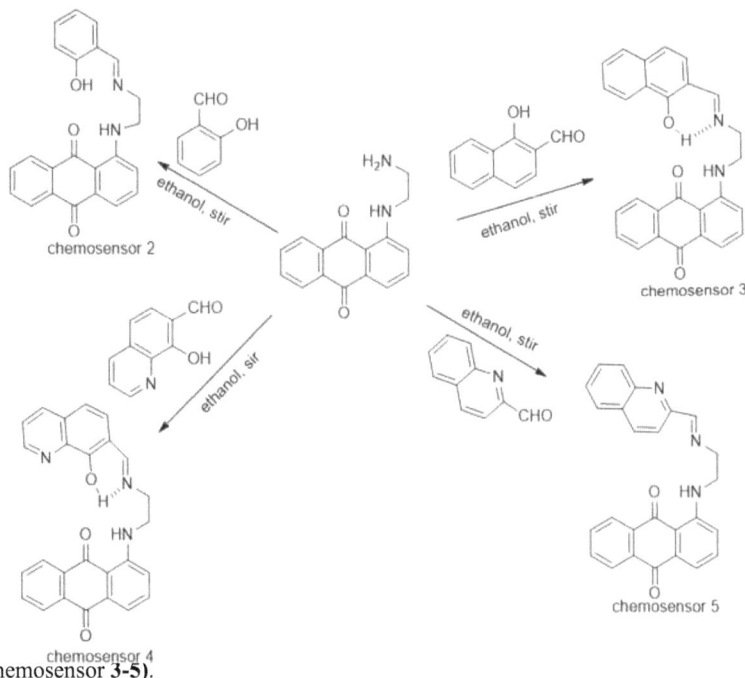

Scheme (23).   nd azo-methine derivatives (chemosensor **3-5**).

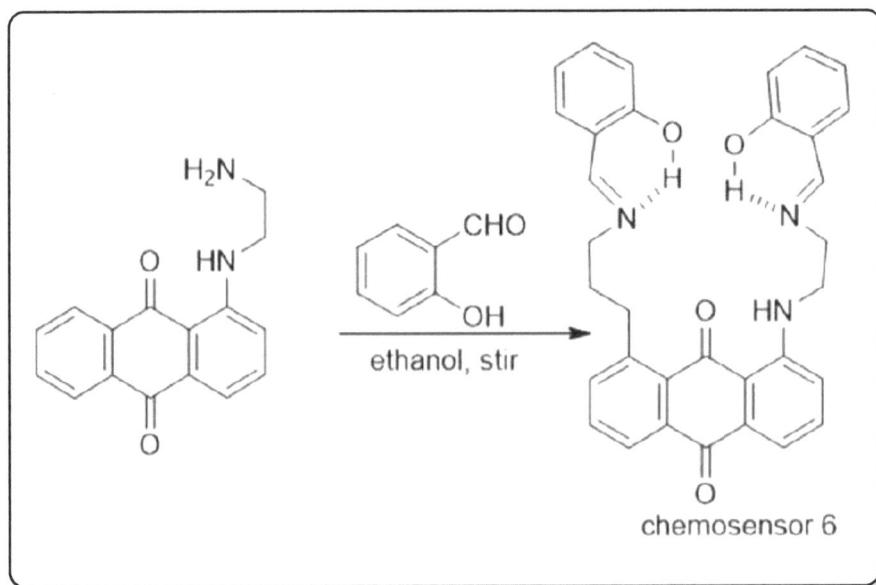

Scheme (24). Development of 1,8-di-(2-aminoehylamino)anthracene-9,10-dione with 2-hydroxybenzaldehyde in ethanol; formation of chemosensor **6**.

Pentacenequinone Derivative

In 2013, Bhalla and her research team created a pentacenequinone derivative that possesses aggregation-induced emission (AIE) characteristics [93]. This derivative can form fluorescent organic nano aggregates in aqueous media. Pd ions can be found at the nanogram level by these nanoaggregates. These nanoaggregates may also serve as reactors in the synthesis of Pd nanoparticles. By combining them with $NaBH_4$, these nanoparticles can efficiently reduce 4-nitrophenol to 4-aminophenol Scheme (25).

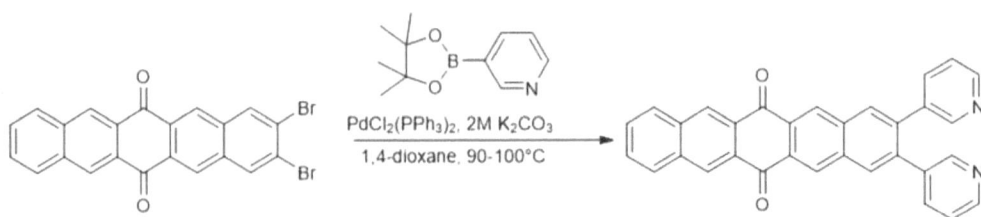

Scheme (25). Development of Pentacenequinone derivative.

Naphthoquinone Derivatives

Naphthoquinones are secondary metabolites found in plants, animals, and fungi, which serve a variety of biological functions [94]. Naphthoquinones, usually exhibiting variations of orange or brown, have a crucial function in pigmentation.

Plants that include the naphthoquinone ring are commonly utilized in conventional healthcare [27, 95, 96].

Bayrak *et al.* discovered cyclic 1,4-naphthoquinone derivatives containing heteroatoms that exhibit important biological activity, particularly against fungi and bacteria. These derivatives include both known and unknown compounds. Various 2-(aryl/alkyl)thio-3-chloro-1,4-naphthoquinones and 2,3-(aryl/alkyl)thi--1,4-naphthoquinones were produced by combining a variety of thiols with 2,3-dichloro-1,4-naphthoquinone.

These compounds were subsequently utilized as foundational components for the production of 2-(arylthio)-3-amino-1,4-naphthoquinones [97]. Except for one cyclized molecule, the researchers got 2-arylthio-3-amino-1,4-naphthoquinones as the only recognizable results from the reaction of substituted naphthoquinones with sodium azide in dimethylformamide Scheme (**26**).

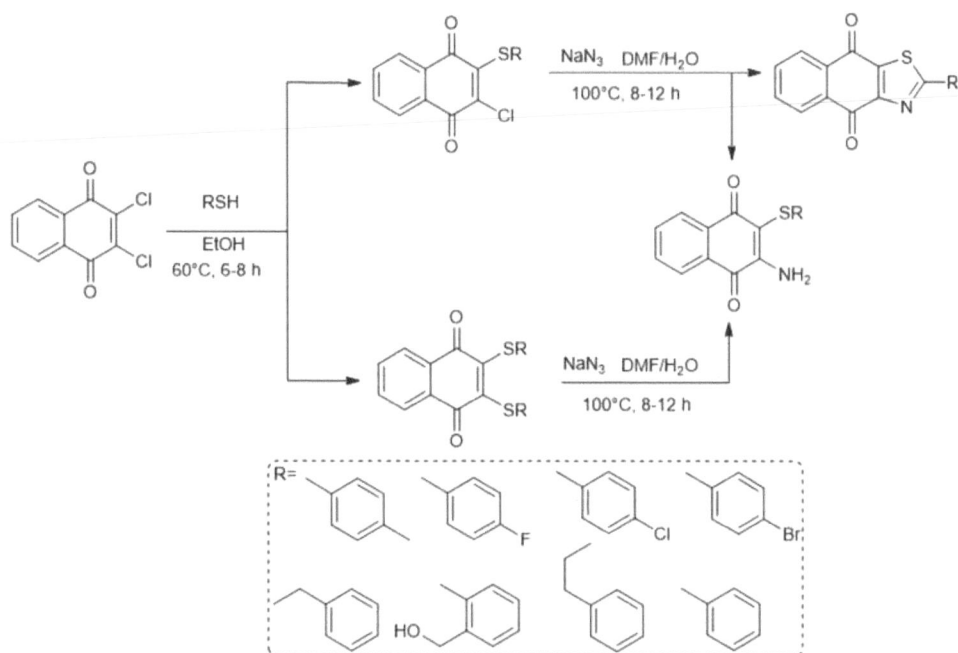

Scheme (26). Development of 2-arylthio-3-amino-1,4-naphthoquinones.

The development of novel derivatives of naphthoquinones is a significant area of research aimed at improving their pharmaceutical properties. The synthesis, physicochemical characteristics, and antibacterial activity assessment of novel 2-mercapto-3-substituted-1,4-naphthoquinones have been reported by Rau *et al.* For the synthesis, they utilized numerous 2,3-disubstituted derivatives of 1,4-

naphthoquinone and thiourea. Using dichlone (2,3-dichloro-1,4-naphthoquinone) and amines (3-aminophenol, 2-aminosulphathiazole, 4-aminosalicylic acid, or 2,4-diaminophenylhydrazine), they established a one-step synthesis to produce 2-chloro-substituted-1,4-naphthoquinones.   2-Mercapto-3-substituted-1,4-na-htho-quinones were produced by synthesizing 2-chloro-3-substituted-1,4-naphthoquinones through the use of a three-step process containing acetic acid, sodium hydroxide, and thiourea Scheme (**27** & **28**) [98].

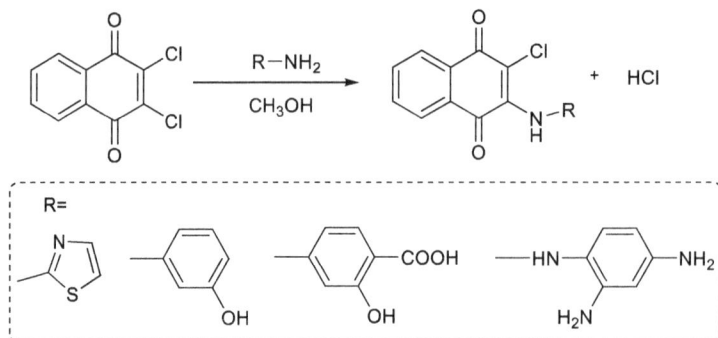

Scheme (27). Development of 2-chloro-substituted-1,4-naphthoquinones.

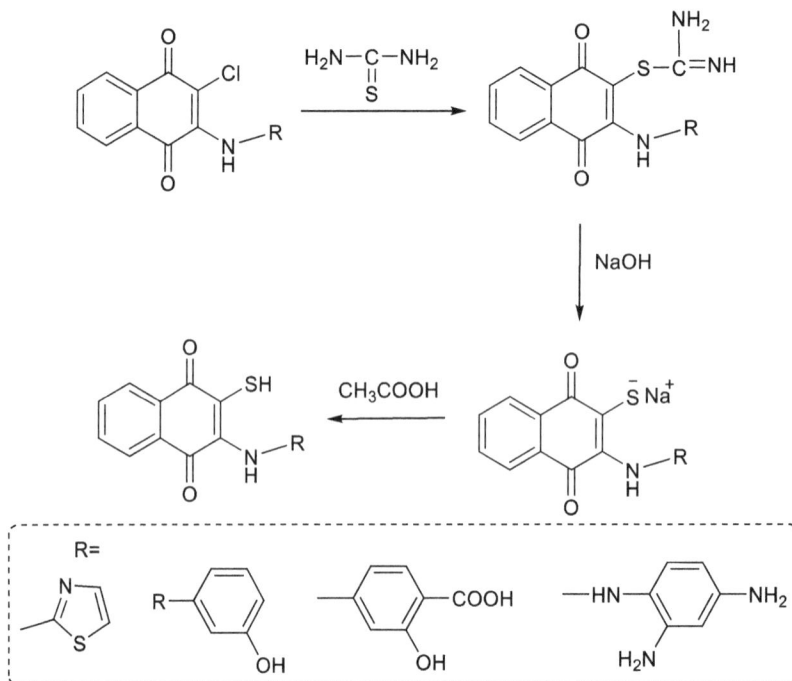

Scheme (28). Development of 2-Mercapto-3-substituted-1,4-naphtho-quinones.

The sulfanyl 1,4-naphthoquinones, containing an arylamine with a -CF_3 group at 2, 3, or 4 positions, and also 2,3-disulfanyl 1,4-naphthoquinone were produced at room temperature. This was achieved by performing a nucleophilic substitution reaction between aminonaphthoquinones and aryl- and alkyl thiols in CH_2Cl_2, with the addition of Et_3N (1.1 eq.) as a base [99]. All synthesized compounds were evaluated for antibacterial activity as well as antifungal properties. The antibacterial tests of the synthesized compounds demonstrated that they exhibited robust antibacterial properties Scheme (**29** & **30**).

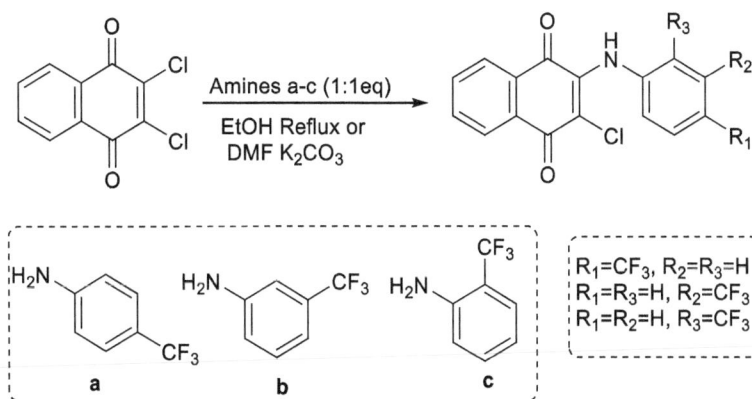

Scheme (29). Development of sulfanyl 1,4-naphthoquinones, containing an arylamine with a -CF3 group at 2, 3, or 4 positions, and also 2,3-disulfanyl 1,4-naphthoquinone.

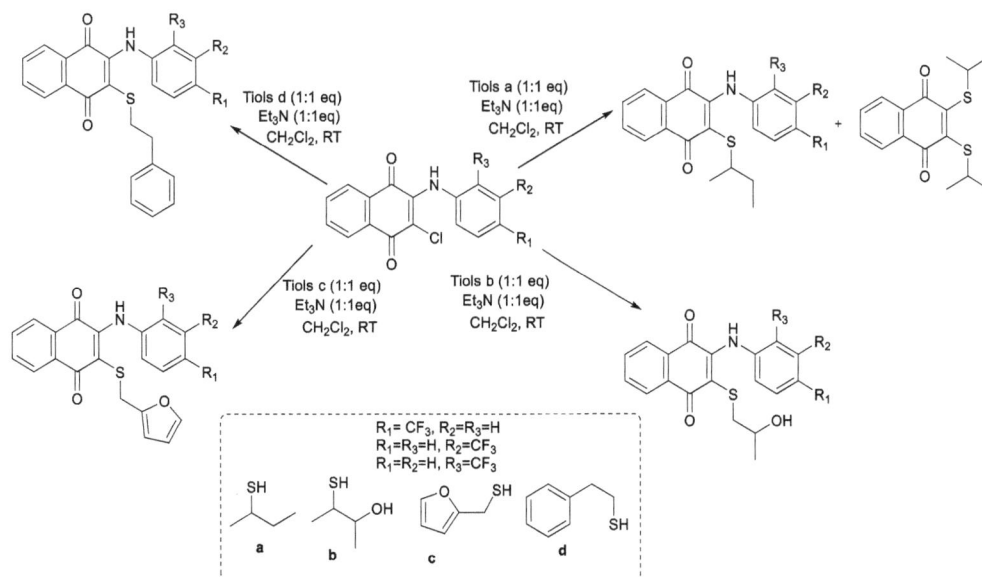

Scheme (30). Development of sulfanyl 1,4-naphthoquinones derivatives.

Using microwave irradiation, Novais and his coworkers developed 12 novel analogs of 2-hydroxy-3-phenylsulfanylmethyl- [1, 4]-naphthoquinones [100]. To synthesize these analogs, they combined a thiol as well as various substituents with a quinone methide. These analogs show *in vitro* efficacy against both Gram-negative and Gram-positive bacterial strains and are also used to combat bacterial biofilm formation Scheme (**31**).

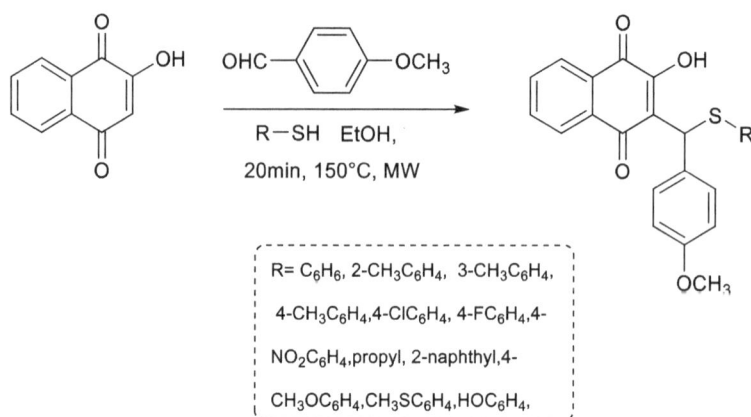

R= C_6H_6, 2-$CH_3C_6H_4$, 3-$CH_3C_6H_4$, 4-$CH_3C_6H_4$,4-ClC_6H_4, 4-FC_6H_4,4-$NO_2C_6H_4$,propyl, 2-naphthyl,4-$CH_3OC_6H_4$,$CH_3SC_6H_4$,HOC_6H_4,

Scheme (31).   Development of 12 novel analogs of 2-hydroxy-3-phenylsulfanylmethyl- [1, 4]-naphthoquinones.

Zhou *et al.* conducted a study to create a set of new anthraquinones by modifying the structure of anthraquinone, which is an active component of various Chinese medicinal products [101]. The newly synthesized molecule had the highest inhibitory effect on HCT116 cell activity and proved to effectively eliminate tumor cells by activating the ROS-JNK pathway, leading to an increase in ROS levels, JNK phosphorylation, and mitochondrial stress. The process proceeded to the release of Cytochrome-C into the cytoplasm, activating the cysteine protease pathway and eventually causing tumor cell apoptosis. These findings indicate that this compound has the potential to be used for colon cancer treatment Scheme (**32**).

Azaanthraquinones are a group of naturally occurring chemicals that exhibit diverse biological applications. Wang *et al.* and their team recently synthesized a collection of 6-substituted azaanthraquinone analogs to create a multi-targe--directed ligand (MTDL) that could potentially affect critical targets implicated in the neurodegeneration of Alzheimer's Disease (AD). The synthesized analogs exhibited substantial inhibitory effects on self-induced Aβ42 aggregation, Aβ42 secretion, and the synthesis of pro-inflammatory cytokines (TNF-α, IL-1β, and IL-6) in LPS-stimulated macrophages. Additionally, the synthesized derivatives exhibited the potential for acetylcholinesterase (AChE) and butyrylcholinesterase

(BChE), with a slight preference for the inhibition of AChE, and showed the aptitude to penetrate the blood-brain barrier with low toxicity. The synthesized compounds displayed the most potent anti-inflammatory activity, with a high degree of inhibition against Aβ42 aggregation and secretion. Additionally, they exhibited significant neuroprotective characteristics, excellent capacity to cross the blood-brain barrier (BBB), and minimal toxicity, positioning them as a highly acceptable prospect for Alzheimer's disease (AD) treatment Scheme (**33**).

Lawsonone, 6-hydroxy-1,4-naphthoquinone, and juglone were all used as building blocks for 1,4-naphthoquinone derivatives through acylation, sulfonylation, and alkylation reactions. Type A lawsone derivatives had a yield of 52-99%, type B had a yield of 53-96%, and type C had a yield of 28-95%. They looked at the structure-activity relationship and tested each drug's cytotoxicity *in vitro* against HeLa and KB cells, which are human cervical epithelioid carcinoma and oral epidermoid carcinoma, respectively. The compound showed topoisomerase inhibitory action with IC50 values ranging from 8.3 to 91 μM among other compounds that were examined for their potential to inhibit DNA topoisomerase I Scheme (**34**) [102].

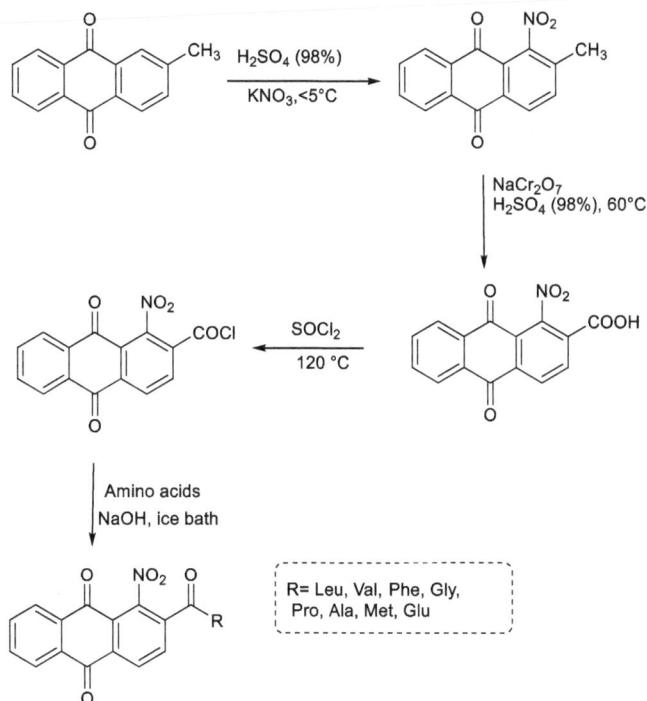

Scheme (32). Development of a set of new anthraquinones.

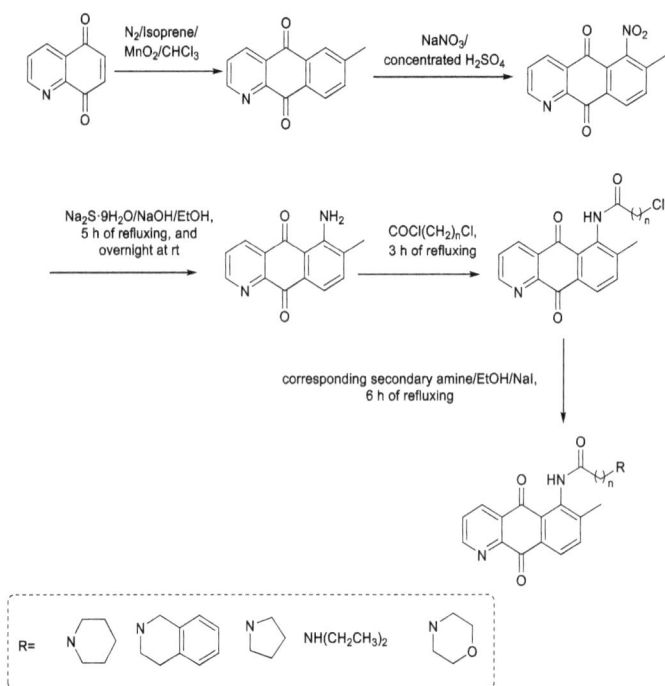

Scheme (33). Development of Azaanthraquinones.

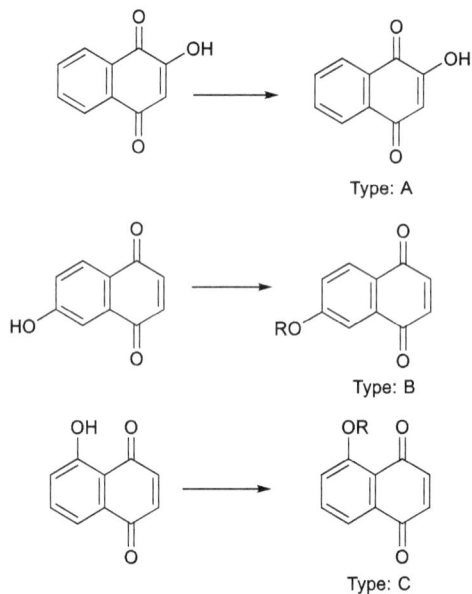

Scheme (34). Development of 1,4-naphthoquinone derivatives.

CONCLUDING REMARKS

Synthesis of a variety of novel quinones and derivatives, including naphthoquinones, benzoquinones, and anthraquinones, is the topic of discussion in this chapter. These quinones have several applications in the field of biomedicine and can be employed in various diagnostic processes. As a result of the fact that the analysis of quinones and their derivatives has revealed substantial biological activity, it is intriguing to design and synthesize further quinones and derivatives in order to investigate the biological applications of these compounds. These investigations have the potential to serve as a source of motivation for future therapeutic breakthroughs.

REFERENCES

[1]   López López LI, Nery Flores SD, Silva Belmares SY. SÁENZ GALINDO, A. Naphthoquinones: biological properties and synthesis of lawsone and derivatives-a structured review. Vitae 2014; 21(3): 248-58.
[http://dx.doi.org/10.17533/udea.vitae.17322]

[2]   Vukic MD, Vukovic NL, Djelic GT, *et al.* Antibacterial and cytotoxic activities of naphthoquinone pigments from Onosma visianii Clem. EXCLI J 2017; 16: 73-88.
[PMID: 28435429]

[3]   Tandon VK, Chhor RB, Singh RV, Rai S, Yadav DB. Design, synthesis and evaluation of novel 1,4-naphthoquinone derivatives as antifungal and anticancer agents. Bioorg Med Chem Lett 2004; 14(5): 1079-83.
[http://dx.doi.org/10.1016/j.bmcl.2004.01.002] [PMID: 14980639]

[4]   Kim BH, Yoo J, Park SH, Jung JK, Cho H, Chung Y. Synthesis and evaluation of antitumor activity of novel 1,4-Naphthoquinone derivatives (IV). Arch Pharm Res 2006; 29(2): 123-30.
[http://dx.doi.org/10.1007/BF02974272] [PMID: 16526275]

[5]   Chaudhary A, Khurana M. J. 2-Hydroxy-1, 4-Naphthoquinone: A versatile synthon in organic synthesis. Curr Org Chem 2016; 20(12): 1314-44.
[http://dx.doi.org/10.2174/1385272820666151125231522]

[6]   Ryu CK, Kim A, Im HA, Kim JY. Synthesis and antifungal activity of 1-thia-4b--za-cyclopenta[b]fluorene-4,10-diones. Bioorg Med Chem Lett 2012; 22(18): 5777-9.
[http://dx.doi.org/10.1016/j.bmcl.2012.07.097] [PMID: 22902652]

[7]   El-Najjar N, Gali-Muhtasib H, Ketola RA, Vuorela P, Urtti A, Vuorela H. The chemical and biological activities of quinones: overview and implications in analytical detection. Phytochem Rev 2011; 10(3): 353-70.
[http://dx.doi.org/10.1007/s11101-011-9209-1]

[8]   Monks TJ, Hanzlik RP, Cohen GM, Ross D, Graham DG. Quinone chemistry and toxicity. Toxicol Appl Pharmacol 1992; 112(1): 2-16.
[http://dx.doi.org/10.1016/0041-008X(92)90273-U] [PMID: 1733045]

[9]   Yang S, Wang W, Ling T, *et al.* α-tocopherol quinone inhibits β-amyloid aggregation and cytotoxicity, disaggregates preformed fibrils and decreases the production of reactive oxygen species, NO and inflammatory cytokines. Neurochem Int 2010; 57(8): 914-22.
[http://dx.doi.org/10.1016/j.neuint.2010.09.011] [PMID: 20933033]

[10]   Woo CC, Kumar AP, Sethi G, Tan KHB. Thymoquinone: Potential cure for inflammatory disorders and cancer. Biochem Pharmacol 2012; 83(4): 443-51.
[http://dx.doi.org/10.1016/j.bcp.2011.09.029] [PMID: 22005518]

[11]   Savarino L, Fioravanti A, Leo G, Aloisi R, Mian M. Anthraquinone-2,6-disulfonic acid as a disease-modifying osteoarthritis drug: an *in vitro* and *in vivo* study. Clin Orthop Relat Res 2007; 461(461): 231-7.
[http://dx.doi.org/10.1097/BLO.0b013e3180533b5c] [PMID: 17806152]

[12]   Lown JW. The mechanism of action of quinone antibiotics. Mol Cell Biochem 1983; 55(1): 17-40.
[http://dx.doi.org/10.1007/BF00229240] [PMID: 6353197]

[13]   Fritsch VN, Loi VV, Busche T, *et al.* The MarR-type repressor MhqR confers quinone and antimicrobial resistance in Staphylococcus aureus. Antioxid Redox Signal 2019; 31(16): 1235-52.
[http://dx.doi.org/10.1089/ars.2019.7750] [PMID: 31310152]

[14]   Atia A, Alrawaiq N, Abdullah A. A review of NAD (P) H: Quinone oxidoreductase 1 (NQO1); A multifunctional antioxidant enzyme. J Appl Pharm Sci 2014; 4(12): 118-22.

[15]   Asaduzzaman Khan M, Tania M, Fu S, Fu J. Thymoquinone, as an anticancer molecule: from basic research to clinical investigation. Oncotarget 2017; 8(31): 51907-19.
[http://dx.doi.org/10.18632/oncotarget.17206] [PMID: 28881699]

[16]   Colucci MA, Couch GD, Moody CJ. Natural and synthetic quinones and their reduction by the quinone reductase enzyme NQO1: from synthetic organic chemistry to compounds with anticancer potential. Org Biomol Chem 2008; 6(4): 637-56.
[http://dx.doi.org/10.1039/B715270A] [PMID: 18264564]

[17]   Frydman B, Marton LJ, Sun JS, *et al.* Induction of DNA topoisomerase II-mediated DNA cleavage by β-lapachone and related naphthoquinones. Cancer Res 1997; 57(4): 620-7.
[PMID: 9044837]

[18]   Enguita F J, Leitão A L. Hydroquinone: environmental pollution, toxicity, and microbial answers. Bio Med Research International 2013; 2013.
[http://dx.doi.org/10.1155/2013/542168]

[19]   Kishi S, Saito K, Kato Y, Ishikita H. Redox potentials of ubiquinone, menaquinone, phylloquinone, and plastoquinone in aqueous solution. Photosynth Res 2017; 134(2): 193-200.
[http://dx.doi.org/10.1007/s11120-017-0433-4] [PMID: 28831654]

[20]   Pink JJ, Planchon SM, Tagliarino C, Varnes ME, Siegel D, Boothman DA. NAD(P)H:Quinone oxidoreductase activity is the principal determinant of β-lapachone cytotoxicity. J Biol Chem 2000; 275(8): 5416-24.
[http://dx.doi.org/10.1074/jbc.275.8.5416] [PMID: 10681517]

[21]   Kamo S, Yoshioka K, Kuramochi K, Tsubaki K. Total syntheses of juglorescein and juglocombins A and B. Angew Chem Int Ed 2016; 55(35): 10317-20.
[http://dx.doi.org/10.1002/anie.201604765] [PMID: 27460486]

[22]   Petronico A, Bassett KL, Nicolau BG, Gewirth AA, Nuzzo RG. Toward a Four-Electron Redox Quinone Polymer for High Capacity Lithium Ion Storage. Adv Energy Mater 2018; 8(5): 1700960.
[http://dx.doi.org/10.1002/aenm.201700960]

[23]   Farrell MM. Electroanalysis in the nanodomain: quinone monolayers and nanometer dimensioned electrodes. Dublin City University 2003.

[24]   Zurro M, Maestro A. Asymmetric Catalytic Transformations of Aza- *ortho* - and Aza- *para* -Quinone Methides. ChemCatChem 2023; 15(13): e202300500.
[http://dx.doi.org/10.1002/cctc.202300500]

[25]   Tandon VK, Maurya HK, Mishra NN, Shukla PK. Design, synthesis and biological evaluation of novel nitrogen and sulfur containing hetero-1,4-naphthoquinones as potent antifungal and antibacterial agents. Eur J Med Chem 2009; 44(8): 3130-7.
[http://dx.doi.org/10.1016/j.ejmech.2009.03.006] [PMID: 19349095]

[26]   Ryu CK, Kim DH. The synthesis and antimicrobial activities of some 1,4-naphthoquinones (II). Arch

Pharm Res 1992; 15(3): 263-8.
[http://dx.doi.org/10.1007/BF02974067]

[27] Tandon VK, Maurya HK, Verma MK, Kumar R, Shukla PK. 'On water' assisted synthesis and biological evaluation of nitrogen and sulfur containing hetero-1,4-naphthoquinones as potent antifungal and antibacterial agents. Eur J Med Chem 2010; 45(6): 2418-26.
[http://dx.doi.org/10.1016/j.ejmech.2010.02.023] [PMID: 20207052]

[28] Abraham I, Joshi R, Pardasani P, Pardasani RT. Recent advances in 1,4-benzoquinone chemistry. J Braz Chem Soc 2011; 22(3): 385-421.
[http://dx.doi.org/10.1590/S0103-50532011000300002]

[29] Dandawate PR, Vyas AC, Padhye SB, Singh MW, Baruah JB. Perspectives on medicinal properties of benzoquinone compounds. Mini Rev Med Chem 2010; 10(5): 436-54.
[http://dx.doi.org/10.2174/138955710791330909] [PMID: 20370705]

[30] Kumagai Y, Shinkai Y, Miura T, Cho AK. The chemical biology of naphthoquinones and its environmental implications. Annu Rev Pharmacol Toxicol 2012; 52(1): 221-47.
[http://dx.doi.org/10.1146/annurev-pharmtox-010611-134517] [PMID: 21942631]

[31] Caro Y, Anamale L, Fouillaud M, Laurent P, Petit T, Dufossé L. Natural hydroxyanthraquinoid pigments as potent food grade colorants: an overview. Nat Prod Bioprospect 2012; 2(5): 174-93.
[http://dx.doi.org/10.1007/s13659-012-0086-0]

[32] Duval J, Pecher V, Poujol M, Lesellier E. Research advances for the extraction, analysis and uses of anthraquinones: A review. Ind Crops Prod 2016; 94: 812-33.
[http://dx.doi.org/10.1016/j.indcrop.2016.09.056]

[33] Takeya T, Motegi S, Itoh T, Tobinaga S. TOBINAGA, S. Utility of Weitz'aminium salt for obtaining quinones as potential synthetic precursors of quassinoids. Chem Pharm Bull (Tokyo) 1997; 45(4): 613-9.
[http://dx.doi.org/10.1248/cpb.45.613]

[34] Feldman KS, Quideau S, Appel HM. Galloyl-derived orthoquinones as reactive partners in nucleophilic additions and Diels— Alder dimerizations: A novel route to the dehydrodigalloyl linker unit of agrimoniin-type ellagitannins. J Org Chem 1996; 61(19): 6656-65.
[http://dx.doi.org/10.1021/jo961043u] [PMID: 11667537]

[35] Murahashi SI, Naota T, Miyaguchi N, Noda S. Ruthenium-catalyzed oxidation of phenols with alkyl hydroperoxides. A novel, facile route to 2-substituted quinones. J Am Chem Soc 1996; 118(10): 2509-10.
[http://dx.doi.org/10.1021/ja954009q]

[36] Suresh S, Skaria S, Ponrathnam S. Polymer supported vanadium salt as a catalyst for the oxidation of phenols. Synth Commun 1996; 26(11): 2113-7.
[http://dx.doi.org/10.1080/00397919608003569]

[37] Hashemi MM, Beni YA. Oxidation of phenols to quinones by oxygen catalysed by a mixture of cobalt and manganese salts of p-aminobenzoic acid supported on silica gel. J Chem Res Synop 1998; (3): 138-9.
[http://dx.doi.org/10.1039/a705855a]

[38] Akai S, Takeda Y, Iio K, Takahashi K, Fukuda N, Kita Y. Novel ipso-Substitution of p-Sulfinylphenols through the Pummerer-Type Reaction: A Selective and Efficient Synthesis of p-Quinones and Protected p-Dihydroquinones. J Org Chem 1997; 62(16): 5526-36.
[http://dx.doi.org/10.1021/jo970418o]

[39] Guan J, Brossi A, Zhu XK, Wang HK, Lee KH. Oxidation products of phenolic thiocolchicines: Ring a quinones and dienones. Synth Commun 1998; 28(9): 1585-91.
[http://dx.doi.org/10.1080/00397919808006862]

[40] Palmgren A, Thorarensen A, Bäckvall JE. Efficient synthesis of symmetrical 2, 5-disubstituted

benzoquinones *via* palladium-catalyzed double Negishi coupling. J Org Chem 1998; 63(11): 3764-8.
[http://dx.doi.org/10.1021/jo9721812]

[41]   Yao Z, Tang W, Wang X, Wang C, Yang C, Fan C. Synthesis of 1,4-benzoquinone dimer as a high-capacity (501 mA h g−1) and high-energy-density (>1000 Wh kg−1) organic cathode for organic Li-Ion full batteries. J Power Sources 2020; 448: 227456.
[http://dx.doi.org/10.1016/j.jpowsour.2019.227456]

[42]   Ryu CK, Lee JY. Synthesis and antifungal activity of 6-hydroxycinnolines. Bioorg Med Chem Lett 2006; 16(7): 1850-3.
[http://dx.doi.org/10.1016/j.bmcl.2006.01.005] [PMID: 16434193]

[43]   Gusakov EA, Topchu IA, Mazitova AM, *et al.* Design, synthesis and biological evaluation of 2-quinolyl-1,3-tropolone derivatives as new anti-cancer agents. RSC Advances 2021; 11(8): 4555-71.
[http://dx.doi.org/10.1039/D0RA10610K] [PMID: 33996031]

[44]   Bekaert A, Andrieux J, Plat M, Brion JD. A convenient synthesis of monpain trimethylether. Tetrahedron Lett 1997; 38(24): 4219-20.
[http://dx.doi.org/10.1016/S0040-4039(97)00860-5]

[45]   Miguel del Corral J, Gordaliza M, Angeles Castro M, Mahiques MM, San Feliciano A, García-Grávalos MD. Further antineoplastic terpenylquinones and terpenylhydroquinones. Bioorg Med Chem 1998; 6(1): 31-41.
[http://dx.doi.org/10.1016/S0968-0896(97)10007-4] [PMID: 9502103]

[46]   Carreño MC, García Ruano JL, Toledo MA, *et al.* Influence of the Sulfinyl Group on the Chemoselectivity and π-Facial Selectivity of Diels−Alder Reactions of *(S)* -2-(*p* -Tolylsulfinyl)-1-4-benzoquinone. J Org Chem 1996; 61(2): 503-9.
[http://dx.doi.org/10.1021/jo951438y] [PMID: 11666967]

[47]   Engler TA, Iyengar R. Lewis acid-directed reactions of quinones with styrenyl systems: the case of 2-methoxy-3-methyl-1, 4-benzoquinone. J Org Chem 1998; 63(6): 1929-34.
[http://dx.doi.org/10.1021/jo971937u]

[48]   Thapliyal PC. Iodine catalyzed chlorination of naphthoquinones using metal (II) chlorides. Synth Commun 1998; 28(7): 1123-6.
[http://dx.doi.org/10.1080/00397919808005952]

[49]   Bansal V, Kanodia S, Thapliyal PC, Khanna RN. Microwave induced selective bromination of 1, 4-quinones and coumarins. Synth Commun 1996; 26(5): 887-92.
[http://dx.doi.org/10.1080/00397919608003692]

[50]   Kidwai M, Kohli S, Kumar P. Microwave-induced Selective Mercuration of 1,4-Naphthoquinone. J Chem Res Synop 1998; (1): 52-3.
[http://dx.doi.org/10.1039/a705428i]

[51]   de Oliveira RA, Carazza F, Pereira MOS. Synthesis of 2,6-Dimethoxy-3-(3-methyl-2-buten-l)-1,4-benzoquinone Using Organometallic Reagents. Synth Commun 1997; 27(10): 1743-9.
[http://dx.doi.org/10.1080/00397919708004086]

[52]   Echavarren AM, de Frutos Ó, Tamayo N, Noheda P, Calle P. Palladium-catalyzed coupling of naphthoquinone triflates with stannanes. Unprecedented nucleophilic aromatic substitution on a hydroxynaphthoquinone triflate. J Org Chem 1997; 62(13): 4524-7.
[http://dx.doi.org/10.1021/jo9621027] [PMID: 11671788]

[53]   de Frutos Ó, Echavarren AM. Syntheses of fenanthroviridone, gilvocarcin BE-12406X2, and antibiotic ws 5995b based on the palladium and copper catalyzed coupling of organostannanes with bromoquinones. Tetrahedron Lett 1996; 37(49): 8953-6.
[http://dx.doi.org/10.1016/S0040-4039(96)02056-4]

[54]   Echavarren AM, Tamayo N, de Frutos Ó, García A. Synthesis of benzo[b]carbazoloquinones by coupling of organostannanes with bromoquinones. Tetrahedron 1997; 53(49): 16835-46.

[http://dx.doi.org/10.1016/S0040-4020(97)10085-0]

[55]   Maeda H, Kraus GA. A direct asymmetric synthesis of juglomycin A. J Org Chem 1996; 61(9): 2986-7.
       [http://dx.doi.org/10.1021/jo952077p] [PMID: 11667158]

[56]   Kraus GA, Liu P. A Racemic Synthesis of the Novel Antibacterial Agent Juglomycin A. Synth Commun 1996; 26(23): 4501-6.
       [http://dx.doi.org/10.1080/00397919608003852]

[57]   Liu F, Liebeskind LS. *tert* -Butyl Substituent as a Regiodirecting and Novel C−H Protecting Group in Cyclobutenedione-Based Benzannulation Chemistry. J Org Chem 1998; 63(9): 2835-44.
       [http://dx.doi.org/10.1021/jo971565p]

[58]   Heileman MJ, Tiedemann R, Moore HW. New metathesis methodology leading to angularly-fused polycyclic quinones and related compounds. J Am Chem Soc 1998; 120(15): 3801-2.
       [http://dx.doi.org/10.1021/ja980039s]

[59]   Behforouz M, Haddad J, Cai W, *et al.* Highly efficient and practical syntheses of lavendamycin methyl ester and related novel quinolindiones. J Org Chem 1996; 61(19): 6552-5.
       [http://dx.doi.org/10.1021/jo960794t] [PMID: 11667519]

[60]   Behforouz M, Haddad J, Cai W, Gu Z. Chemistry of Quinoline-5,8-diones. J Org Chem 1998; 63(2): 343-6.
       [http://dx.doi.org/10.1021/jo971823i]

[61]   Zhang D, Llorente I, Liebeskind LS. Versatile Synthesis of Dihydroquinolines and Quinoline Quinones Using Cyclobutenediones. Construction of the Pyridoacridine Ring System. J Org Chem 1997; 62(13): 4330-8.
       [http://dx.doi.org/10.1021/jo970039v] [PMID: 11671755]

[62]   Tödter C, Lackner H. Synthesis of Azabenzisochromanequinone Antibiotics, II: 9(6)-Hydroxy-6(-)-Azabenzisochromanequinones *via* Aminoisochromanes and Meldrum's Acid. Synthesis 1997; 1997(5): 567-72.
       [http://dx.doi.org/10.1055/s-1997-1222]

[63]   Molina P, Vidal A, Tovar F. Electrocyclization of β-Arylvinyl Ketenimines: Formal Syntheses of the Alkaloid from Marine Origin, 5,8-Dihydro-7-methoxy-1,6-dimethylisoquinoline-5,8-dione, and 3-Ethoxycarbonylrenierol. Synthesis 1997; 1997(8): 963-6.
       [http://dx.doi.org/10.1055/s-1997-1277]

[64]   Kita Y, Takada T, Ibaraki M, *et al.* An intramolecular cyclization of phenol derivatives bearing aminoquinones using a hypervalent iodine reagent. J Org Chem 1996; 61(1): 223-7.
       [http://dx.doi.org/10.1021/jo951439q]

[65]   Chang P. A Facile Synthesis of A Naphtho[2,3-f]-Quinoxaline-7, 12-Dione From Mitoxantrone. Synth Commun 1996; 26(21): 3929-35.
       [http://dx.doi.org/10.1080/00397919608003814]

[66]   Xiong Y, Moore HW. Ring expansion of 4-alkynylcyclobutenones. Synthesis of piperidinoquinones, highly substituted dihydrophenanthridines, benzophenanthridines, and the naturally occurring pyrrolophenanthridine, assoanine. J Org Chem 1996; 61(26): 9168-77.
       [http://dx.doi.org/10.1021/jo9613803]

[67]   Wang W, Breining T, Li T, Milburn R, Attardo G. Dehydrogenation by air: Preparation of 1,3-disubstituted-5,1-dioxo-5,10-dihydro-1H-benzo[g] isochromene scaffold. Tetrahedron Lett 1998; 39(17): 2459-62.
       [http://dx.doi.org/10.1016/S0040-4039(98)00287-1]

[68]   Brimble MA, Nairn MR. Reductive thioalkylation of a kalafungin analogue. Tetrahedron Lett 1998; 39(27): 4879-82.
       [http://dx.doi.org/10.1016/S0040-4039(98)00884-3]

[69]   Swenton JS, Freskos JN, Dalidowicz P, Kerns ML. A Facile Entry into Naphthopyran Quinones *via* an Annelation Reaction of Levoglucosenone. The Total Synthesis of (−)-Hongconin. J Org Chem 1996; 61(2): 459-64.
[http://dx.doi.org/10.1021/jo951607e] [PMID: 11666961]

[70]   Green IR, Hugo VI, Oosthuizen F, Giles RGF. A high yielding synthesis of racemic hongconin. Synth Commun 1996; 26(5): 867-80.
[http://dx.doi.org/10.1080/00397919608003690]

[71]   Deshpande PP, Price KN, Baker DC. A Concise, Enantioselective Synthesis of (−)- and (+)-Hongconin. J Org Chem 1996; 61(2): 455-8.
[http://dx.doi.org/10.1021/jo951602h] [PMID: 11666960]

[72]   Onofrey TJ, Gomez D, Winters M, Moore HW. A New Photoannulation Reaction of 2-Aryl-3-alk-xy-1,4-naphthquinones. Synthesis of Dimethylnaphthgeranine E. J Org Chem 1997; 62(17): 5658-9.
[http://dx.doi.org/10.1021/jo970385c]

[73]   Stuhr-Hansen N, Henriksen L. Syntheses of 9, 10-phenanthrenequinone and 9-methoxyphenanthrene by oxidation of phenanthrene with dihydroxy phenylselenonium benzenesulfonate. Synth Commun 1997; 27(1): 89-94.
[http://dx.doi.org/10.1080/00397919708004809]

[74]   Zippel S, Boldt P. Part 15.(1, 2: 5, 6)-Anthradiquinones by Oxidation of 2, 6-Dihydroxyanthracenes. ChemInform 1997; 28(30): no-no.

[75]   Kraus GA, Zhao G. Direct Synthesis of G-2N. J Org Chem 1996; 61(8): 2770-3.
[http://dx.doi.org/10.1021/jo9517609] [PMID: 11667111]

[76]   Al Hariri M, Jouve K, Pautet F, Domard M, Fenet B, Fillion H. Generation and Trapping of 4-Methylene-5-(bromomethylene)-4,5-dihydrothiazole with Dienophiles. J Org Chem 1997; 62(2): 405-10.
[http://dx.doi.org/10.1021/jo961457n] [PMID: 11671416]

[77]   Bingham SJ, Tyman JHP. The synthesis of kermesic acid and isokermesic acid derivatives and of related dihydroxyanthraquinones. J Chem Soc, Perkin Trans 1 1997; (24): 3637-42.
[http://dx.doi.org/10.1039/a704317a]

[78]   Carreño MC, Mahugo J, Urbano A. Improved synthesis of 1, 4-phenanthrenequinones from Diels-Alder cycloadditions of 2-(p-tolylsulfinyl)-1, 4-benzoquinone. Tetrahedron Lett 1997; 38(17): 3047-50.
[http://dx.doi.org/10.1016/S0040-4039(97)00505-4]

[79]   Carreño MC, García Ruano JL, Urbano A. Remote Regiocontrol by a Thioether Group in Diels−Alder Reactions of Naphthazarin: Regioselective Access to Tetracyclic Polyhydroxyquinones. J Org Chem 1996; 61(18): 6136-8.
[http://dx.doi.org/10.1021/jo960855n] [PMID: 11667447]

[80]   Zhang X, Fox BW, Hadfield JA. Preparation of naturally occurring anthraquinones. Synth Commun 1996; 26(1): 49-62.
[http://dx.doi.org/10.1080/00397919608003861]

[81]   Dienes Z, Vogel P. Asymmetric Synthesis and DNA Intercalation of (−)--[[(Aminoalkyl)oxy]methyl]-4-demethoxy-6,7- dideoxydaunomycinones [1]. J Org Chem 1996; 61(20): 6958-70.
[http://dx.doi.org/10.1021/jo960606z] [PMID: 11667593]

[82]   Acosta JC, Caballero E, Grávalos DG, *et al.* New 7-aryl analogues of anthracyclines: Synthesis and cytotoxic activity of (±)-7-(3,4,5-trimethoxyphenyl)-7-deoxyidarubicinone. Bioorg Med Chem Lett 1997; 7(23): 2955-8.
[http://dx.doi.org/10.1016/S0960-894X(97)10122-6]

[83]   Adeva M, Caballero E, García F, Medarde M, Sahagún H, Tomé F. Diels-alder reactivity of 1-

alkoxyphenyl-3-trialkylsiloxy-1,3-dienes. Tetrahedron Lett 1997; 38(39): 6893-6.
[http://dx.doi.org/10.1016/S0040-4039(97)01588-8]

[84]   Krohn K, Böker N, Flörke U, Freund C. Synthesis of angucyclines. 8. Biomimetic-type synthesis of rabelomycin, tetrangomycin, and related ring B aromatic angucyclinones. J Org Chem 1997; 62(8): 2350-6.
[http://dx.doi.org/10.1021/jo9622587] [PMID: 11671566]

[85]   Krohn K, Böker N, Gauhier A, Schäfer G, Werner F. Highly substituted anthraquinones by anionic cyclization reactions. J Prakt Chem Chem-Zeitung 1996; 338(1): 349-54.
[http://dx.doi.org/10.1002/prac.19963380168]

[86]   Almeida WP, Costa PRR. Orthobromodiphenylmethane Derivatives as Starting Materials for the Total Synthesis of Anthraquinones. Synth Commun 1996; 26(23): 4507-18.
[http://dx.doi.org/10.1080/00397919608003853]

[87]   Son EJ, Kim JH, Kim K, Park CB. Quinone and its derivatives for energy harvesting and storage materials. J Mater Chem A Mater Energy Sustain 2016; 4(29): 11179-202.
[http://dx.doi.org/10.1039/C6TA03123D]

[88]   Monks T, Jones D. The metabolism and toxicity of quinones, quinonimines, quinone methides, and quinone-thioethers. Curr Drug Metab 2002; 3(4): 425-38.
[http://dx.doi.org/10.2174/1389200023337388] [PMID: 12093358]

[89]   Sahoo PMS, Behera S, Behura R, *et al.* A brief review: antibacterial activity of quinone derivatives. Biointerface Res Appl Chem 2022; 12(3): 3247-58.

[90]   Jali BR. A mini-review: quinones and their derivatives for selective and specific detection of specific cations. Biointerface Res Appl Chem 2021; 11: 11679-99.

[91]   Kaur N, Kumar S. Single molecular colorimetric probe for simultaneous estimation of Cu2+ and Ni2+. Chem Commun (Camb) 2007; (29): 3069-70.
[http://dx.doi.org/10.1039/b703529b]

[92]   Kaur N, Kumar S. Aminoanthraquinone-based chemosensors: colorimetric molecular logic mimicking molecular trafficking and a set–reset memorized device. Dalton Trans 2012; 41(17): 5217-24.
[http://dx.doi.org/10.1039/c2dt12201d] [PMID: 22426303]

[93]   Bhalla V, Gupta A, Kumar M. Nanoaggregates of a pentacenequinone derivative as reactors for the preparation of palladium nanoparticles. Chem Commun (Camb) 2012; 48(97): 11862-4.
[http://dx.doi.org/10.1039/c2cc36667c] [PMID: 23042509]

[94]   Babula P, Adam V, Havel L, Kizek R. Noteworthy secondary metabolites naphthoquinones-their occurrence, pharmacological properties and analysis. Curr Pharm Anal 2009; 5(1): 47-68.
[http://dx.doi.org/10.2174/157341209787314936]

[95]   Al-Hiari YM, Shakya AK, Alzweiri MH, Aburjai T, Abu-Dahab R. Synthesis and biological evaluation of substituted tetrahydro-1H-quino [7, 8-b][1, 4] benzodiazepine-3-carboxylic derivatives. Farmacia 2014; 62(3): 570-88.

[96]   Stasevych MV, Plotnikov MY, Platonov MO, Sabat SI, Musyanovych RY, Novikov VP. Sulfur-containing derivatives of 1,4-naphthoquinone, part 1: Disulfide synthesis. Heteroatom Chem 2005; 16(3): 205-11.
[http://dx.doi.org/10.1002/hc.20112]

[97]   Heteroatoms NDC. Synthesis, biological, and computational study of naphthoquinone derivatives containing heteroatoms. J Chem Soc Pak 2016; 38(06): 1211.

[98]   Răn G, Crețu FM, Andrei AM, *et al.* Synthesis and evaluation of antimicrobial activity of new 2-mercapto-3-substituted-1, 4-naphthoquinones (I). Farmacia 2015; 63(5): 665-9.

[99]   Yıldırım H, Bayrak N, Tuyun AF, Kara EM, Çelik BÖ, Gupta GK. 2,3-Disubstituted-1-4-naphthoquinones containing an arylamine with trifluoromethyl group: synthesis, biological

evaluation, and computational study. RSC Advances 2017; 7(41): 25753-64.
[http://dx.doi.org/10.1039/C7RA00868F]

[100] Novais JS, Moreira CS, Silva ACJA, *et al.* Antibacterial naphthoquinone derivatives targeting resistant strain Gram-negative bacteria in biofilms. Microb Pathog 2018; 118: 105-14.
[http://dx.doi.org/10.1016/j.micpath.2018.03.024] [PMID: 29550501]

[101] Li Y, Guo F, Guan Y, *et al.* Novel anthraquinone compounds inhibit colon cancer cell proliferation *via* the reactive oxygen species/JNK pathway. Molecules 2020; 25(7): 1672.
[http://dx.doi.org/10.3390/molecules25071672] [PMID: 32260423]

[102] Shen CC, Afraj SN, Hung CC, *et al.* Synthesis, biological evaluation, and correlation of cytotoxicity *versus* redox potential of 1,4-naphthoquinone derivatives. Bioorg Med Chem Lett 2021; 41: 127976.
[http://dx.doi.org/10.1016/j.bmcl.2021.127976] [PMID: 33766765]

CHAPTER 3

Identification Techniques of Natural and Synthetic Quinones Using Various Methods

Satyanarayana Battula[1,*] and **Ashutosh Kumar Dash**[2]

[1] *Department of Chemistry, Central University of Jammu, Jammu & Kashmir, 181143, India*

[2] *Senior Research Scientist (R&D), Drug Discovery Division, Macleod Pharmaceuticals Ltd, Mumbai, India*

Abstract: Quinones are intriguing substances with distinctive properties and several significant biological and chemical functions and applications. Quinones are found in many parts of nature, including the tissues of plants and animals. They have several important roles in biological systems, for example, in the electron transport process to preserve plants' and animals' biological processes, in the form of plastoquinone and phylloquinone to be a part of photosynthesis in plants, and in the posttranslational modification of proteins and others. On essentiality grounds, they need to be detected and determined from the natural and synthetic samples. This chapter incorporates the detection and determination methods for various natural and synthetic quinones, viz., titrimetric methods, spectrophotometric methods, HPLC-based methods, and GC-M--based methods.

Keywords: GC-MS, HPLC, Titrimetric methods, Quinones.

INTRODUCTION

A special class of chemical molecules known as quinones is generated from aromatic compounds such as naphthalene or benzene. Quinones are composed of two carbonyl bonds formed when two oxygen atoms are replaced by two hydrogen atoms in a six-membered core benzene ring [1]. Quinones are a class of biological pigments that are present in many different types of living things, including fungi, bacteria, higher plants, and a few mammals [2]. They can be found in nature in a variety of forms, including polycyclic quinones, benzoquinones, naphthoquinones, and anthraquinones. Quinones have displayed multiple applications, including biological (antibacterial, anticancer, antimalarial, antioxidant, and anti-inflammatory properties) [3]. They are used as natural colorants in the fabric industry as they exert antifungal, anti-insecticide, anti-

---

* **Corresponding author Satyanarayana Battula:** Department of Chemistry, Central University of Jammu, Jammu & Kashmir, 181143, India; E-mail: satyamssd@gmail.com

Ashutosh Kumar Dash & Deepak Kumar (Eds.)

bacterial, and anti-UV properties to the fabric, particularly for the textile industry [2]. Their low cost, sustainability, and strong environmental stability make them an attractive material for supercapacitors [4]. They are used as an oxidant in several organic oxidations in the form of *p*-quinone oxidations (DDQ and chloranil for hydride abstraction) [5]. They also have biological functions (oxidative phosphorylation [6], electron transport, and bioenergetic transport processes) [7] and are used as cathodic materials for lithium-ion batteries as their ability to undergo reversible self-redox reaction makes them indispensable for efficient energy storage [8].

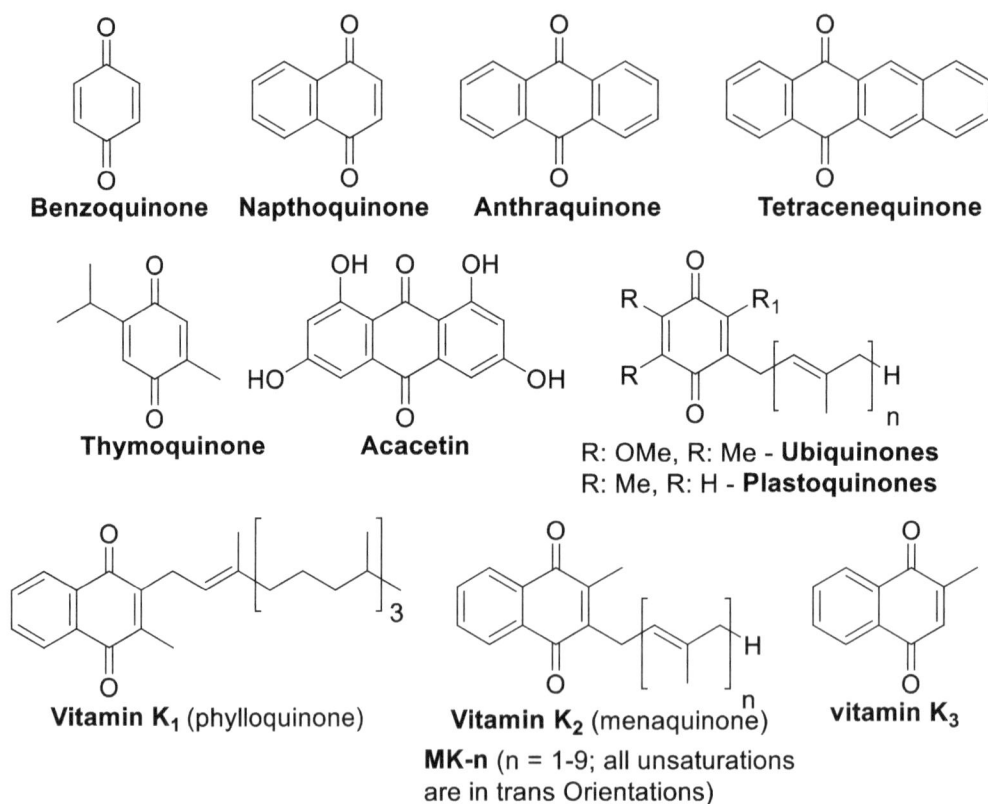

Fig. (1). Different quinone structures.

THE BIOLOGICAL, SYNTHETIC, AND INDUSTRIAL IMPORTANCE OF QUINONES

The quinones are one of the important classes of natural molecules with a variety of useful applications in biological systems. Almost all types of aerobic species, including bacteria, higher plants, and animals, contain ubiquinones (n = 1–12). They are present in mitochondria and play a major role in the electron transport mechanism in the respiratory chain [9]. On the other hand, chloroplasts of green plants encompass plastoquinones (plastoquinone; n=9), which are generally involved in electron transport pathways during photosynthesis [10]. In addition, vitamin K consists of a structurally related class of 2-methyl-1,4-naphthoquinone derivatives with the side chains containing either isoprenoid units (menaquinones (MKs), vitamin K$_2$) or a side chain containing phytyl unit (phylloquinone; vitamin K$_1$) [11]. It was previously established that vitamin K is advantageous for bone formation, metabolism, and blood coagulation [12]. Additionally, vitamin K displays imperative clinical applications like treating osteoporosis, arterial calcification [13], and vitamin K insufficiency. There are other anthraquinone molecules, for example, doxorubicin (DXR) antibiotic, which have been utilized in the clinical treatment of malignant tumors [14]. Rhein (the main active ingredient in rhubarb, a traditional Chinese herb) is an immunosuppressive and anti-inflammatory molecule [15].

Adversely, quinones have also been considered a class of toxins that can have a wide range of harmful effects on living cells; for instance, they produce reactive oxygen species (ROS) in biological systems through their redox cycle, initiating several types of oxidative damage; for example, to DNA, proteins, and others [16, 17]. Moreover, the atmosphere contains polycyclic aromatic hydrocarbon quinones (PAHQ), as it is believed that the photo-oxidation of polycyclic aromatic hydrocarbons takes place, which are generally discharged by motor vehicle engines into the environment. These PAHQs cause the pathogenesis of respiratory diseases [18].

Apart from the wide spectrum of biological interests, quinones and their derivatives have beenproven to exhibit extensive applications in diverse fields owing to their special chemical characteristics. Quinone has been employed as a dienophile in a stream of Diels-Alder reactions [19] as Michael donors/acceptors and 1,3-dipolarophiles [20] for decades and used in the synthesis of several natural products and stereo-selective complex molecules. In addition, ortho-quinone methides are imperative synthetic intermediates and used in enantioselective nucleophilic addition reactions [21]. As quinones have an additional nature to undergo reversible reduction and oxidation reactions, they are essential for effective energy storage devices and battery making [22]. Anaquinone, 1,4-naphthoquinone (NQ), and 1,4-benzoquinone are important organic cathodes thathave already been used in a number of metal-organic systems, and they are capable materials for the making of multivalent batteries such as Li, Na, K, Mg, Al, and others [23].

ANALYTICAL METHODS FOR THE DETERMINATION OF QUINONES

All these factors suggest that the techniques for determining the presence of quinones are essential either in biological or environmental samples to evaluate various parameters related to quinones, such as the study of quinone's physiological characteristics, the therapeutic monitoring of quinone-containing medications, and the assessment of the potential harm that toxic quinones may cause to humans. Here, this chapter incorporates the titrimetric methods, spectroscopic methods, and chromatographic techniques to determine the natural and synthetic quinones.

TITRIMETRIC METHODS FOR THE DETERMINATION OF QUINONES

There are several methods to determine quinones quantitatively; in general, the titrimetric methods involve the conversion of quinones to their equivalent hydroquinones using organic reducing reagents like sodium borohydride. The other method is the metal-mediated method, viz., chromium (II), tin (II), titanium (III), vanadium (II), and iron (II), wherein the amount of quinones is estimated in their acidic solution [24].

Sodium borohydride ($NaBH_4$) performs a selective reduction of quinones to hydroquinones. Organic quinones, such as 1,6-benzoquinone, 1,2-naphthoquinones, 9,10-anthraquinone, 1,2-benzanthraquinone, and anthanthrone, were studied to determine redox titrations (Fig. **2**). In this method, a particular amount of 1,4-naphthoquinone was added in a reaction vessel filled with N_2 gas, and an excess amount of known $NaBH_4$ was added and subjected to stirring for a while; the amount of quinone estimated by determining unreacted $NaBH_4$ was estimated by the evolved amount of hydrogen through acidification by adding sulfuric acid [25].

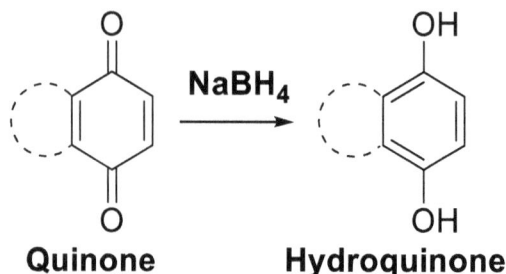

Fig. (2). $NaBH_4$ conversion of quinone to hydroquinone.

Iron salts are mild reducing agents under acidic conditions and show different potential for the couple Fe(II)/Fe(III) in different acidic conditions. They are utilized for the determination of a few quinones, viz., tetrachloro-1,- -benzoquinone, 2,3-dichloro-5,6-dicyano-1,4-benzoquinone (DDQ), methyl-1,- -benzoquinone, and 2,6-Dimethyl-1,4-benzoquinone [26]. In this process, methylene blue, methylene green, Azure A, Azure C or Azure-2-eosin thionine, and toluidine blue are used as redox indicators. Otherwise, an excess amount of iron (II) can be addedto quinone, and the formed iron (III) is determined calorimetrically with thiocyanate. The same authors also studied the application of Ti (III) chloride as a determining agent for the same quinones potentiometrically in HCl and H_2SO_4 media, wherein they also studied the redox potential of quinone/hydroquinone in different acidic mediums (HCl, H_2SO_4, and acetic acid) [27].

SPECTROPHOTOMETRIC METHODS FOR THE DETERMINATION OF QUINONES

M.T.M. Zaki and co-workers employed 3-phenylthiazolidine-2,4-dione as a selective and sensitive agent for the identification and estimation of quinone molecules in the basic media of ammonia (Fig. **3**). 2/3 drops of 3-phenylthiazolidine-2,4-dione solution and a drop of ammonia solution were added to the ethanolic quinone solution. The appearance of green color was because of tetrachloro-p-benzoquinone, while in the case of p-benzoquinone and 1,4-naphthoquinone, Prussian blue color was developed. The spectrophotometric method was used for the determination of the above-mentioned quinones using 3-phenylthiazolidine-2,4-dione at different absorption maxima for different quinones. 695, 795, and 685 nm were used for p-benzoquinone, 1,4-naphthoquinone, and tetrachloro-p-benzoquinone, respectively.[24] To detect and determine the quinones spectrophotometrically, the reaction of 3-phenylthiazolidine-2,4-dione with p-benzoquinone, tetrachloro-p-benzoquinone, and I,4-naphthoquinone in ammoniacal media was utilized.

3-Phenylthiazolidine -2,4-dione　　　　　**Quinoid moities**

Fig. (3). Reaction between quinone and 3-phenylthiazolidine-2,4-dione.

The quinoid moieties obtained in the above reactions are varied for different quinones; thereby, their molar absorptivity values are made different and utilized in the estimation processes. Owing to the crowdedness of the groups in tetrachloro-p-benzoquinone, it could not react with the 3-phenylthiazolidine-2-4-dione under conditions.

In another method of spectrophotometric determination of quinones, ethanolic piperidine is utilized to produce a colored solution for several quinones; the color is generated because of the interaction between the tested quinone and piperidine, and its intensity depends on the nature of quinone and its concentration. The quinones, 1,4-napthaquinone, menadione (vitamin K3), p-benzoquinone, and tetrachloro-p-benzoquinone, react with piperidine in ethanol and produce an intense color after 10 min at an ambient temperature. The quantitative variations in the respective quinone-piperidine complex color intensities and their variations with respect to diverse temperatures and piperidine concentrations are studied; thus, estimations of quinones were done [28].

Another protocol includes barbituric acid reaction with quinones, which establishes color compounds and shows absorption maxima between 485 and 555 nm in a 50% methyl alcohol-water mixture. At these wavelengths, the product absorption holds good the Beer-Lamberts law within the 0.025-0.5 mM range of product concentrations. By using this sensitive spectrophotometric method, the determination of p-benzoquinone, p-chloranil, and 1,4-naphthoquinone was done [29]. Another reagent, N,N-diethy-1,4-phenylenediamine was established as a spectrophotometric protocol for the determination of p-quinones. For 2,3-dimethoxy-5-methyl-1,4-benzoquinone determination, $0.1\square1.5$ µg/ml concentration ranges of the products were best suited for the estimation by Beer's law. The molar absorptivity value was 1.1×10^5 l.mol^{-1}cm^{-1} at an absorption maxima of 552 nm. The relative standard deviation was 0.48% for six replicate determinations for 0.18 µg/ml [30].

HPLC-BASED METHODS FOR THE DETERMINATION OF QUINONES

Cumulatively, high-performance liquid chromatography (HPLC)-electrospray ionization (ESI)-tandem mass spectrometry (MS) could be a significant detection technique for the estimation of methoxy-substituted quinones [31]. During this ESI process, the ionization proficiency can be efficiently enhanced by introducing methoxy groups into quinones, such as p-benzoquinone, methyl-p-benzoquinone, 1,4-naphthoquinone, 1,2-naphthoquinone, and 1,4-anthraquinones; the derivatization of quinones is performed with methanol. It offers a limit to the determination of the 5 quinones up to <0.02 – 2.06 pg by adjusting either the reaction time or solvent composition (less reaction times were observed with a 1:1 methanol and water solvent system). This method was successfully applied to the determination of quinones in the airborne particles.

HPLC, along with chemiluminescence, assists in the detection of ubiquinone in plasma samples. The technique relies on the detection of superoxide anion by luminol chemiluminescence, which is produced by the ubiquinone and dithiothreitol redox cycle reaction. An octyl column with methanol as the mobile phase was used in the HPLC system. After ubiquinone was eluted from the column, it was combined simultaneously with luminol and dithiothreitol solutions, and the chemiluminescence that resulted was observed using a chemiluminescence detector. The peak of ubiquinone in human plasma could be easily seen on the chromatogram using the suggested HPLC protocol, and it was free from interference from other plasma constituents [32].

Fat-soluble vitamin-based quinones menadione and menaquinones were simultaneously estimated by using a rapid reverse-phase HPLC method in biofluids like blood serum and urine [33]. At room temperature, the Phenomenex Luna C18 (150 mm X 4.6 mm) 3 μm analytical column was in operation. The mobile phase was a 50–50% v/v mixture of $CH_3OH–CH_3CN$ that was provided *via* a linear gradient at a flow rate of 1.3 ml/min. The composition of the mixture ended at 30–70%. As the internal standard, xanthophyll (2 ng/μl) was employed. 280 nm was used for the monitoring of the vitamin, whereas internal standard monitoring was done at 450 nm. For each vitamin, quantification was carried out at its maximal wavelength. The range of 1.4-6.6 ng per 20 μl injected samples was found to be the detection limit. Solid-phase extraction methods were used to treat the biological fluids (the sample volumes were 100 μl of blood serum and 100 μl of urine) to eliminate any endogenous interferences from the sample matrix. Retention and elution were optimized in the solid-phase extraction procedure. Using Cyclohexyl J.T. Baker SPE cartridges with methanol as the eluent, high extraction recoveries from biological fluids were observed.

HPLC-fluorescence-based method was established for the determination of vitamin K derivatives from the plasma, such as Vitamin K1 (phylloquinone) and Vitamin K2 (menaquinones, MK-n; MK-4 and MK-7), using post-column reduction and internal standards [34]. The use of these synthetic internal standards allowed for the attainment of sufficient precision and accuracy while optimizing chromatographic settings to improve the selectivity and reproducibility of the results. Hexane and ethanol were used to extract the lipids from plasma samples after internal standards were added. Isomatic reverse phase separation was used for chromatography on a C_{18} column. Vitamin K compounds were found at 430 nm, with MK-4 excitation occurring at 320 nm and phylloquinone and MK-7 excitation occurring at 240 nm. To assess the clinical and nutritional status of Vitamin K, this protocol was absolutely suitable to determine their levels. In another procedure, the determination of phylloquinone from serum microsamples (50 L) was performed with high-performance liquid chromatography with a nonaqueous eluent, wherein they used solid-phase extraction with C_8 Bond-Elut columns. Photodiode array identification with absorbance ratio was utilized for peak homogeneity. The data was obtained at 248 nm over a range of concentrations of the compound, from 20-200 ng/mL to 200-4000 ng/mL. The sensitivity here was increased twice as compared to the conventional columns [35].

GC-MS-BASED METHODS FOR THE DETERMINATION OF QUINONES

Gas spectrometry, along with MS, was utilized for the determination of anthraquinone, alkyl anthraquinones, 9-fluoranone, and benz[a]anthracene-7,1--dione from sediment, which was obtained from an aluminum smelter subsiding in a pond contaminated with polycyclic aromatic hydrocarbons (PAH) [36]. Many of these target compounds were either undetectable or had questionable confirmations due to matrix interferences when analyzed using traditional GC/MS techniques. However, by employing the GC/MS/MS process, their detection and identification were significantly enhanced. To conduct GC/MS/MS studies, the molecular ion of a target chemical was broken with collision-induced dissociation (CID) to produce product ions that, in the case of unsubstituted compounds, correspond to the loss of CO or in the case of alkylated compounds, to the loss of CO plus CH3. Using anthraquinone and 2-methylanthraquinone standards, the CID conditions were adjusted by adjusting the RF storage levels and CID excitation energy to produce the ideal amounts of fragment ions.

Quinones, along with the polycyclic aromatic compounds, were determined in surface and groundwater samples by employing GC–MS after single-drop microextraction. The optimized SDME conditions were determined for the samples, such as a drop volume of 1.0 μL. Here toluene was used as the extraction solvent, which was stirred for 30 minutes at 200 rpm. The detected limits ranged from 0.01 to 0.03 μg L^{-1}. The suggested approach was quick, reliable, thorough, effective, successfully implemented, and well-determined for the quinones and PAHs. Nitro-PAHs in water samples were demonstrated with good sensitivity, linearity, precision, and accuracy [37].

In another protocol, the GC–MS method was used for the direct determination of quinones, including 1,2-naphthoquinone, 1,4-naphthoquinone, 1,4-benzoquinone, 9,10-phenanthraquinone, and 9,10-anthraquinone in the fine atmospheric particulate matter [38]. To assess the determination of the quinones, they were evaluated in both nonderivatized and acetylated derivatized forms of quinones. The linear range, linearity, accuracy, limit of detection (LOD), and limit of quantification (LOQ) were evaluated for all these molecules during their determination. The quinones in the nonderivatized form had a detection range of 0.01–2.18 mg L^{-1}, while those in the acetylated derivatized form had limits of detection of 0.05–0.20 mg L^{-1}. For quinones, the quantitative limits were between 0.05 and 4.37 mg L^{-1}. For quinones found in the nonderivatized form, the concentration levels varied from 0.32 to 3.38 ng m^{-3} and from 0.29 to 4.75 ng m^{-3} for those found in the acetylated derivatized form. The determination process is very compatible with all the quinones, irrespective of whether they possess substitutions or not.

CONCLUSION

It is a high demand to estimate and detect quinones in natural and synthetic samples owing to their important roles in biology and chemistry. This chapter incorporates the detection techniques of a few quinones from natural and synthetic sources, including biofluids (blood serum, urine, plasma, and others), groundwater samples under certain situations, airborne particles in the environment, and others. The quinones in the above-mentioned samples were determined by several processes, which include titrimetric methods, spectrophotometric methods, and chromatographic methods (TLC, HPLC, and GC, including MS).

REFERENCES

[1]   Colucci MA, Couch GD, Moody CJ. Natural and synthetic quinones and their reduction by the quinone reductase enzyme NQO1: from synthetic organic chemistry to compounds with anticancer potential. Org Biomol Chem 2008; 6(4): 637-56.
        [http://dx.doi.org/10.1039/B715270A] [PMID: 18264564]

[2]   Dulo B, Phan K, Githaiga J, Raes K, De Meester S. Natural Quinone Dyes: A Review on Structure, Extraction Techniques, Analysis and Application Potential. Waste Biomass Valoriz 2021; 12(12): 6339-74.
        [http://dx.doi.org/10.1007/s12649-021-01443-9]

[3]   El-Najjar N, Gali-Muhtasib H, Ketola RA, Vuorela P, Urtti A, Vuorela H. The chemical and biological activities of quinones: overview and implications in analytical detection. Phytochem Rev 2011; 10(3): 353-70.
        [http://dx.doi.org/10.1007/s11101-011-9209-1]

[4]   Ega SP, Srinivasan P. Quinone materials for supercapacitor: Current status, approaches, and future directions. J Energy Storage 2022; 47: 103700.
        [http://dx.doi.org/10.1016/j.est.2021.103700]

[5]   Wendlandt AE, Stahl SS. Quinone☐Catalyzed Selective Oxidation of Organic Molecules. Angew Chem Int Ed 2015; 54(49): 14638-58.
        [http://dx.doi.org/10.1002/anie.201505017] [PMID: 26530485]

[6]   Jana S, Sinha M, Chanda D, *et al.* Mitochondrial dysfunction mediated by quinone oxidation products of dopamine: Implications in dopamine cytotoxicity and pathogenesis of Parkinson's disease. Biochim Biophys Acta Mol Basis Dis 2011; 1812(6): 663-73.
        [http://dx.doi.org/10.1016/j.bbadis.2011.02.013] [PMID: 21377526]

[7]   Sarewicz M, Osyczka A. Electronic connection between the quinone and cytochrome C redox pools and its role in regulation of mitochondrial electron transport and redox signaling. Physiol Rev 2015;

95(1): 219-43.
[http://dx.doi.org/10.1152/physrev.00006.2014] [PMID: 25540143]

[8]   Hiltermann TW, Sarkar S, Thangadurai V, Sutherland TC. Diamino-Substituted Quinones as Cathodes for Lithium-Ion Batteries. ACS Appl Mater Interfaces 2024; 16(7): 8580-8.
[http://dx.doi.org/10.1021/acsami.3c14123] [PMID: 38320233]

[9]   Kurosu M, Begari E. Vitamin K2 in electron transport system: are enzymes involved in vitamin K2 biosynthesis promising drug targets? Molecules 2010; 15(3): 1531-53.
[http://dx.doi.org/10.3390/molecules15031531] [PMID: 20335999]

[10]   Liu M, Lu S. Plastoquinone and Ubiquinone in Plants: Biosynthesis, Physiological Function and Metabolic Engineering. Front Plant Sci 2016; 7: 1898.
[http://dx.doi.org/10.3389/fpls.2016.01898] [PMID: 28018418]

[11]   Yerramsetti N, Dampanaboina L, Mendu V, Battula S. Synergistic factors ensue high expediency in the synthesis of menaquinone [K2] analogue MK-6: Application to access an efficient one-pot protocol to MK-9. Tetrahedron 2020; 76(49): 131696.
[http://dx.doi.org/10.1016/j.tet.2020.131696]

[12]   Akbari S, Rasouli-Ghahroudi AA. Vitamin K and Bone Metabolism: A Review of the Latest Evidence in Preclinical Studies. BioMed Res Int 2018; 2018: 1-8.
[http://dx.doi.org/10.1155/2018/4629383] [PMID: 30050932]

[13]   Adams J, Pepping J. Vitamin K in the treatment and prevention of osteoporosis and arterial calcification. Am J Health Syst Pharm 2005; 62(15): 1574-81.
[http://dx.doi.org/10.2146/ajhp040357] [PMID: 16030366]

[14]   Bellance N, Furt F, Melser S, *et al.* Doxorubicin Inhibits Phosphatidylserine Decarboxylase and Modifies Mitochondrial Membrane Composition in HeLa Cells. Int J Mol Sci 2020; 21(4): 1317.
[http://dx.doi.org/10.3390/ijms21041317] [PMID: 32075281]

[15]   Wang H, Yang D, Li L, Yang S, Du G, Lu Y. Anti-inflammatory Effects and Mechanisms of Rhein, an Anthraquinone Compound, and Its Applications in Treating Arthritis: A Review. Nat Prod Bioprospect 2020; 10(6): 445-52.
[http://dx.doi.org/10.1007/s13659-020-00272-y] [PMID: 33128198]

[16]   Zhang Q, Tu T, d'Avignon DA, Gross ML. Balance of beneficial and deleterious health effects of quinones: a case study of the chemical properties of genistein and estrone quinones. J Am Chem Soc 2009; 131(3): 1067-76.
[http://dx.doi.org/10.1021/ja806478b] [PMID: 19115854]

[17]   Bolton JL, Dunlap T. Formation and Biological Targets of Quinones: Cytotoxic *versus* Cytoprotective Effects. Chem Res Toxicol 2017; 30(1): 13-37.
[http://dx.doi.org/10.1021/acs.chemrestox.6b00256] [PMID: 27617882]

[18]   Låg M, Øvrevik J, Refsnes M, Holme JA. Potential role of polycyclic aromatic hydrocarbons in air pollution-induced non-malignant respiratory diseases. Respir Res 2020; 21(1): 299.
[http://dx.doi.org/10.1186/s12931-020-01563-1] [PMID: 33187512]

[19]   Nawrat CC, Moody CJ. Quinones as dienophiles in the Diels-Alder reaction: history and applications in total synthesis. Angew Chem Int Ed 2014; 53(8): 2056-77.
[http://dx.doi.org/10.1002/anie.201305908] [PMID: 24446164]

[20]   Hosamani B, Ribeiro MF, da Silva Júnior EN, Namboothiri INN. Catalytic asymmetric reactions and synthesis of quinones. Org Biomol Chem 2016; 14(29): 6913-31.
[http://dx.doi.org/10.1039/C6OB01119E] [PMID: 27337246]

[21]   Pathak TP, Sigman MS. Applications of ortho-quinone methide intermediates in catalysis and asymmetric synthesis. J Org Chem 2011; 76(22): 9210-5.
[http://dx.doi.org/10.1021/jo201789k] [PMID: 21999240]

[22]   Pooja; Mudila, H.; Kumar, A., Quinone based conducting materials for efficient energy storage. AIP

Conf Proc 2023; 2800(1)

[23]   Bitenc J, Pavčnik T, Košir U, Pirnat K. Quinone Based Materials as Renewable High Energy Density Cathode Materials for Rechargeable Magnesium Batteries. Materials (Basel) 2020; 13(3): 506.
[http://dx.doi.org/10.3390/ma13030506] [PMID: 31973193]

[24]   Zaki MTM, Abdel-Rehiem AG. New method for detection and spectrophotometric determination of quinones. Microchem J 1984; 29(1): 44-8.
[http://dx.doi.org/10.1016/0026-265X(84)90085-7]

[25]   Matsumura Y, Takahashi H. Potentiometric redox titration of quinone in carbon black with NaBH4 and I2. Carbon 1979; 17(2): 109-14.
[http://dx.doi.org/10.1016/0008-6223(79)90016-2]

[26]   Murty NK, Dakshina Murty PM. Quantitative study of the reaction between quinones and iron(II) in phosphoric acid medium. Talanta 1982; 29(3): 234-6.
[http://dx.doi.org/10.1016/0039-9140(82)80101-X] [PMID: 18963119]

[27]   Murty NK, Dakshina Murty PM. Potential & visual estimation of some quinones with TiCl$_3$. Indian J Chem 1982; 21A: 756-7.

[28]   Iskander ML, Medien HAA, Khalil LH. Spectrophotometric Determination of Some Quinones. Anal Lett 1995; 28(8): 1513-23.
[http://dx.doi.org/10.1080/00032719508006410]

[29]   Medien HAA. New method for spectrophotometric determination of quinones and barbituric acid through their reaction. A kinetic study. Spectrochim Acta A Mol Biomol Spectrosc 1996; 52(12): 1679-84.
[http://dx.doi.org/10.1016/0584-8539(96)01713-8]

[30]   Fujimoto Y, Fujimoto T, Yamaguchi T, Fujita Y. Spectrophotometric determination of p-quinones with N,N-diethy-1,4-phenylenediamine. Bunseki Kagaku 2004; 53(10): 1093-6.
[http://dx.doi.org/10.2116/bunsekikagaku.53.1093]

[31]   Pei J, Wang Y, Yu K. Sensitive Determination of Quinones by High-Performance Liquid Chromatography-Electrospray Ionization-Tandem Mass Spectrometry with Methanol Derivatization. Anal Sci 2018; 34(3): 335-9.
[http://dx.doi.org/10.2116/analsci.34.335] [PMID: 29526902]

[32]   Kishikawa N, Ohkubo N, Ohyama K, Nakashima K, Kuroda N. Selective determination of ubiquinone in human plasma by HPLC with chemiluminescence reaction based on the redox cycle of quinone. Anal Bioanal Chem 2011; 400(2): 381-5.
[http://dx.doi.org/10.1007/s00216-011-4662-7] [PMID: 21246189]

[33]   Chatzimichalakis PF, Samanidou VF, Papadoyannis IN. Development of a validated liquid chromatography method for the simultaneous determination of eight fat-soluble vitamins in biological fluids after solid-phase extraction. J Chromatogr B Analyt Technol Biomed Life Sci 2004; 805(2): 289-96.
[http://dx.doi.org/10.1016/j.jchromb.2004.03.009] [PMID: 15135103]

[34]   Kamao M, Suhara Y, Tsugawa N, Okano T. Determination of plasma Vitamin K by high-performance liquid chromatography with fluorescence detection using Vitamin K analogs as internal standards. J Chromatogr B Analyt Technol Biomed Life Sci 2005; 816(1-2): 41-8.
[http://dx.doi.org/10.1016/j.jchromb.2004.11.003] [PMID: 15664332]

[35]   Kirk EM, Fell AF. Analysis of supplemented vitamin K1(20) in serum microsamples by solid-phase extraction and narrow-bone HPLC with multichannel ultraviolet detection. Clin Chem 1989; 35(7): 1288-92.
[http://dx.doi.org/10.1093/clinchem/35.7.1282] [PMID: 2758573]

[36]   Mosi A, Reimer KJ, Eigendorf GK. Analysis of polyaromatic quinones in a complex environmental matrix using gas chromatography ion trap tandem mass spectrometry. Talanta 1997; 44(6): 985-1001.

[http://dx.doi.org/10.1016/S0039-9140(96)02172-8] [PMID: 18966830]

[37] Santos LO, dos Anjos JP, Ferreira SLC, de Andrade JB. Simultaneous determination of PAHS, nitro-PAHS and quinones in surface and groundwater samples using SDME/GC-MS. Microchem J 2017; 133: 431-40.
[http://dx.doi.org/10.1016/j.microc.2017.04.012]

[38] Sousa ET, Cardoso MP, Silva LA, de Andrade JB. Direct determination of quinones in fine atmospheric particulate matter by GC–MS. Microchem J 2015; 118: 26-31.
[http://dx.doi.org/10.1016/j.microc.2014.07.013]

CHAPTER 4

Quinone in Traditional Therapy and Nutraceutical Use

Santosh Kumar Rath[1,*] and **Ashutosh Kumar Dash**[2]

[1] *School of Pharmaceuticals and Population Health Informatics, Faculty of Pharmacy, DIT University, Dehradun, Uttarakhand-248009, India*

[2] *Senior Research Scientist (R&D), Drug Discovery Division, Macleod Pharmaceuticals Ltd, Mumbai, India*

Abstract: Quinones are a distinct group in chemistry, having a wide range of chemical and biological properties. These are extensively cast off as traditional medicines, such as anticancer, anti-inflammatory, antibacterial, *etc*. Plants such as Henna, Rhubarb, and Aloe vera possess quinones as active ingredients, which developed diverse medicinal possessions. Traditional uses and nutraceutical ethics have been enriched owing to the molecule. The biological application of quinones is discussed.

Keywords: Biological use, Nutraceuticals, Traditional use, Quinone.

INTRODUCTION

Quinones are a prominent class of organic compounds that hold significant importance in a multitude of biological processes. They are characterized by their fully conjugated cyclic dione structure, which consists of a ring system with two ketone (carbonyl) groups. This unique structure allows quinones to participate in various redox reactions, making them essential in biochemical pathways [1]. Quinones are naturally abundant, especially in the plant kingdom, where they play critical roles in photosynthesis, respiration, and defense mechanisms.

Historically, quinones have been utilized in traditional medicine for centuries. Their presence in medicinal plants has been exploited for their therapeutic properties long before the advent of modern pharmaceuticals. For example, quinones like coenzyme Q10 are vital for cellular energy production, while others, such as vitamin K, are crucial for blood clotting processes [2].

---

* **Corresponding author Santosh Kumar Rath:** School of Pharmaceuticals and Population Health Informatics, Faculty of Pharmacy, DIT University, Dehradun, Uttarakhand-248009, India; E-mails: skrath1985@gmail.com and santoshk.rath@dituniversity.edu.in

Ashutosh Kumar Dash & Deepak Kumar (Eds.)
All rights reserved-© 2025 Bentham Science Publishers

In recent years, the scientific community has shown a growing interest in the potential of quinones as nutraceuticals. These compounds are widely distributed

in nature and found in various plants, fungi, bacteria, and marine organisms. The natural occurrence and biological significance of quinones make them valuable candidates for nutraceutical applications, offering potential health benefits beyond basic nutrition [3]. Nutraceuticals are food-derived products that offer health benefits beyond basic nutrition. The interest in quinones is largely due to their impressive range of bioactive properties, including antioxidant, anti-inflammatory, and anticancer activities. Ongoing research and development are essential to fully understand their mechanisms of action, optimize their bioavailability, and integrate them effectively into nutraceutical products. As science continues to uncover the therapeutic potential of quinones, their role in promoting health and preventing disease is likely to expand, making them an exciting area of focus in the nutraceutical industry [4].

ANTIOXIDANT PROPERTIES

Quinones are renowned for their ability to neutralize free radicals, thereby preventing oxidative stress and cellular damage and protecting biological systems from damage. This antioxidant property is particularly crucial in defending cells from the harmful effects of reactive oxygen species (ROS), which are linked to aging and various chronic diseases [5]. Quinones can substitute between their oxidized (quinone) and reduced (hydroquinone or semiquinone) forms. This redox cycling allows quinones to act as electron acceptors and donors, neutralizing ROS and preventing oxidative damage to cellular components. Quinones can directly scavenge free radicals, such as superoxide anions, hydroxyl radicals, and peroxyl radicals [6]. By donating electrons or hydrogen atoms, quinones neutralize these reactive species, reducing their potential to cause cellular damage. Some quinones can chelate transition metals like iron and copper, which are catalysts in the formation of highly reactive hydroxyl radicals *via* the Fenton reaction. By binding these metals, quinones prevent the catalysis of ROS production. The ability of quinones to undergo redox cycling, scavenge free radicals, and chelate metals underpins their effectiveness as antioxidants.

ANTI-INFLAMMATORY EFFECTS

Inflammation is a biological response to harmful stimuli, but chronic inflammation can lead to various health issues, including autoimmune diseases and cancer. Quinones have been found to exhibit anti-inflammatory effects by modulating pathways that reduce inflammation and inhibit the production of pro-inflammatory cytokines. Quinones can suppress the production of pro-inflammatory cytokines such as tumor necrosis factor-alpha (TNF-α), interleukins

(IL-1β, IL-6), and interferon-gamma (IFN-γ) [7, 8]. This inhibition helps reduce the overall inflammatory response. NF-κB is a key transcription factor that regulates the expression of various inflammatory genes. Quinones can inhibit the activation of NF-κB, thereby reducing the expression of pro-inflammatory cytokines, chemokines, and adhesion molecules [9]. Quinones can inhibit the activity of COX and LOX enzymes, which are involved in the synthesis of pro-inflammatory eicosanoids such as prostaglandins and leukotrienes [10]. This suppression leads to reduced inflammation and pain. The nuclear factor erythroid 2–related factor 2 (Nrf2) pathway plays a critical role in the cellular antioxidant response. Quinones can activate Nrf2, leading to the upregulation of antioxidant enzymes and suppression of inflammation. Quinones can affect the MAPK signaling pathways, which are involved in the regulation of inflammatory responses [11]. By modulating these pathways, quinones help in reducing the expression of inflammatory mediators. Their ability to modulate key inflammatory pathways, such as NF-κB, COX, LOX, Nrf2, and MAPK, underpins their effectiveness as anti-inflammatory agents.

ANTICANCER POTENTIAL

The anticancer properties of quinones are among the most promising. They can induce apoptosis (programmed cell death) in cancer cells, inhibit cell proliferation, and interfere with tumor growth and metastasis. These effects are mediated through various mechanisms, including the generation of ROS to selectively target cancer cells and the inhibition of key signaling pathways involved in cancer progression. Due to these multifaceted properties, quinones are being extensively studied for their potential applications in health and medicine. Their role as antioxidants, anti-inflammatory agents, and anticancer compounds highlights their importance in the development of new therapeutic strategies and health supplements [12, 13]. As research continues to uncover the diverse benefits of quinones, their incorporation into modern healthcare and nutraceutical products is likely to expand, offering new avenues for enhancing human health and well-being. Some quinones can intercalate into the DNA double helix, disrupting the DNA structure and interfering with DNA replication and transcription. Certain quinones can form covalent bonds with DNA, causing DNA alkylation. This can lead to DNA cross-linking and strand breaks, further inhibiting DNA synthesis and triggering cell death mechanisms. Topoisomerases are enzymes that regulate the overwinding or underwinding of DNA during replication and transcription [14, 15]. Quinones, such as anthraquinones like doxorubicin, can inhibit topoisomerase II, preventing the enzyme from re-ligating DNA strands after they have been cut. This inhibition results in the accumulation of DNA breaks, leading to apoptosis [16]. Quinones can modulate the cellular redox balance by interacting with cellular thiols and other antioxidant systems. This disruption can deplete cellular antioxidants like glutathione, making cells more susceptible to oxidative damage. The imbalance in redox status can lead to the activation of stress signaling pathways, such as the MAPK and JNK pathways, promoting cell death [13, 17]. The mechanism of action of quinones in cancer therapy is given in Fig. (**2**).

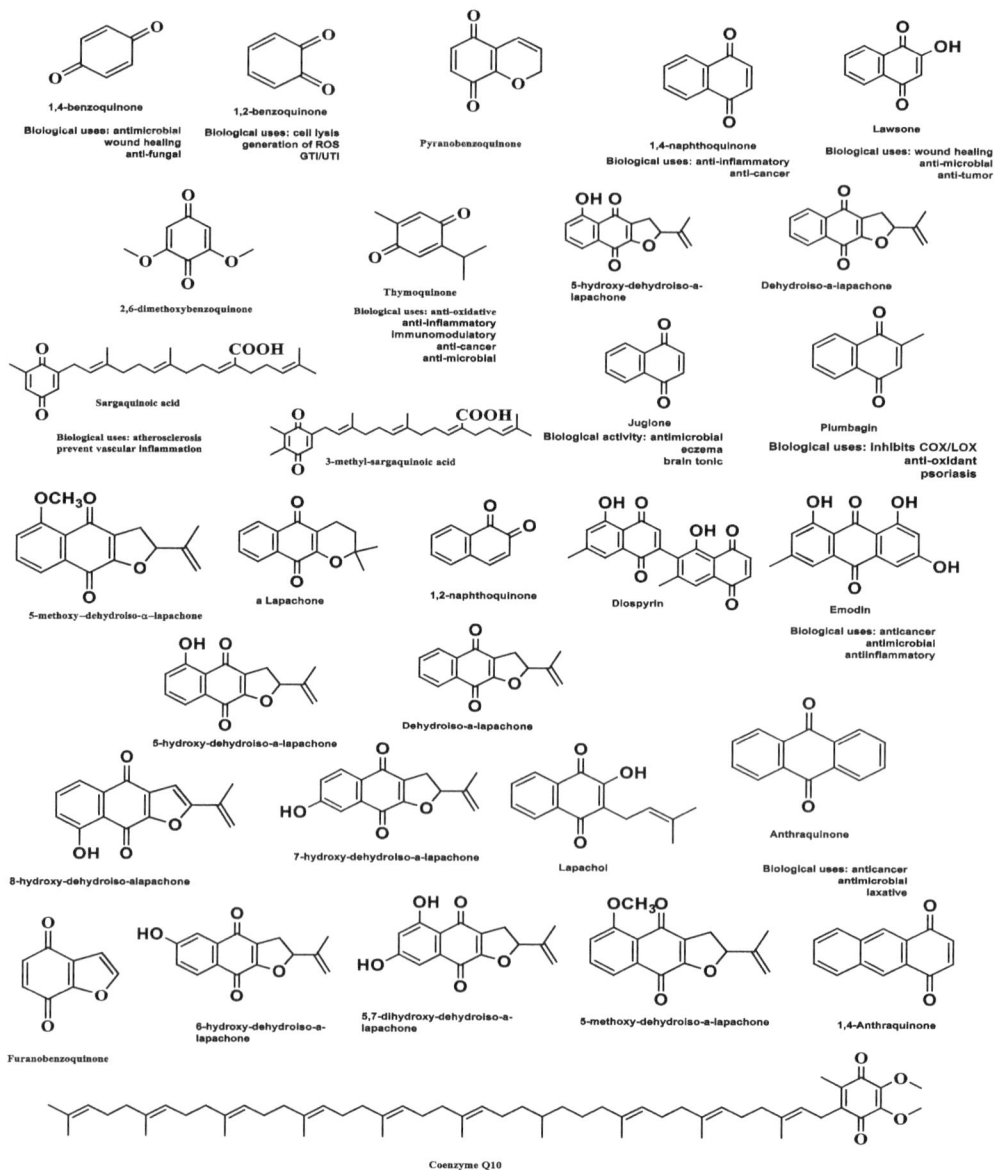

Fig. (1). Natural products bearing quinone scaffold.

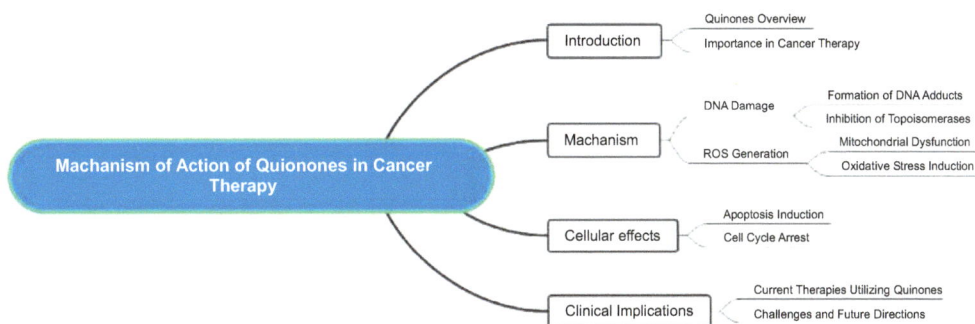

Fig. (2). Mechanism of Action of Quinones in Cancer Therapy [41, 42].

EXAMPLES OF QUINONE-CONTAINING PLANTS

Several plants known for their medicinal properties contain benzoquinones. Natural products bearing quinones scaffold are given in Fig. (**1**). Some examples include:

1. **Henna (*Lawsonia inermis*)**: Henna leaves contain lawsone, a benzoquinone with strong antimicrobial properties. Henna has been traditionally used for its wound healing and antimicrobial effects. Lawsone is primarily known for its use as a dye, especially in traditional body art and hair coloring; its nutritional value and potential health benefits have also been studied [18].
2. **Black Walnut (*Juglans nigra*)**: The hulls of black walnut contain juglone, a benzoquinone that exhibits antimicrobial activity. Black walnut has been used in traditional medicine for its ability to treat fungal and bacterial infections [19].
3. **Aloe Vera (*Aloe barbadensis*)**: Aloe vera contains aloesin, a benzoquinone derivative. Aloe vera gel has been traditionally applied to wounds and burns for its antimicrobial and healing properties [20].
4. ***Plumbago zeylanica* (Chitrak, Leadwort)**: This plant is widely used in Ayurvedic medicine for its anti-inflammatory and anticancer properties. It also treats skin diseases, digestive disorders, and respiratory issues [21].
5. **Rhubarb (*Rheum officinale* and *Rheum palmatum*):** Rhubarb roots have been used in traditional Chinese medicine as a laxative and purgative. They are also used to treat digestive disorders, liver problems, and skin conditions [22].
6. ***Cascara Sagrada* (*Rhamnus purshiana*):***Cascara sagrada* bark is used as a natural laxative to treat chronic constipation. It has also been used to promote liver and gallbladder health [23].
7. ***Flacourtia Jangomas***: The dichloromethane (DCM) fraction of the organic leaf extract of *Flacourtia Jangomas* was reported as a rich source of 2,6-

dimethoxy benzoquinone. The potential inhibitory activity of 2,6-dimethoxy benzoquinone was identified in an inhibition zone size of 21.6 ± 0.6 to 21.7 ± 0.58 mm against *Staphylococcus aureus* (MTCC 737 and MTCC 96 strains) [24].

8. *Newbouldia laevis*: Four novel (6-hydroxydehydroiso-α-lapachone, 7-hydroxydehydroiso-α-lapachone, 5,7-dihydroxydehydroiso-α-lapachone, and 3-hydroxy-5-methoxydehydroiso-α-lapachone) and six known naphthoquinones isolated from this species have been shown to have antifungal and antibacterial properties against *Escherichia coli*, *Candida albicans*, *Cladosporium cucumerinum*, and *Bacillus subtilis* [25, 26].

9. *Bulbine spp.*: It was discovered that newly identified isofuranonaphthoquinones and novel phenyl anthraquinones from *Bulbine spp.* had antioxidant and antiparasitic properties [27].

10. **Mendoncia cowanii:** Two new naphthoquinones, Avicequinones D and E, were isolated from *Mendoncia cowanii* root and stem extracts using bioassay-guided fractionation [28].

TYPES OF QUINONES

Quinones can be classified into several types based on their structure and natural sources. The major types include:

Benzoquinones: These are classes of substances that have two carbonyl groups, often in ortho or para positions (monocyclic), on a saturated hexacyclic aromatic ring system (benzene ring). They are found in various plants and used for their antimicrobial properties.

Naphthoquinones: They are commonly present in the roots of certain plants and known for their anticancer activity.

Anthraquinones: They are widely distributed in the plant kingdom and used for their laxative effects.

Ubiquinones (Coenzyme Q): They are essential for cellular respiration and energy production in humans.

TRADITIONAL THERAPEUTIC USES

BENZOQUINONES

Benzoquinones, a subset of quinones, have been utilized in traditional medicine for their potent antimicrobial properties. These compounds are characterized by a benzene ring with two ketone substitutions, forming a conjugated cyclic dione structure. Their effectiveness against a wide range of bacterial and fungal infections has been recognized for centuries, long before the advent of modern antibiotics.

ANTIMICROBIAL PROPERTIES

Benzoquinones are particularly valued for their ability to inhibit the growth of various microorganisms. This antimicrobial activity makes them effective in treating infections caused by bacteria and fungi. The mechanisms through which benzoquinones exert their antimicrobial effects include:

DISRUPTION OF CELL MEMBRANES

Benzoquinones can integrate into the cell membranes of bacteria and fungi, disrupting their integrity and causing cell lysis. This disruption is often lethal to the microorganisms.

INHIBITION OF ENZYMATIC ACTIVITY

Many benzoquinones can inhibit critical enzymes involved in microbial metabolism. For instance, they can interfere with enzymes essential for the synthesis of nucleic acids and proteins, thereby inhibiting microbial growth and reproduction.

GENERATION OF REACTIVE OXYGEN SPECIES (ROS)

Benzoquinones can induce the production of ROS within microbial cells. These reactive molecules cause oxidative stress, damaging cellular components such as DNA, proteins, and lipids, ultimately leading to cell death.

TRADITIONAL APPLICATIONS

In traditional medicine systems, benzoquinones have been extracted from various plants and used in different formulations to treat infections. Some notable traditional applications include:

WOUND HEALING

Benzoquinone-containing plants have been used to treat wounds and prevent infections. The antimicrobial properties help to keep the wound area sterile, promoting faster healing.

TOPICAL TREATMENTS

Preparations containing benzoquinones have been applied topically to treat skin infections, such as fungal infections (*e.g.*, ringworm) and bacterial infections (*e.g.*, impetigo). Their ability to penetrate the skin and reach the site of infection makes them effective in these applications.

INTERNAL USE

In some traditional practices, extracts containing benzoquinones have been administered internally to treat systemic infections. For example, decoctions and infusions of benzoquinone-rich plants have been used to treat respiratory infections, gastrointestinal infections, and urinary tract infections.

PRESERVATION OF FOOD AND NATURAL PRODUCTS

The antimicrobial properties of benzoquinones have also been exploited in the preservation of food and natural products. Traditional methods often involved the use of benzoquinone-containing plant extracts to extend the shelf life of perishable items by preventing microbial spoilage.

NAPHTHOQUINONES

Naphthoquinones are a class of quinones characterized by a naphthalene ring fused with a quinone structure. These compounds are renowned for their diverse therapeutic properties, including anti-inflammatory and anticancer effects. One of the most well-known naphthoquinones is plumbagin, which is extracted from the roots of the plant *Plumbago zeylanica*. This plant, commonly known as chitrak or leadwort, is widely used in Ayurvedic medicine.

ANTI-INFLAMMATORY PROPERTIES

Plumbagin and other naphthoquinones have been traditionally used in Ayurvedic medicine to manage inflammatory conditions. Their anti-inflammatory effects are mediated through various mechanisms:

INHIBITION OF PRO-INFLAMMATORY ENZYMES

Plumbagin inhibits key enzymes involved in the inflammatory process, such as cyclooxygenase (COX) and lipoxygenase (LOX). By blocking these enzymes, plumbagin reduces the production of pro-inflammatory mediators like prostaglandins and leukotrienes.

SUPPRESSION OF INFLAMMATORY CYTOKINES

Plumbagin can modulate the immune response by suppressing the production of inflammatory cytokines, such as tumor necrosis factor-alpha (TNF-α) and interleukins (IL-1, IL-6). This suppression helps in reducing inflammation and alleviating symptoms associated with inflammatory diseases.

ANTIOXIDANT ACTIVITY

The antioxidant properties of plumbagin contribute to its anti-inflammatory effects. By neutralizing reactive oxygen species (ROS), plumbagin reduces oxidative stress, which is a major contributor to inflammation.

TRADITIONAL ANTI-INFLAMMATORY APPLICATIONS

In Ayurvedic medicine, plumbagin and *Plumbago zeylanica* have been used to treat various inflammatory conditions, including:

ARTHRITIS

Preparations containing plumbagin are used to alleviate the symptoms of arthritis, including joint pain, swelling, and stiffness. The anti-inflammatory properties help in reducing joint inflammation and improving mobility. At a dosage of $1 \sim 3.5$ µM, plumbibagin decreased the viability of human fibroblast-like synoviocytes (HFLS). The medication employed as the positive control, methotrexate, exhibited a similar inhibitory effect on cell proliferation when 1 µM plumbagin was added. Plumbagin inhibited the activation of IκB and nuclear factor kappa-B (NF-κB), as well as the entry of p65 into the nucleus, and downregulated the levels of inflammatory cytokines and matrix metalloproteinases (MMPs) in IL-1β-treated HFLS. Moreover, plumbagin was shown to reduce the activation of the NF-κB pathway, downregulate TNF-α, IL-6, and MMPs, and lessen joint injury in mice with CIA-like models. These findings were also shown in animal trials [29].

SKIN INFLAMMATION

Plumbagin-rich extracts are applied topically to treat skin conditions characterized by inflammation, such as eczema, psoriasis, and dermatitis. These preparations help in reducing redness, itching, and swelling [30, 31].

RESPIRATORY INFLAMMATION

Plumbago zeylanica is used in formulations to manage respiratory conditions like bronchitis and asthma, where inflammation of the airways plays a significant role [32].

ANTICANCER PROPERTIES

Naphthoquinones, particularly plumbagin, have garnered attention for their potential anticancer properties. These effects are attributed to several mechanisms:

INDUCTION OF APOPTOSIS

Plumbagin can induce apoptosis (programmed cell death) in cancer cells. It activates pathways that lead to cell death, thereby inhibiting the growth and proliferation of cancer cells.

INHIBITION OF CANCER CELL PROLIFERATION

Plumbagin disrupts cell cycle progression, preventing cancer cells from dividing and multiplying. It can arrest the cell cycle at various stages, leading to growth inhibition.

ANTIMETASTATIC EFFECTS

Plumbagin inhibits the processes involved in cancer metastasis, including cell migration and invasion. By targeting these pathways, it helps in preventing the spread of cancer to other parts of the body.

MODULATION OF SIGNALING PATHWAYS

Plumbagin interferes with key signaling pathways involved in cancer progression, such as the NF-κB, STAT3, and PI3K/Akt pathways. By modulating these pathways, plumbagin exerts its anticancer effects.

TRADITIONAL ANTICANCER APPLICATIONS

In Ayurvedic medicine, plumbagin and *Plumbago zeylanica* have been used to support cancer treatment and overall health:

CANCER SUPPORT

Ayurvedic formulations containing plumbagin are used as adjuncts to conventional cancer treatments. These formulations are believed to enhance the efficacy of treatments and reduce side effects.

TUMOR REDUCTION

Plumbagin extracts are traditionally used to reduce the size of tumors and prevent their growth. This is often done in conjunction with other herbal treatments to maximize efficacy.

GENERAL HEALTH TONIC

Plumbago zeylanica is also used as a general health tonic to boost the immune system and enhance overall vitality, which is crucial for patients undergoing cancer treatment.

ANTHRAQUINONES

Anthraquinones are a class of naturally occurring organic compounds characterized by an anthracene ring with two ketones (quinone) substitutions. These compounds are widely 111distributed in the plant kingdom and are known for their diverse biological activities. One of the most well-known and widely utilized properties of anthraquinones is their laxative effect, but they also possess other therapeutic uses.

LAXATIVE EFFECTS

Anthraquinones are commonly found in plants such as aloe, senna, rhubarb, and cascara sagrada. These compounds act as stimulant laxatives, promoting bowel movements through various mechanisms:

STIMULATION OF PERISTALSIS

Anthraquinones stimulate the smooth muscles of the colon, enhancing peristalsis (the wave-like contractions that move contents through the digestive tract). This action helps to accelerate the passage of stool through the intestines.

INCREASED WATER AND ELECTROLYTE SECRETION

Anthraquinones increase the secretion of water and electrolytes into the intestinal lumen, softening the stool and making it easier to pass. This effect is achieved by inhibiting the absorption of water and electrolytes from the intestines back into the bloodstream.

IRRITATION OF THE INTESTINAL MUCOSA

These compounds mildly irritate the mucosal lining of the intestines, which further stimulates bowel movements.

OTHER THERAPEUTIC USES

While the laxative effects of anthraquinones are their most widely recognized use, these compounds also possess other therapeutic properties:

ANTICANCER

Some anthraquinones, such as emodin, have shown potential anticancer properties by inhibiting the growth and proliferation of cancer cells and inducing apoptosis (programmed cell death).

ANTIMICROBIAL

Anthraquinones exhibit antimicrobial activity against a range of bacteria, fungi, and viruses. This property makes them useful in treating infections and in the preservation of food and herbal products.

ANTI-INFLAMMATORY

Anthraquinones have anti-inflammatory effects that can help reduce inflammation in various conditions, such as skin diseases, arthritis, and gastrointestinal disorders.

ANTIOXIDANT

The antioxidant properties of anthraquinones help protect cells from oxidative stress and damage, which is beneficial in preventing chronic diseases and aging-related conditions.

NUTRACEUTICAL USES

Quinones are potent antioxidants and have been incorporated into various nutraceutical products to promote health and prevent diseases. CoQ10 is essential for the production of adenosine triphosphate (ATP), the primary energy carrier in cells. Supplementation can help improve energy levels, particularly in individuals with deficiencies or conditions that impair mitochondrial function. CoQ10 supports cardiovascular health by improving energy production in heart cells and reducing oxidative damage. It has been shown to help in the management of conditions like heart failure, angina, and hypertension [32]. Some studies suggest that CoQ10 supplementation can improve symptoms and quality of life in patients with heart failure. CoQ10 can enhance physical performance by increasing energy production and reducing oxidative stress in muscles during exercise [33, 34]. It may help improve endurance and reduce fatigue.

ANTIOXIDANT PROPERTIES

Ubiquinones (Coenzyme Q10) are widely used as dietary supplements for their role in energy production and their antioxidant properties. They help in reducing oxidative stress and improving heart health.

ANTI-INFLAMMATORY AND ANTICANCER PROPERTIES

Quinones, including naphthoquinones and anthraquinones, are well-recognized for their potent anti-inflammatory and anticancer activities. These properties have led to increased interest in their inclusion in nutraceuticals—food-derived products that offer health benefits beyond basic nutrition. The goal is to harness these therapeutic benefits in a natural, non-toxic manner, providing a safer alternative to synthetic drugs.

ANTI-INFLAMMATORY PROPERTIES

Inflammation is a biological response to harmful stimuli, such as pathogens, damaged cells, or irritants. While acute inflammation is a protective mechanism, chronic inflammation can contribute to various diseases, including autoimmune disorders, cardiovascular diseases, and cancer. Quinones exhibit anti-inflammatory effects through several mechanisms:

INHIBITION OF PRO-INFLAMMATORY ENZYMES

Quinones can inhibit key enzymes involved in the inflammatory response, such as cyclooxygenase (COX) and lipoxygenase (LOX). By blocking these enzymes, quinones reduce the production of pro-inflammatory mediators like prostaglandins and leukotrienes.

SUPPRESSION OF INFLAMMATORY CYTOKINES

Quinones modulate the immune response by suppressing the production of inflammatory cytokines, such as tumor necrosis factor-alpha (TNF-α) and interleukins (IL-1, IL-6). This suppression helps to alleviate inflammation and reduce tissue damage.

ANTIOXIDANT ACTIVITY

Quinones possess antioxidant properties, which help to neutralize reactive oxygen species (ROS) and reduce oxidative stress, a major contributor to inflammation. By protecting cells from oxidative damage, quinones help to mitigate inflammatory processes.

ANTICANCER PROPERTIES

Cancer is characterized by uncontrolled cell growth and the potential to invade or spread to other parts of the body. Quinones exhibit anticancer properties through various mechanisms:

INDUCTION OF APOPTOSIS: Quinones can trigger apoptosis (programmed cell death) in cancer cells. This is achieved by activating specific pathways that lead to cell death, thereby inhibiting the growth and proliferation of cancer cells.

INHIBITION OF CELL PROLIFERATION: Quinones interfere with cell cycle progression, preventing cancer cells from dividing and multiplying. By arresting the cell cycle at different stages, quinones inhibit tumor growth.

ANTIMETASTATIC EFFECTS: Quinones inhibit the processes involved in cancer metastasis, such as cell migration and invasion. By targeting these pathways, quinones help to prevent the spread of cancer to other parts of the body.

MODULATION OF SIGNALING PATHWAYS: Quinones interfere with key signaling pathways involved in cancer progression, such as the NF-κB, STAT3, and PI3K/Akt pathways. By modulating these pathways, quinones exert their anticancer effects.

EXAMPLES OF QUINONES WITH ANTI-INFLAMMATORY AND ANTICANCER PROPERTIES

NAPHTHOQUINONES

PLUMBAGIN: Extracted from the roots of *Plumbago zeylanica*, plumbagin has been shown to possess significant anti-inflammatory and anticancer properties. It inhibits the NF-κB signaling pathway, which is involved in inflammation and cancer progression.

SHIKONIN: Found in the roots of *Lithospermum erythrorhizon*, shikonin exhibits strong anti-inflammatory and anticancer activities. It induces apoptosis in cancer cells and suppresses inflammation by inhibiting pro-inflammatory cytokines.

ANTHRAQUINONES

EMODIN: Present in rhubarb (*Rheum officinale*), emodin has demonstrated both anti-inflammatory and anticancer effects. It inhibits COX-2, a key enzyme in inflammation, and induces apoptosis in various cancer cell lines [35].

ALOIN: Found in aloe vera (*Aloe vera*), aloin possesses anti-inflammatory properties by inhibiting LOX and reducing the production of pro-inflammatory mediators [36]. It also exhibits anticancer effects by inducing apoptosis and inhibiting cancer cell proliferation. *in vitro*, aloin dramatically reduced the migration, proliferation, and tube formation of HUVECs. Aloin inhibited the activation of VEGF receptor (VEGFR) 2 and STAT3 phosphorylation in endothelial cells, according to Western blotting. Furthermore, in human SW620 cancer cells, the constitutively active STAT3 protein, as well as the expression of STAT3-regulated proliferative (c-Myc), angiogenic (VEGF), and antiapoptotic (Bcl-xL) proteins, was down-regulated in response to AL. In line with the previously mentioned results, aloin significantly decreased tumor sizes and weight *in vivo* in mouse xenografts while also inhibiting tumor cell viability and inducing cell apoptosis *in vitro*—all without harmful effects [37].

INCLUSION IN NUTRACEUTICALS

The presence of quinones like naphthoquinones and anthraquinones in nutraceuticals aims to provide therapeutic benefits in a natural and non-toxic manner. Nutraceuticals are designed to offer health benefits beyond basic nutrition and are typically derived from food sources or medicinal plants. The advantages of using quinones in nutraceuticals include:

1. **SAFETY AND TOLERABILITY**: As naturally occurring compounds, quinones are generally considered safe and well-tolerated when consumed in appropriate amounts. This makes them a preferable alternative to synthetic drugs, which may have significant side effects [38, 39]. A strong coenzyme antioxidant pyrroloquinoline quinone (PQQ), which is found in food, has been shown to preserve brain cells by promoting the production of nerve growth factors (NGF) and NGF receptors and inhibiting amyloid β fibril formation and aggressiveness. The researchers developed a new PQQ disodium salt called mnemoPQQ® and evaluated its safety in toxicity tests that complied with GLP regulations. MnemoPQQ®'s acute toxicity experiments in Wistar rats showed that, although its acute dermal LD_{50} was >2000 mg/kg bw, its LD_{50} in male and female rats was 1825 and 1410 mg/kg body weight (bw), respectively. In an acute dermal irritation/corrosion investigation, mnemoPQQ® was shown to be nonirritating to rabbit skin; in an acute ocular irritation/corrosion research, it was determined that mnemoPQQ® was nonirritating to rabbit eyes. The non-mutagenic potential was demonstrated by the Ames bacterial reverse mutation experiment and the *in vitro* Mammalian cell gene mutation test. Mammalian *in vivo* erythrocyte micronucleus testing indicated that mnemoPQQ® was neither mutagenic nor clonogenic. There was no indication of systemic toxicity in a 90-day sub-chronic toxicity study, which was carried out at and up to the maximum daily dose of 600 mg/kg body weight. No significant abnormal clinical signs or changes in hematology, clinical chemistry, neurological evaluation, thyroid functions, reproductive hormone levels, sperm evaluations, vaginal cytology, endocrine functions, organ weight, or gross and microscopic pathology findings were observed in any of the rats that survived the treatment.

MnemoPQQ® was determined to have a no-observed-adverse-effect level (NOAEL) of more than 600 mg/kg body weight. The broad range safety of mnemoPQQ® for human intake is confirmed by these investigations [38].

2. **MULTIFACETED BENEFITS**: Quinones provide a range of health benefits, including anti-inflammatory, antioxidant, and anticancer effects. Their inclusion in nutraceuticals can help to address multiple health concerns simultaneously. While ubiquinones have been identified in most plants and animals in general, phytoquinones, attocopherolquinones, and phylloquinones are primary metabolites that are likely present in all tissues that participate in photosynthesis. The anthranoid chemicals have a laxative action. Chemically speaking, they are also known as dihydroxy-anthraquinones, -dianthrones, and -anthrones. These compounds are frequently referred to as vegetable laxatives because they are the ingredients of several plants and their extracts, including aloe, cascara, frangula, rhubarb, and senna [4].

3. **PREVENTIVE HEALTH**: Nutraceuticals containing quinones can be used for preventive health, helping to reduce the risk of chronic diseases associated with inflammation and oxidative stress, such as cardiovascular diseases, diabetes, and cancer. Products and preparations made from natural quinones and their synthetic mimics have therapeutic, medical, and technical uses [4]. In technology, materials of interest span from dyes and wood to semiconductors. Quinones are among the potential novel materials for microelectronics that offer a variety of noteworthy benefits. In a similar vein, polymers featuring quinone activity are biodegradable and show promise as future functional material options [40].

4. **ENHANCED BIOAVAILABILITY**: Formulating quinones in nutraceuticals can enhance their bioavailability, ensuring that they are effectively absorbed and utilized by the body.

5. SAFETY AND TOXICITY

Quinones, including naphthoquinones and anthraquinones, have garnered significant attention for their therapeutic properties, such as anti-inflammatory and anticancer effects. However, like any bioactive compounds, their safety and potential toxicity are crucial considerations to ensure they provide health benefits without causing harm. Proper dosage and formulation are essential to mitigate adverse effects and maximize therapeutic outcomes [43].

POTENTIAL TOXICITY OF QUINONES
1. OXIDATIVE STRESS

Mechanism: Quinones can participate in redox cycling, leading to the production of reactive oxygen species (ROS). While low levels of ROS can play a role in cell signaling and defense mechanisms, excessive ROS can cause oxidative stress, damaging cellular components such as DNA, proteins, and lipids.

IMPLICATIONS: Prolonged oxidative stress can contribute to chronic diseases, including neurodegenerative disorders, cardiovascular diseases, and cancer.

2. CYTOTOXICITY

MECHANISM: Quinones can induce cell death through apoptosis (programmed cell death) or necrosis (uncontrolled cell death). While this property is beneficial for targeting cancer cells, it can also affect healthy cells if the concentration is too high.

IMPLICATIONS: High doses of quinones may lead to toxicity in healthy tissues, necessitating precise dosing to avoid harmful side effects.

3. GASTROINTESTINAL IRRITATION

MECHANISM: Anthraquinones, especially those used as laxatives, can irritate the gastrointestinal mucosa, leading to increased intestinal motility and water secretion.

IMPLICATIONS: Overuse of anthraquinone-based laxatives can result in abdominal cramps, diarrhea, and dehydration. Chronic use may lead to conditions such as "cathartic colon," characterized by reduced bowel function.

4. HEPATOTOXICITY

MECHANISM: Some quinones have been associated with liver toxicity, potentially leading to liver enzyme elevation, jaundice, and liver damage.

IMPLICATIONS: Long-term or high-dose use of quinones necessitates monitoring of liver function to prevent serious liver conditions.

5. ALLERGIC REACTIONS

MECHANISM: Quinones can cause allergic reactions in some individuals, manifesting as skin rashes, itching, and respiratory symptoms.

IMPLICATIONS: Identifying and avoiding quinones in sensitive individuals is crucial to prevent allergic reactions.

ENSURING SAFETY: PROPER DOSAGE AND FORMULATION

1. DOSAGE REGULATION

THERAPEUTIC WINDOW: Determining the therapeutic window and the range of doses that provide therapeutic benefits without causing toxicity is essential. Dosage recommendations should be based on clinical studies and tailored to individual patient needs, considering factors such as age, weight, and overall health.

AVOIDING OVERDOSE: Ensuring that patients do not exceed the recommended dosage is critical to prevent toxic effects.

2. STANDARDIZATION

CONSISTENCY: Herbal extracts containing quinones should be standardized to ensure consistent potency and quality. Standardization helps deliver a precise amount of active quinones, reducing the risk of variability that could lead to underdosing or overdosing [44, 45].

QUALITY CONTROL: Implementing rigorous quality control measures in the production of quinone-containing products is essential to ensure safety and efficacy [46].

3. FORMULATION

BIOAVAILABILITY: Formulating quinones in a way that maximizes their bioavailability and minimizes potential side effects is essential. This can include using protective coatings, controlled-release formulations, or combining quinones with other compounds that enhance their efficacy and reduce toxicity [47, 48].

COMBINATION THERAPIES: Using quinones in combination with other therapeutic agents can enhance their efficacy and reduce the required dose, potentially lowering the risk of toxicity [49].

4. MONITORING AND GUIDELINES

REGULAR MONITORING: Regular monitoring of patients using quinone-based treatments is important to detect any signs of toxicity early [49]. Healthcare providers should follow established guidelines for the use of quinones, including recommendations for duration of use, dosage adjustments, and periodic health evaluations [50].

PATIENT EDUCATION: Educating patients about the correct use of quinone-containing products is vital. Patients should be informed about the potential side effects, the importance of adhering to prescribed dosages, and the need to report any adverse reactions promptly.

5. RESEARCH AND DEVELOPMENT

Ongoing Research: Continuous research is necessary to better understand the pharmacokinetics, pharmacodynamics, and long-term effects of quinones. This knowledge will help refine dosage recommendations and improve safety profiles [51, 52].

Innovation in Formulation: Developing innovative formulations that enhance the safety and efficacy of quinones, such as nanoformulations or targeted delivery systems, can further mitigate the risk of adverse effects [53].

Table 1. Safety Profile of Common Quinones.

Compound	Toxicity Level	Safe Dosage
Plumbagin	Moderate	2-5 mg/kg
Coenzyme Q10	Low	30-200 mg/day

CONCLUSION

Quinones, with their diverse and potent biological activities, hold significant promise in both traditional therapy and modern nutraceutical applications. Their ability to modulate inflammation, combat cancer, and provide other health benefits makes them invaluable in promoting overall well-being. Ongoing research continues to uncover new insights into their mechanisms of action, optimal formulations, and therapeutic potential. By ensuring proper dosage, standardization, and safety measures, quinones can be effectively and safely incorporated into health products, offering natural and potent solutions for enhancing human health. Plants high in quinones are used to treat a wide range of ailments in traditional medicine around the globe. Coenzyme Q10, idobenone, mitoquinone, plastoquinone, vatiquinone, vitamins K, embelin, APX-3330, cannabinoid-derived quinones, asterriquinones, pyrroloquinolinequinone, geldanamycin, rifampicin quinone, memoquin, and their analogs are just a few examples of the many natural and artificial quinones that exhibit neuroprotective, anti-inflammatory, anti-cancer, antimicrobial, antifungal and nutraceutical potential against diverse diseases.

REFERENCES

[1]   Mbala-Mavinga B. Synthesis of quinoid natural products and analogues. Ghent University 2011.

[2]   Garrido-Maraver J, Cordero MD, Oropesa-Ávila M, *et al.* Coenzyme Q_{10} Therapy. Mol Syndromol 2014; 5(3-4): 187-97.
[http://dx.doi.org/10.1159/000360101] [PMID: 25126052]

[3]   Zheng L, Jin J, Shi L, *et al.* Gamma tocopherol, its dimmers, and quinones: Past and future trends. Crit Rev Food Sci Nutr 2020; 60(22): 3916-30.
[http://dx.doi.org/10.1080/10408398.2020.1711704] [PMID: 31957471]

[4]   Martínez MJA. Biological activity of quinones. 2005; 30: 303-66.

[5]   Klotz LO, Hou X, Jacob C. 1,4-naphthoquinones: from oxidative damage to cellular and inter-cellular signaling. Molecules 2014; 19(9): 14902-18.
[http://dx.doi.org/10.3390/molecules190914902] [PMID: 25232709]

[6]   Erlank H, Elmann A, Kohen R, Kanner J. Polyphenols activate Nrf2 in astrocytes via H2O2, semiquinones, and quinones. Free Radic Biol Med 2011; 51(12): 2319-27.
[http://dx.doi.org/10.1016/j.freeradbiomed.2011.09.033] [PMID: 22037513]

[7]   Mukherjee S, Pal M. Quinolines: a new hope against inflammation. 2013; 18(7-8): 389-98.
[PMID: 23159484]

[8]   Xin D, Li H, Zhou S, Zhong H, Pu W. Effects of anthraquinones on immune responses and inflammatory diseases. Molecules 2022; 27(12): 3831.
[http://dx.doi.org/10.3390/molecules27123831] [PMID: 35744949]

[9]   Gwon WG, Lee B, Joung EJ, *et al.* Sargaquinoic acid inhibits TNF-α-induced NF-κB signaling, thereby contributing to decreased monocyte adhesion to human umbilical vein endothelial cells (HUVECs). J Agric Food Chem 2015; 63(41): 9053-61.
[http://dx.doi.org/10.1021/acs.jafc.5b04050] [PMID: 26437568]

[10]   Sisa M, Dvorakova M, Temml V, Jarosova V, Vanek T, Landa P. Synthesis, inhibitory activity and in silico docking of dual COX/5-LOX inhibitors with quinone and resorcinol core. Eur J Med Chem 2020; 204112620
[http://dx.doi.org/10.1016/j.ejmech.2020.112620] [PMID: 32738413]

[11]   Škandík M, Mrvová N, Bezek Š, Račková L. Semisynthetic quercetin-quinone mitigates BV-2 microglia activation through modulation of Nrf2 pathway. 2020; 152: 18-32.
[PMID: 32142880]

[12]   Asche CJMrimc. Antitumour quinones. 5 (5):449-467.

[13]   Bolton JL, Dunlap T. Formation and biological targets of quinones: cytotoxic versus cytoprotective effects. Chem Res Toxicol 2017; 30(1): 13-37.
[http://dx.doi.org/10.1021/acs.chemrestox.6b00256] [PMID: 27617882]

[14]   Ho SHS, Sim MY, Yee WLS, Yang T, Yuen SPJ, Go ML. Antiproliferative, DNA intercalation and redox cycling activities of dioxonaphtho[2,3-d]imidazolium analogs of YM155: A structure–activity relationship study. Eur J Med Chem 2015; 104: 42-56.
[http://dx.doi.org/10.1016/j.ejmech.2015.09.026] [PMID: 26433618]

[15]   Khisamutdinov E. Part I Nucleic Acid Site-Selective Binding Studies of Isomers of Dihydrodioxin-Masked Ortho-Quinones as Potential Antitumor Drugs Part II The Role of Non-Watson-Crick Base Pairs in Stabilizing Recurrent RNA Motif. Bowling Green State University 2012.

[16]   van der Zanden SY, Qiao X, Neefjes J. New insights into the activities and toxicities of the old anticancer drug doxorubicin. FEBS J 2021; 288(21): 6095-111.
[http://dx.doi.org/10.1111/febs.15583] [PMID: 33022843]

[17]   Cross JV, Deak JC, Rich EA, *et al.* Quinone reductase inhibitors block SAPK/JNK and NFkappaB pathways and potentiate apoptosis. J Biol Chem 1999; 274(44): 31150-4.

[http://dx.doi.org/10.1074/jbc.274.44.31150] [PMID: 10531305]

[18]   A review on phytochemistry, pharmacological and coloring potential of lawsonia inermis. 2018; 2: 169.

[19]   Sharma M, Sharma M. A comprehensive review on ethnobotanical, medicinal and nutritional potential of walnut (Juglans regia L.). 2022; 88(4): 601-16.

[20]   Egbuna C, Gupta E, Ezzat SM, *et al.* Nutraceuticals: Bioactive Components F, Innovations (2020) Aloe species as valuable sources of functional bioactives. 2020, 337-387.

[21]   Goel S, Parihar PS. Meshram VJBnpidd Plant-derived quinones as a source of antibacterial and anticancer agents. 2020, 245-279.

[22]   Chen JQ, Li DW, Chen YY, *et al.* Elucidating dosage-effect relationship of different efficacy of rhubarb in constipation model rats by factor analysis. J Ethnopharmacol 2019; 238111868 [http://dx.doi.org/10.1016/j.jep.2019.111868] [PMID: 30981706]

[23]   Santucci NR, Chogle A, Leiby A, *et al.* Non-pharmacologic approach to pediatric constipation. 2021; 59102711
[PMID: 33737146]

[24]   Tomar R, Mishra SS, Sahoo J, Rath SK. Isolation, chemical characterization, antimicrobial activity, and molecular docking studies of 2,6-dimethoxy benzoquinone isolated from medicinal plant *Flacourtia jangomas.* 3 Biotech 2024; 14(6): 156.
[http://dx.doi.org/10.1007/s13205-024-04002-w] [PMID: 38766321]

[25]   Gafner S, Wolfender JL, Nianga M, Stoeckli-Evans H, Hostettmann K. Antifungal and antibacterial naphthoquinones from Newbouldia laevis roots. Phytochemistry 1996; 42(5): 1315-20.
[http://dx.doi.org/10.1016/0031-9422(96)00135-5] [PMID: 9397206]

[26]   Eyong KO, Krohn K, Hussain H, *et al.* Newbouldiaquinone and newbouldiamide: a new naphthoquinone-anthraquinone coupled pigment and a new ceramide from Newbouldia laevis. Chem Pharm Bull (Tokyo) 2005; 53(6): 616-9.
[http://dx.doi.org/10.1248/cpb.53.616] [PMID: 15930769]

[27]   Abegaz BMJPR. Novel phenylanthraquinones, isofuranonaphthoquinones, homoisoflavonoids, and biflavonoids from African plants in the genera Bulbine, Scilla, Ledebouria, and Rhus. 2002; 1: 299-310.

[28]   Williams R, Norris A, Miller J, *et al.* Two new cytotoxic naphthoquinones from Mendoncia cowanii from the rainforest of Madagascar. Planta Med 2006; 72(6): 564-6.
[http://dx.doi.org/10.1055/s-2006-931554] [PMID: 16773542]

[29]   Shu C, Chen J, Lv M, Xi Y, Zheng J, Xu X. Plumbagin relieves rheumatoid arthritis through nuclear factor kappa-B (NF-κB) pathway. Bioengineered 2022; 13(5): 13632-42.
[http://dx.doi.org/10.1080/21655979.2022.2081756] [PMID: 35653787]

[30]   Tabassum N. Hamdani MJPr Plants used to treat skin diseases. 2014, 8 (15):52

[31]   Touitou E, Natsheh H. Topical administration of drugs incorporated in carriers containing phospholipid soft vesicles for the treatment of skin medical conditions. Pharmaceutics 2021; 13(12): 2129.
[http://dx.doi.org/10.3390/pharmaceutics13122129] [PMID: 34959410]

[32]   Bhatia M, Chaudhary J, Jain A, Dhingra A, Chopra BJCTM. A Recent Update on Ayurvedic Anti-asthmatic Formulations: Highlighting the Role of Major Anti-asthmatic Plants. 2024; 10(6): 22-33.

[33]   Yang YK, Wang LP, Chen L, *et al.* Coenzyme Q10 treatment of cardiovascular disorders of ageing including heart failure, hypertension and endothelial dysfunction. Clin Chim Acta 2015; 450: 83-9.
[http://dx.doi.org/10.1016/j.cca.2015.08.002] [PMID: 26254995]

[34]   Kumar A, Kaur H, Devi P, Mohan V. Role of coenzyme Q10 (CoQ10) in cardiac disease, hypertension and Meniere-like syndrome. Pharmacol Ther 2009; 124(3): 259-68.

[http://dx.doi.org/10.1016/j.pharmthera.2009.07.003] [PMID: 19638284]

[35]   Huang Q, Lu G, Shen HM, Chung MCM, Ong CN. Anti□cancer properties of anthraquinones from rhubarb. Med Res Rev 2007; 27(5): 609-30.
[http://dx.doi.org/10.1002/med.20094] [PMID: 17022020]

[36]   Park MY, Kwon HJ, Sung MK. Dietary aloin, aloesin, or aloe-gel exerts anti-inflammatory activity in a rat colitis model. Life Sci 2011; 88(11-12): 486-92.
[http://dx.doi.org/10.1016/j.lfs.2011.01.010] [PMID: 21277867]

[37]   Pan Q, Pan H, Lou H, Xu Y, Tian L. Inhibition of the angiogenesis and growth of Aloin in human colorectal cancer in vitro and in vivo. Cancer Cell Int 2013; 13(1): 69.
[http://dx.doi.org/10.1186/1475-2867-13-69] [PMID: 23848964]

[38]   Shiojima Y, Deshmukh N, Moriyama H, *et al.* Safety assessment of a novel, dietary pyrroloquinoline quinone disodium salt (mnemoPQQ ®). Toxicol Mech Methods 2022; 32(9): 662-77.
[http://dx.doi.org/10.1080/15376516.2022.2076635] [PMID: 35546737]

[39]   Malik EM, Müller CE. Anthraquinones as pharmacological tools and drugs. Med Res Rev 2016; 36(4): 705-48.
[http://dx.doi.org/10.1002/med.21391] [PMID: 27111664]

[40]   Jia Z, Wen M, Cheng Y, Zheng YJAFM. Strategic advances in spatiotemporal control of bioinspired phenolic chemistries in materials science. 2021; 31(14)2008821

[41]   Verrax J, Beck R, Dejeans N, *et al.* Redox-active quinones and ascorbate: an innovative cancer therapy that exploits the vulnerability of cancer cells to oxidative stress. Anticancer Agents Med Chem 2011; 11(2): 213-21.
[http://dx.doi.org/10.2174/187152011795255902] [PMID: 21395522]

[42]   Lown JW, Biochemistry C. The mechanism of action of quinone antibiotics. Mol Cell Biochem 1983; 55(1): 17-40.
[http://dx.doi.org/10.1007/BF00229240] [PMID: 6353197]

[43]   Faizan S, Mohsen MMA, Amarakanth C, Justin A, Rahangdale RR, Chandrashekar HR. Quinone scaffolds as potential therapeutic anticancer agents: Chemistry, mechanism of Actions, Structure-Activity relationships and future perspectives. 2024, 101432.

[44]   Chang J. Medicinal herbs: Drugs or dietary supplements? Biochem Pharmacol 2000; 59(3): 211-9.
[http://dx.doi.org/10.1016/S0006-2952(99)00243-9] [PMID: 10609549]

[45]   Chen C-YO, Ribaya-Mercado JD, McKay DL, Croom E, Blumberg JBJFC. Differential antioxidant and quinone reductase inducing activity of American, Asian, and Siberian ginseng. 2010; 119(2): 445-51.

[46]   Bian J, Li X, Wang N, Wu X, You Q, Zhang X. Discovery of quinone-directed antitumor agents selectively bioactivated by NQO1 over CPR with improved safety profile. Eur J Med Chem 2017; 129: 27-40.
[http://dx.doi.org/10.1016/j.ejmech.2017.02.004] [PMID: 28214631]

[47]   Yin Z, Zheng T, Ho C-T, *et al.* Improving the stability and bioavailability of tea polyphenols by encapsulations: A review. 2022; 11(3): 537-56.

[48]   Laddomada B, Caretto S, Mita G. Wheat bran phenolic acids: Bioavailability and stability in whole wheat-based foods. Molecules 2015; 20(9): 15666-85.
[http://dx.doi.org/10.3390/molecules200915666] [PMID: 26343624]

[49]   Bolton J. Quinone methide bioactivation pathway: contribution to toxicity and/or cytoprotection? Curr Org Chem 2014; 18(1): 61-9.
[http://dx.doi.org/10.2174/1385272818011401211123046] [PMID: 25346613]

[50]   Hawi A, Heald S, Sciascia T. Use of an adaptive study design in single ascending-dose pharmacokinetics of A0001 (α-tocopherylquinone) in healthy male subjects. J Clin Pharmacol 2012;

52(1): 65-77.
[http://dx.doi.org/10.1177/0091270010390807] [PMID: 21343342]

[51]   Phillips RM, Hendriks HR, Sweeney JB, Reddy G, Peters GJ. Efficacy, pharmacokinetic and pharmacodynamic evaluation of apaziquone in the treatment of non-muscle invasive bladder cancer. Expert Opin Drug Metab Toxicol 2017; 13(7): 783-91.
[http://dx.doi.org/10.1080/17425255.2017.1341490] [PMID: 28637373]

[52]   Gao M, Wang Z, Yang J, *et al.* Simultaneous determination and pharmacokinetics study of four quinones in rat plasma by ultra high performance liquid chromatography with electrospray ionization tandem mass spectrometry after the oral administration of Qianzhi capsules. J Sep Sci 2018; 41(10): 2161-8.
[http://dx.doi.org/10.1002/jssc.201700981] [PMID: 29436170]

[53]   Ballout F, Habli Z, Rahal ON, Fatfat M, Gali-Muhtasib H. Thymoquinone-based nanotechnology for cancer therapy: promises and challenges. Drug Discov Today 2018; 23(5): 1089-98.
[http://dx.doi.org/10.1016/j.drudis.2018.01.043] [PMID: 29374534]

CHAPTER 5

Efficient Synthesis of Quinone-Based Glycohybrids

Sunil Sharma[1], **Yogesh Yadav**[1], **Ramesh Kumar**[2] and **Ram Sagar**[1,*]

[1] *Glycochemistry Laboratory, School of Physical Sciences, Jawaharlal Nehru University, New Delhi 110067, India*

[2] *Department of Chemistry, Kurukshetra University Kurukshetra, Haryana 136119, India*

Abstract: Quinones are redox-active cyclic chemical compounds with two carbonyl groups in a six-membered ring structure, either contiguous or apart. Quinones are a diverse group of natural compounds that have gained attention for their pharmacological properties. This book chapter focuses on the design and synthesis of natural product-inspired quinone-based glycohybrids. Glycohybrids can have a broad variety of structural and functional properties, including protein-carbohydrate interactions that are essential for the biology of mammals and some disease states. These glycohybrids are designed based on the structures of bioactive aryl glycosides and quinones, aiming to enhance their binding affinity, enhanced bioavailability, high water solubility, low toxicity, and specificity toward cancer-related protein targets. This book chapter consistsof the literature from January 2017 to December 2023 and provides an overview of recent developments in the chemical synthesis of glycohybrids based on natural product scaffold of quinones.

Keywords: 1,4-naphthoquinone, Anticancer, Antiradical, Click chemistry glycohybrids, Cytotoxicity, Glycohybrids, Natural products, Synthetic methods, Quinone.

INTRODUCTION

Quinones are colored substances containing a basic benzoquinone chromophore composed of two carbonyl groups joined by two carbon-carbon double bonds. The quinone dyes are composed of fused benzenoid quinoid ring complexes that have enough conjugation to provide color. The three primary classes of quinones are benzoquinones (**A**), benzoquinones (**B**), and anthraquinones (**C**), which have 1, 2, and 3-ring structures, respectively, as shown in (Fig. **1**). The fundamental building block of quinone molecules is benzoquinone [1]. Chemically, 1,4-benzoquinone, commonly known as para-benzoquinone, is a non-aromatic substance that reduces readily to hydroquinone [2]. Benzoquinone units are

---

[*] **Corresponding author Ram Sagar:** Glycochemistry Laboratory, School of Physical Sciences, Jawaharlal Nehru University, New Delhi 110067, India; E-mail: ram.sagar@jnu.ac.in

Ashutosh Kumar Dash & Deepak Kumar (Eds.)

essential moieties to produce biologically active chemicals and act as building blocks in quinone synthesis [1].

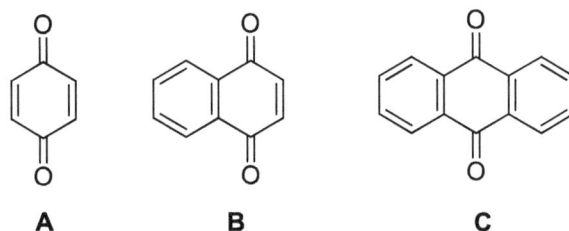

Fig. (1). Chemical structure of benzoquinone **A**, naphthoquinone **B**, and anthraquinone **C**.

Naphthoquinones are compounds that have para-benzoquinones bound to an additional benzene ring at position 2,3-C (carbon). Two carbonyl groups are present on one benzene ring in the naphthoquinone structure (Fig. **1b**), usually in the o- or p-orientation [3]. Naphthoquinones also have α- and β-unsaturated carbonyls. The visible region exhibits significant coloration due to extended electron delocalization across carbonyl groups and double bonds [4].

Nature is full of naphthoquinones [5, 6], which are typically found as glycosides that may be separated from bacteria, fungi, plants, and marine invertebrates [7, 8]. The pharmacological activity [9 - 11] and diverse synthesis techniques of naphthoquinones, including their anticancer, antibacterial, antifungal, and anti-inflammatory properties, have been documented in recent years [12 - 14]. The solubility and activity of naphthoquinones will increase as they convert to naphthoquinone glycosides, and new activity may even develop, offering a new method for obtaining novel compounds with a range of biological activities [15 - 17]. According to reports, the anticancer activities of 1,4-naphthoquinone could be enhanced by the inclusion of acetylated D-glucose and D-galactose residues [18a-b]. One example of this would be the acetylated glycosides of lapachol [19]. Thus, the synthesis of 1,4-naphthoquinone glycosides is a powerful approach to finding novel compounds with strong biological activity [20].

The third class of quinones, known as anthraquinones, are compounds containing the anthracene nucleus with two carbonyl groups. They are derived from the tricyclic aromatic chemical molecule 9,10-dioxoanthracene ($C_{14}H_8O_2$) (Fig. **1**), which has a fundamental structure. Anthraquinones are found in fungi, lichens, and plants. Hydroxyanthraquinoids absorb visible light and are therefore colored. Alizarin is a prominent red dye used in the fabric industry. It has anthraquinone moiety.

There are hundreds of derivatives in nature due to quinone structures' ability to accommodate various substitution sequences, particularly for anthraquinones. A quinone compound's color is often determined by the location, kind, and quantity of hydroxyl and electron-donating/accepting elements, commonly known as auxochromes, as well as by the many rings that affect steric effects and intramolecular hydrogen bonding.

Quinones are important secondary metabolites that play a crucial role in photosynthesis and respiration processes in plants. These activities include electron transport and oxidative phosphorylation. These substances frequently serve as mediators between a plant and its surroundings and oversee energy transduction, color, signaling, defense, scent, and favor. Some of the natural quinone components with antifungal, antibacterial, antioxidant, anti-cancer, anti-inflammatory, laxative, and anti-allergen properties have been employed in pharmacology to cause cytoprotection in humans [21-23a-b].

It is known that glycohybrids are an important class of molecules that exhibit diverse biological activities and are present as structural motifs in many natural products. Glycohybrid structures are formed by linking/connecting heterocyclic rings or hydrocarbon chains and carbohydrate moieties with biologically relevant molecules without changing their initial structure much. These molecules are known as glycohybrids [24a-b]. Linking or merging carbohydrates with bioactive molecules provides a viable source for chemical libraries in drug discovery and development [25]. The glycosylation of bioactive molecules of both synthetic and natural origin most often improves the pharmacological properties and ADMET parameters of the drug. Thus glycoconjugation has emerged as one of the most effective approaches for targeting cancerous cells by linking or merging the pharmacophoric moiety to the glycosyl/carbohydrate unit [25].

Glycohybrid molecules are used in the creation of pharmaceuticals due to their biological activity, high diversity, improved pharmacokinetic and pharmacodynamic properties [26, 27], molecular recognition, intracellular functions, enhanced bioavailability, high water solubility, and low toxicity [28, 29].

Numerous medicinal chemists worldwide have combined organic molecules quinone with carbohydrates, resulting in the production of novel glycohybrids (**D-I**), as shown in (Fig. **2**), with varying structural and functional features [30, 31]. These innovative glycohybrids may exhibit enhanced biological activity or prove to be more efficient, safe, and affordable as potential pharmaceutical candidates. On the basis of these innovations, we have chosen to review and investigate the literature about the recently reported synthesis of quinone-based glycohybrids and their related biological activities. These recent literature reports covering the years 2017-2023 are presented here in this book chapter.

D. 4-dehydro-
deacetylgriseusin A

E. 2a, 8a-epoxy-epi-
deacetylgriseusin A

F. epi-deacetylgriseusin A   **G.** epi-deacetylgriseusin B

H. Cartomarin

I. Safflomin C

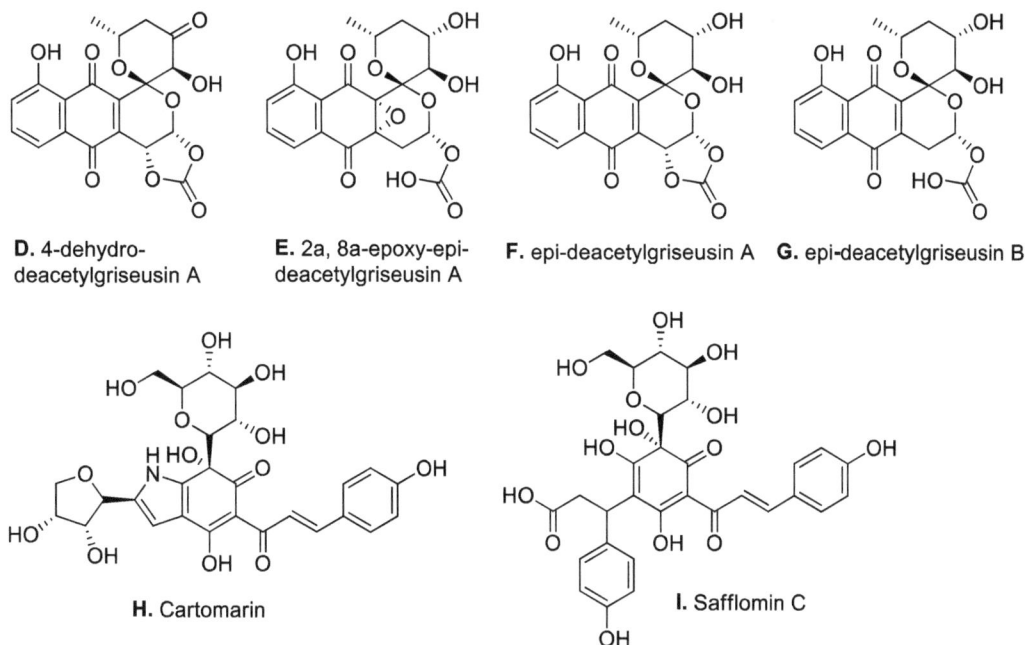

Fig. (2). Quinone-based glycohybrids **D-I**..

SYNTHESIS OF QUINONE-BASED GLYCOHYBRIDS

Nancy O. Huynh *et al.* synthesized a mixture of 2- and 3-amino juglone **3a**, **3b**, and **SF2446-B3 5,** which is also known as quinone-based glycohybrids. In the first step, when quinone derivative juglone **1** is treated with β-1-amino-L rhamnose **2** in the presence of a copper catalyst in a reaction vessel under a microwave condition at higher loadings of catalyst (20 mol %), N-glycoside is formed that undergoes cleavage *in situ* to form mixtures of 2- and 3-amino juglone **3a** and **3b**. Remarkably, glycosidic cleavage can be inhibited at lower loadings of the copper catalyst (5 mol%), allowing the regio isomeric C_2 and C_3 N-glycosides **3a** and **3b** to be extracted in 85% yield as a 3:1 mixture.

Quinone **4** may serve as a doorway to other arenimycins and type II polyketides of the **SF2446 B3 5** family. It was envisaged that quinone **4** would undergo direct amino glycosylation by adding β-1-amino-L-rhamnose **4,** and then the resulting hydroquinone would undergo aerobic oxidation, as shown in Scheme (**1**) [32].

K. Ashish *et al.* synthesized naphthoquinone-based glycohybrids **8a-d** by reacting 3,4,6-tri-O-benzylglycals **7a** and **7b** with diversely substituted 2-hydroxynaphthoquinones **6a-c**. When substrates were dissolved in toluene/AcOH (9:1, v/v) and the reaction mixture was then heated at 80 °C for 20 minutes with the microwave power set at 100 W, naphthoquinone-based glycohybrids **8a-d** were obtained with moderate to good yields, as shown in Scheme (**2**).

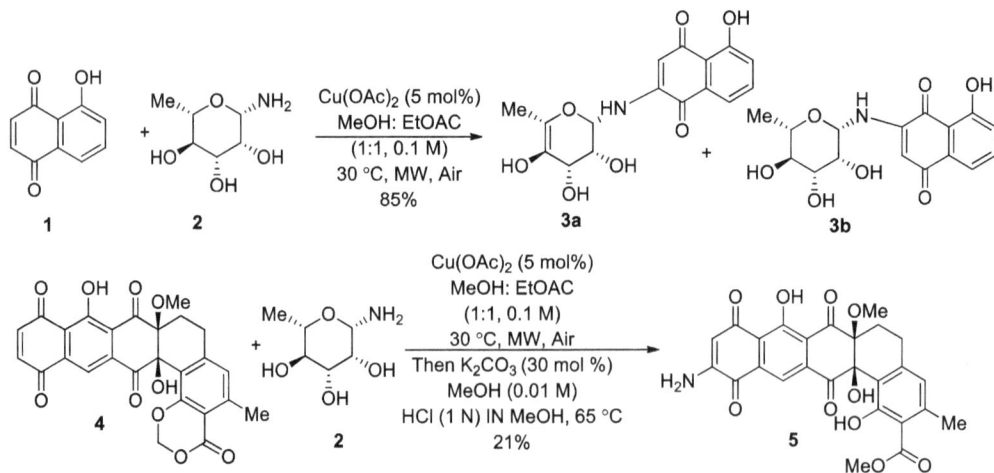

Scheme (1). Synthesis of 2- and 3-amino juglone **3a**, **3b**, and **SF2446-B3 5**.

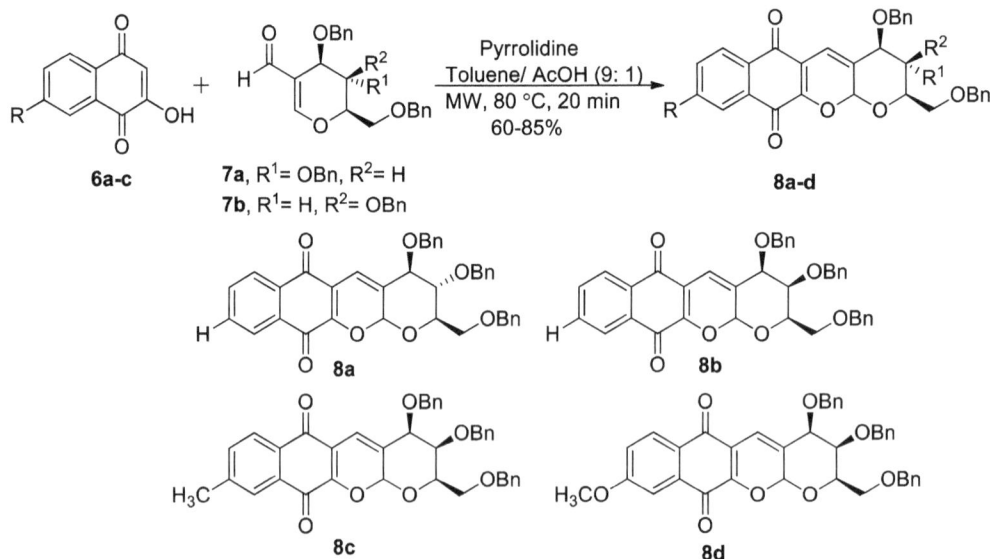

Scheme (2). Synthesis of naphthoquinone-fused glycohybrids **8a-d**.

These compounds exhibit high pharmacological potential and hold promise for therapeutic applications. Additionally, strong evidence has been presented by SAR research and *in silico* docking analyses, indicating that their designed natural product-inspired naphthoquinone-based glycohybrids may function as strong inhibitors of the IRAK1 catalytic site, indicating their potential as a potent anti-inflammatory and anticancer agent [33]. Naphthoquinone-based glycohybrids might be more bioavailable and effective while posing minimal cytotoxicity risks [34].

Shungang Jiao *et al.* synthesized quinone-terpenoid alkaloid alashanine **11**, which is also known as quinone-based glycohybrid, through an intermolecular Diels−Alder reaction of 2-methoxy-1,4-benzoquinone **9** with secoiridoid **10**, as shown in Scheme (**3**).

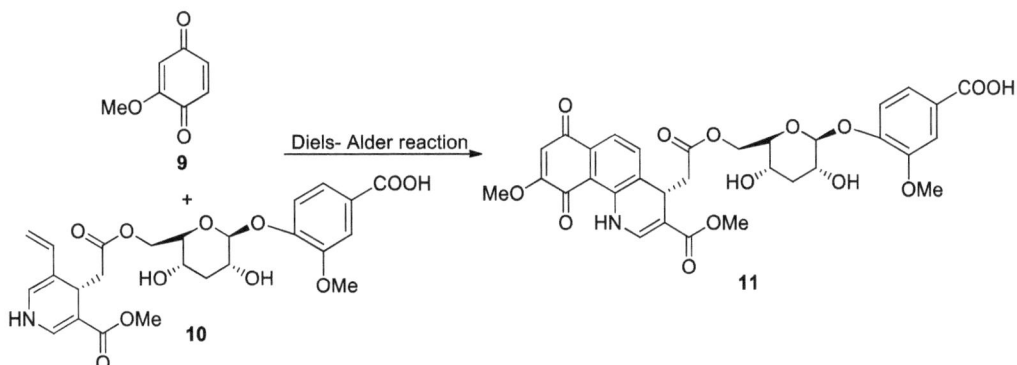

Scheme (3). Synthesis of Quinone-Terpenoid Alkaloid Alashanine **11**.

Alashanine **11** was evaluated using recognized bioassay techniques for its antibacterial activity against Bacillus subtilis and anti-Candida albicans [35, 36]. Alashanine **11**, with a MIC value of 5.31µg/mL, exhibited significant inhibition against Bacillus subtilis. The MTT technique was also used to assess the cytotoxic activity of Alashanine **11** against the growth of HepG2 and MCF-7 human cancer cell lines [37 - 39]. Alashanine **11** was found to possess moderate cytotoxic activity *in vitro*. The IC_{50} values of Alashanine **11** were 5.01µM and 9.16µM, respectively, against HepG2 and MCF-7 cells [40].

Haijuan Liu *et al.* synthesized C-naphthyl ketosides **13a-i,** which are also known as quinone-based glycohybrids, from O-ketosides **12a-i** *via* the Fries-type rearrangement reaction by using Lewis acid $BF_3 \cdot Et_2O$ in dry dichloromethane at - 60 °C under argon. The reaction mixture's temperature was progressively raised to 5 °C over the course of three hours. It was found that the formal O- to C-glycosyl migration is more sensitive to structural changes in the aglycon sections than the similar traditional C-glycosylation process, which employs more reactive aldosyl oxocarbenium ion intermediates. This method could be used to create the angular methyl group-bearing C-naphthyl ketoside building blocks, which are present in every member of the significant anthracycline subclass, as shown in Scheme (**4**) [41].

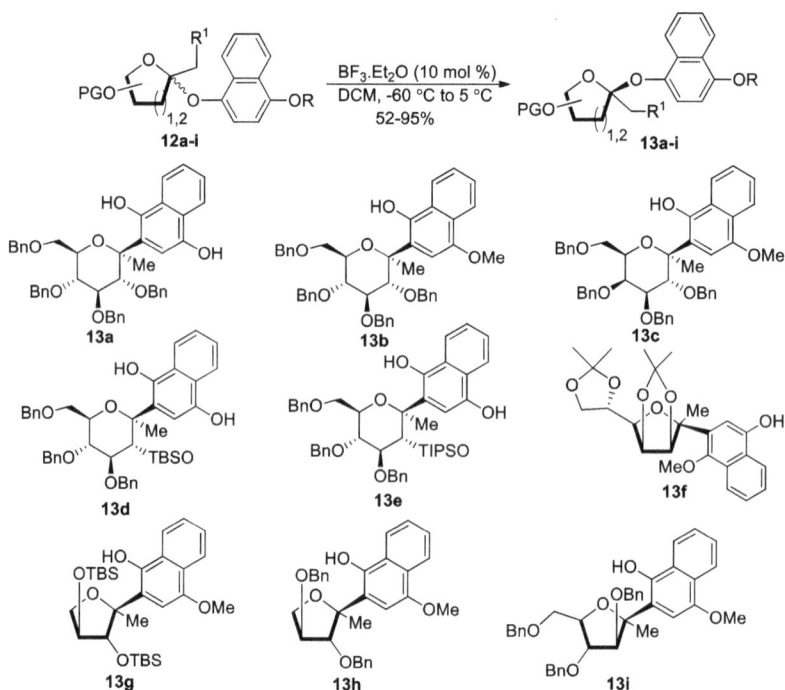

Scheme (4). Synthesis of Quinone-based glycohybrids **13a-i**.

Thaís Barreto Santos *et al.* reported the synthesis of naphthoquinone-based glycohybrid **20**. In the first step, 1, 4- naphthoquinone **14** was treated with L-tryptophan **15** in the presence of ethanol/ water at 23 °C; then, the formation of naphthoquinone compound **16** took place. Naphthoquinone compound **16**undergoes an amide formation reaction with propargylamine, producing **17**. In the terminal alkyne group of **17**, there is a click reaction with azide **18** to form the triazole ring-based naphthoquinone glycohybrid **19**. In the last step, naphthoquinone-based glycohybrid **19** undergoes hydrolysis of the acetate groups in a basic medium to form the naphthoquinone-based glycohybrid **20,** as shown in Scheme (**5**) [42].

Lucas Bonfim Marques *et al.* synthesized naphthoquinone-based glycohybrids LA4A **24** (lapachol-β-glucoside) and LA4C (lapachol-N-acetylglucosamin--β-glucoside) **27**. In the first step, the formation of acetobromo-α-D-glucose **22** takes place when glucose **21** is treated with acetic anhydride and hydrobromic acid in dichloromethane. After the formation of acetobromo-α-D-glucose **22,** it is treated with naphthoquinone derivative Lapachol **23** in the presence of TBAB in dichloromethane solvent, which furnishes naphthoquinone-based glycohybrids LA4A **24** (lapachol-β-glucoside) in excellent yield.

In the second reaction, 1-chloro-tetraacetylated- N- glucosamine **26** was obtained when N-acetylated glucosamine **25** was treated with acyl chloride at room temperature for 48 hours. After the formation of 1-chloro-tetraacetylate--N-glucosamine **26**, it was again treated with naphthoquinone derivative lapachol **23** in the presence of TBAB in dichloromethane solvent, which furnished naphthoquinone-based glycohybrid LA4C **27** (lapachol-N-acetylglucosamin--β-glucoside) in excellent yield.

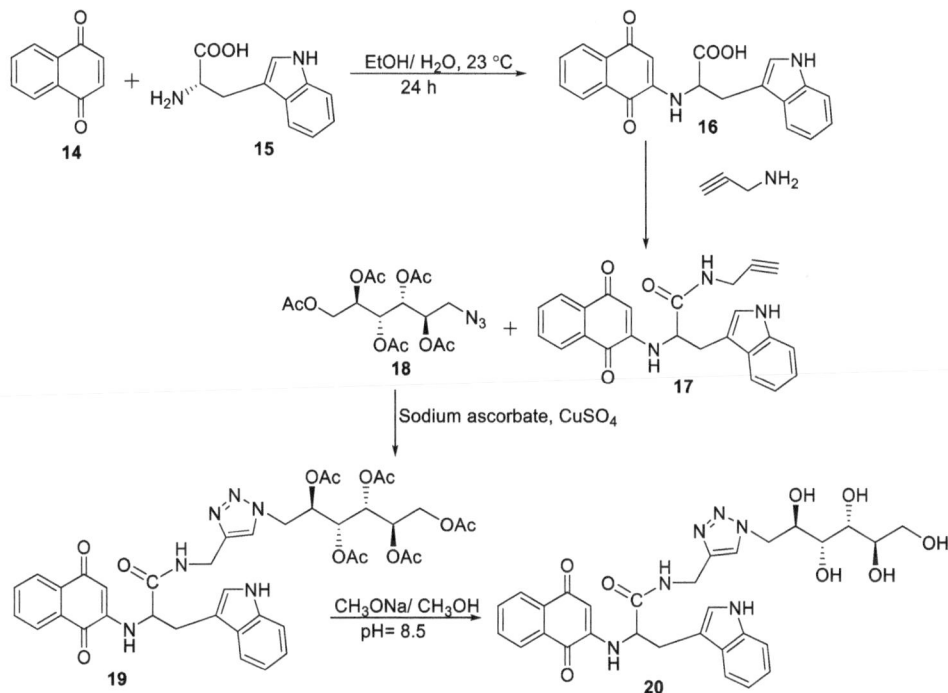

Scheme (5). Synthesis of naphthoquinone-based glycohybrid **20**.

Cytotoxicity of lapachol and its two glycoderivatives, LA4A **24** and LA4C **27,** against HL60, nuclear morphology, and membrane integrity of cells were investigated. Attachment of a β-O-peracetylglycosyl group to lapachol improves the cytotoxic effects of the natural molecule, possibly by enhancing bioavailability. The IC_{50} values (in μM) of lapachol were higher than those of LA4A **24** (5.7) and LA4C **27** (5.3). The classical indicators of apoptosis, including chromatin condensation, DNA fragmentation, exposure of phosphatidylserine on the cell surface, and a drop in the mitochondrial transmembrane potential ($\Delta\Psi_m$) before cell lysis, were elicited by LA4A **24** and LA4C **27**. The study on non-tumor cells was conducted, and the toxicity of lapachol and its derivatives was also examined. The drugs' potential for adverse effects was assessed using human peripheral neurons (Peri Tox test). From this study, it was clear that LA4C **27** was less hazardous than LA4A **24**. They found that LA4C **27** had a low neurotoxicity profile and high toxicity to tumor cells, which was the best for a therapeutic candidate, as shown in Scheme (6) [43].

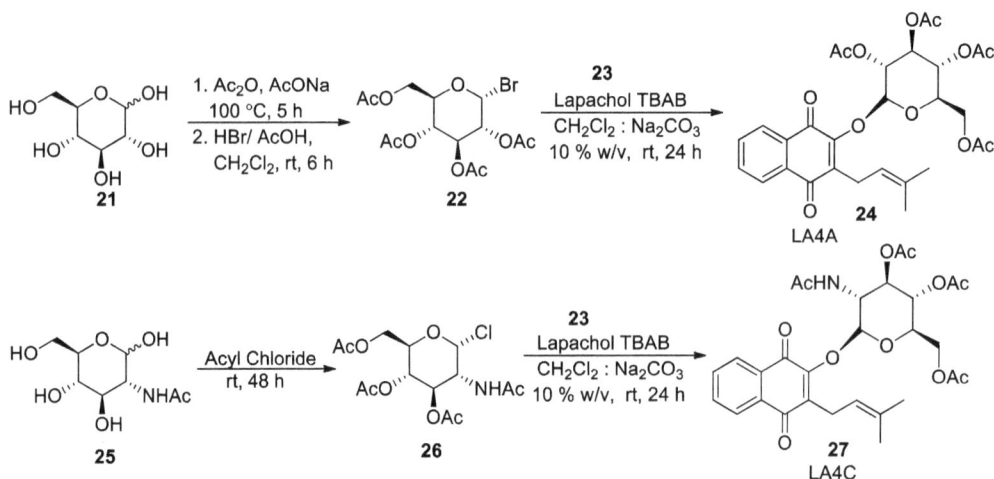

Scheme (6). Synthesis of naphthoquinone-based glycohybrids LA4A **24** and LA4C **27**.

Nishant Pandey *et al.* synthesized hydroxyanthracene triazolyl glycoconjugates **33a-h** and **35a-c** by using click chemistry. In the first step, anthraquinone **28** was treated with lithium (trimethysilyl)acetylide **29** in the presence of n-butyl lithium under an inert condition, giving an acetylide addition product **30**. The desilylation of TMS derivatives **30** was affected by treatment with methanolic KOH solution in the presence of THF to afford the corresponding novel hydroxyanthracene-based terminal alkyne **31** in good yield. The CuAAC reaction of alkynes **31** and **34** was carried out with numerous deoxy-azido-sugars **32a-h** readily prepared from commercially available monosaccharides, which furnished the hydroxyanthracene triazolyl glycoconjugates **33a-c** and **35a-c** in excellent yields, as shown in Scheme (7-9) and Table **1-2** [44].

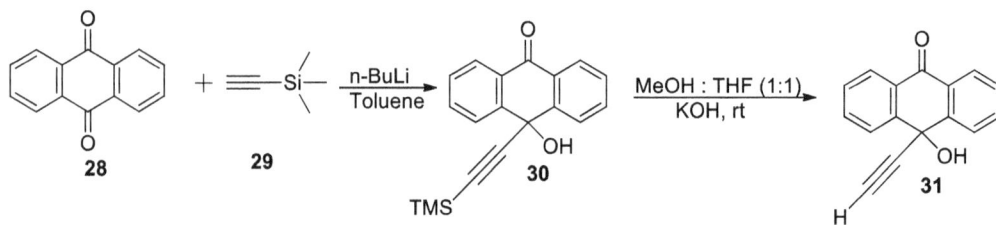

Scheme (7). Synthesis of anthraquinone-based terminal alkyne **31**.

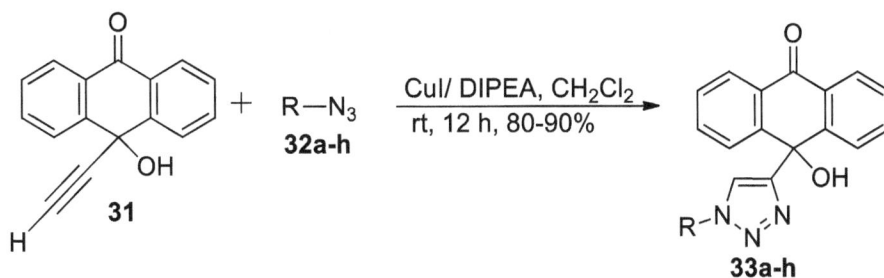

Scheme (8). Synthesis of triazolyl glycoconjugates **33a-h** *via* CuAAC reaction.

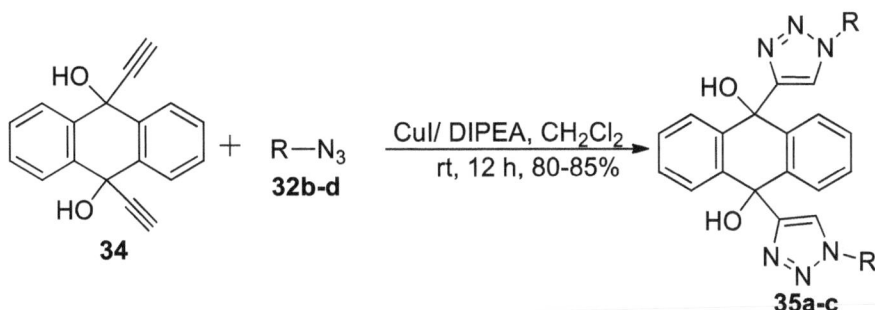

Scheme (9). Synthesis of bis-triazolyl glycoconjugates **35a-c** *via* CuAAC reaction.

Jun Shimura *et al.* synthesized quinone-based glycohybride Saptomycin H **44**. In the first step, anthrapyranone acetal **39** was prepared *via* an aldol reaction between L-vancosamine derivative **36**, compound **37**, and nonracemicynal **38**. Methyl ether **39** was further treated with $MgI_2 \cdot OEt_2$ in acetonitrile to give phenol **40** without touching two acetals. Azide **40** was converted to dimethylamine **41** by employing the Staudinger reaction (PMe_3, H_2O, THF, rt, 24 h), followed by reductive N-dimethylation (HCHO aq, AcOH, $NaBH_3CN$, CH_3CN, rt, 2 h). Thus, phenol **41** was converted to acetate **42**, which was subjected to hydrogenolysis, and the resulting alcohol was acetylated. Selective monodeacetylation of diacetate **42** was achieved by i-$PrNH_2$ (EtOAc, rt, 9 h), removing the acetyl group for the phenol to give the key intermediate **43**. Anthraquinone acetal **43** was subjected to acidic conditions (p-TsOH·H_2O, THF, H2O, 70 °C, 7 h) to prepare for the epoxide synthesis. This hydrolyzed both the dimethyl and isopropylidene acetals. The resulting diol was selectively mesylated at its less hindered sec-hydroxy group ($MeSO_2Cl$, pyridine, CH_2Cl_2, 0 °C, 2 h) to give mesylate product, which was again treated with DBU in dichloromethane allowed clean formation of the oxirane ring without touching the acetyl group, giving (14R,16S)-2 Saptomycin H **44** in excellent yield, as shown in Scheme (**10**) [45].

Table 1. Triazolyl Glycoconjugates 33a-h

S. No.	Azido- sugars	Click Product
33a		
33b		
33c		
33d		
33e		
33f		
33g		
33h		

Table 2. Synthesis of bis-Triazolyl Glycoconjugates 35a-c.

S. No.	Azido- sugars	Click Product
35a		
35b		
35c		

Phenolic O-glycosylated quinone-based glycohybrids **47a-f** were synthesized in good to excellent yields by Haijuan Liu and colleagues using the iron hydride hydrogen atom transfer (HAT) approach. The reaction involved 1,4-quinones **45a-b** interacting with exo-glycals **46a-b**, with $PhSiH_3$ and Na_2HPO_4 acting as buffers in degassed ethanol under argon, as illustrated in Scheme (**11**) [46].

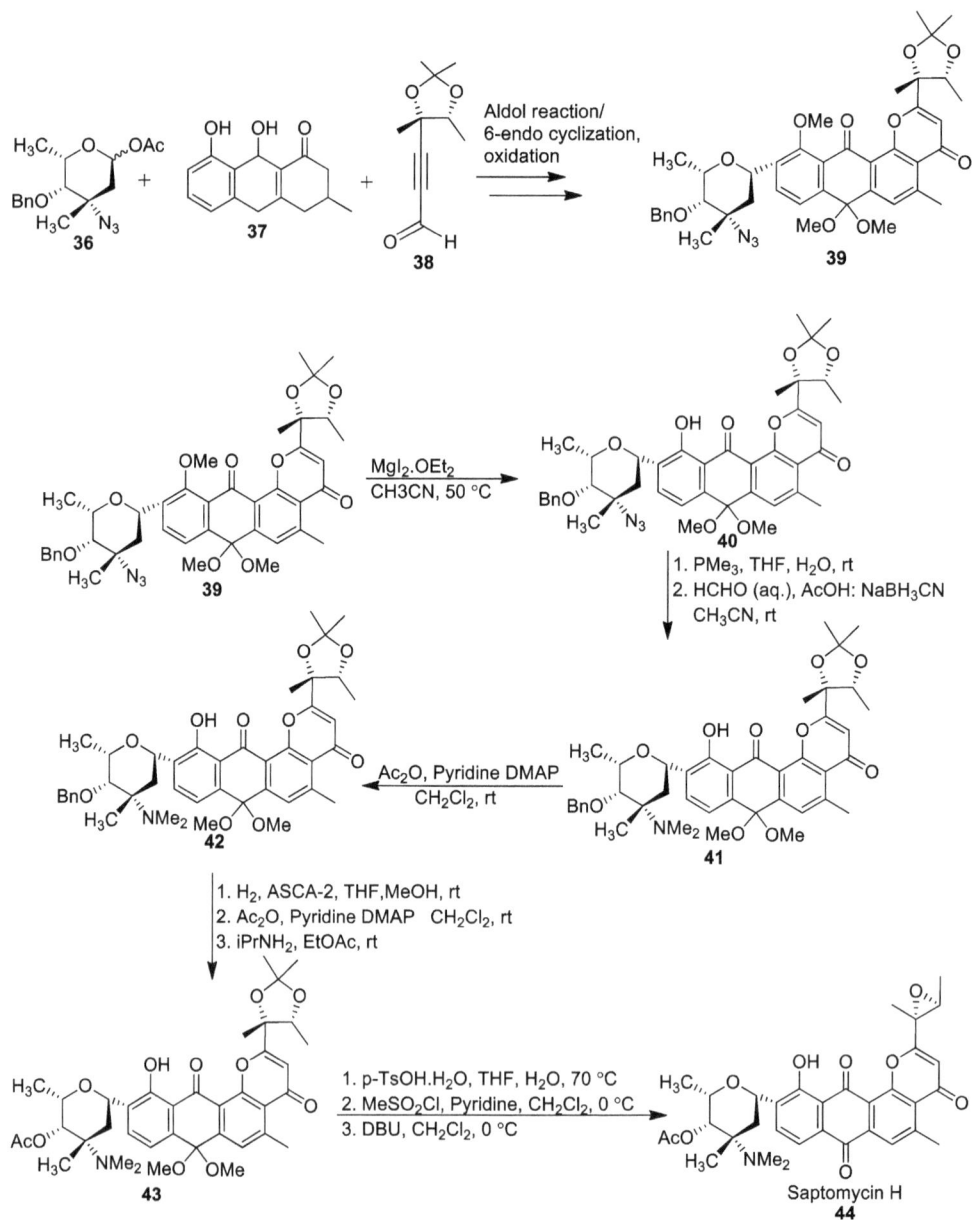

Scheme (10). Synthesized quinone-based glycohybride Saptomycin H **44**.

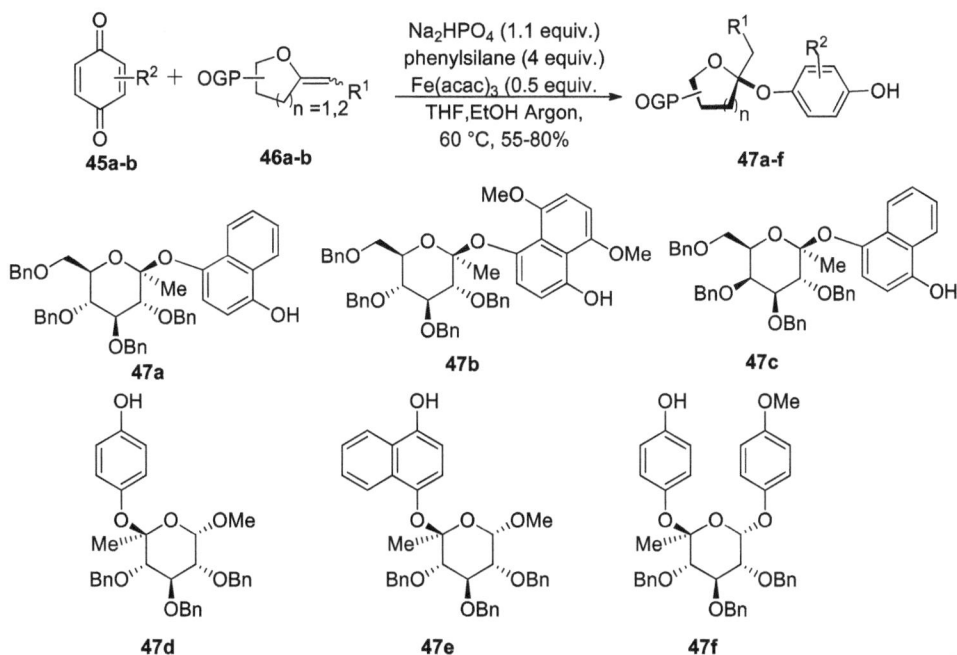

Scheme (11). O-glycosylated quinone-based glycohybrids **47a-f**.

Mingming Yu e. al. determined that the heterologous expression of the sar BGC (biosynthetic gene cluster) led to the production of sarubicin, which is also known as quinone-based glycohybrid. In the first step, the formation of the deoxysugar intermediate dTDP-4-keto-D-olivose **52**, involving four genes (sarS1, sarS2, sarS4, and sarS5), takes place, starting from the sugar moiety **48**. In the next step, the glycosyltransferase SarS3 attached the NDP-sugar **52** to the aromatic intermediate **53** [47] at the C-6 position. The second C–C bond was then established by an intramolecular aldol condensation between the C–5 and the 4-keto carbon of deoxysugar **54**. The cyclized product **54** could be rapidly oxidized in air or by the dehydrogenase SarO to form sarubicin **A 55**, as shown in Scheme **(12)**. In the cytotoxicity assay, we found that quinone-based glycohybrid sarubicin **A 55** exhibited cytotoxicity against cancer cell lines HL-60, SMMC-7721, A-549, MCF-7, and SW480 [48].

Evgeny Pislyagin *et al.* synthesized 1,4-naphthoquinone thioglucosides **58** and **62** and their tetracyclic conjugates **59** and **63**. The acyclic thioglucosides **58** and **62** were synthesized by the condensation of the corresponding 2-chloro-3-meth-xy-1,4-naphthoquinones **56** and **60** with the thioglucose derivatives **57** and **61**. The tetracyclic quinone conjugates **59** and **63**were readily formed by base-catalyzed treatment of the acyclic thioglucosides **58** and **62** [49, 50] in a MeONa/MeOH solution in good yields.

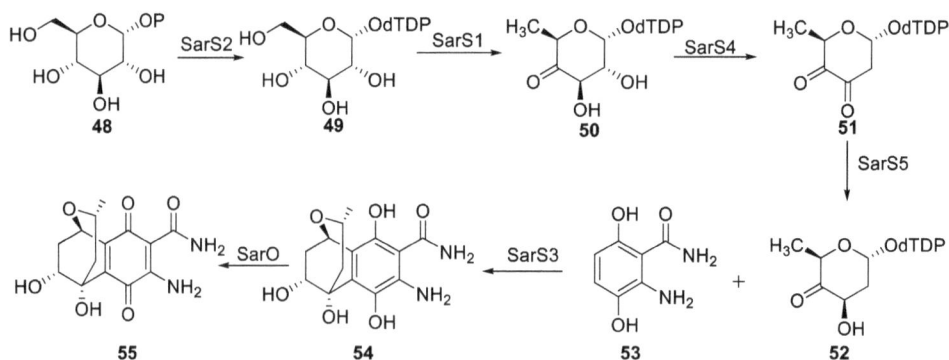

Scheme (12). Synthesis of sarubicin **A**.

The antagonistic effects of these synthesized compounds were investigated against mouse P2X7R. According to biological studies, these substances significantly inhibited murine P2X7R *in vitro*. This restriction led to significant reductions in the formation of ROS and NO, blocking the uptake of ethidium bromide (EtBr) and YO-PRO-1 fluorescent dye and protecting the viability of neuronal cells from the harmful effects of high ATP concentrations. These synthesized 1,4-naphthoquinone thioglucosides showed promising molecular docking results in an *in silico* investigation, suggesting that they may bind in an allosteric location in the extracellular region of P2X7R. These results point to compounds **58, 59, 62,** and **63** as possible building blocks for the development of novel P2X7R inhibitors and drugs that effectively treat neurodegenerative illnesses and neuropathic pain, as shown in Scheme (**13**) [51].

Dorota Narog discussed the formation of glycoconjugates of benzofuranone **68**. It is also clear from the study that quercetin and its derivatives are potent antioxidant flavonoids. An electrochemical reaction forms the glycoconjugate of the oxidized product of quercetin and ip-galpyr. P-quinone is produced when quercetin is electrochemically oxidized **64**. The following stage involves attaching water to the molecule, which tautomerizes to produce **66**. The primary result of the electrochemical glycosylation of quercetin is 2-(3,4- dihydroxybenzoyl)- 2,4,6-trihydroxy-3-(2H)-benzofuranone **68**, which is formed when 1,2,3,4-di-O-diisopropylidene-α-D-galactopyranose is integrated into intermediate product **66,** as shown in Scheme (**14**) [52].

Atul Dubeya *et al.* synthesized diarylmethyl thioglycosides **72a-n** starting from per-O-acetylated sugars **69** with para-Quinone methides **71** *via* S-glycosyl isothiouronium salts **70**. The one-pot reaction conditions involved the rapid conversion of the per-O-acetylated sugar with thiourea in the presence of boron trifluoride etherate as a catalyst. It furnished the corresponding glycosyl isothiouronium salt **70**, which was subsequently treated with a para-quinone methide **71** in the presence of a base that delivered the diarylmethyl thioglycoside **72a-n** in good to moderate yields. The reaction conditions are readily scalable for large-scale preparation, operationally straightforward, gentle, repeatable, and high-yielding. This technique will provide access to novel diarylmethyl thioglycosides, a hitherto undiscovered structural class of glycomimetic chemicals, as shown in Scheme (**15**) [53].

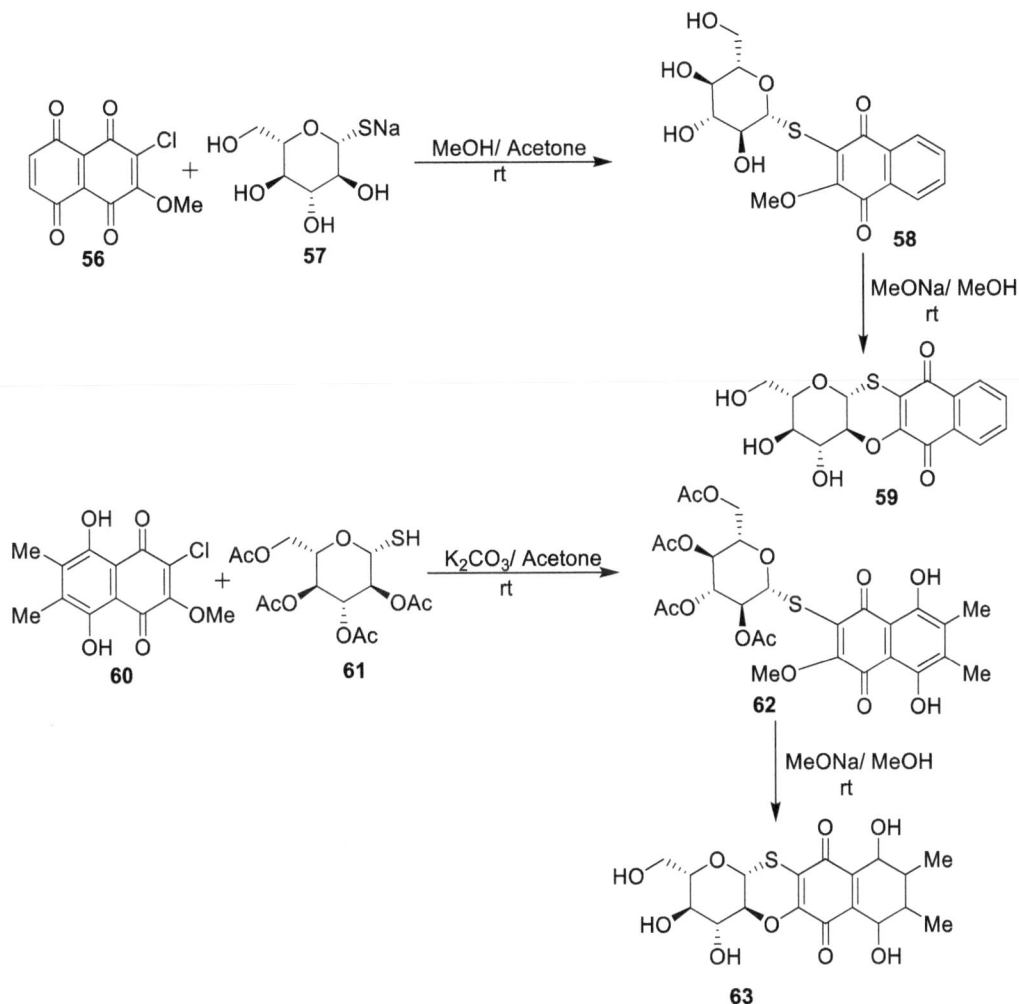

Scheme (13). Synthesis of 1,4-naphthoquinone thioglucosides **58** and **62** and their tetracyclic conjugates **59** and **63**.

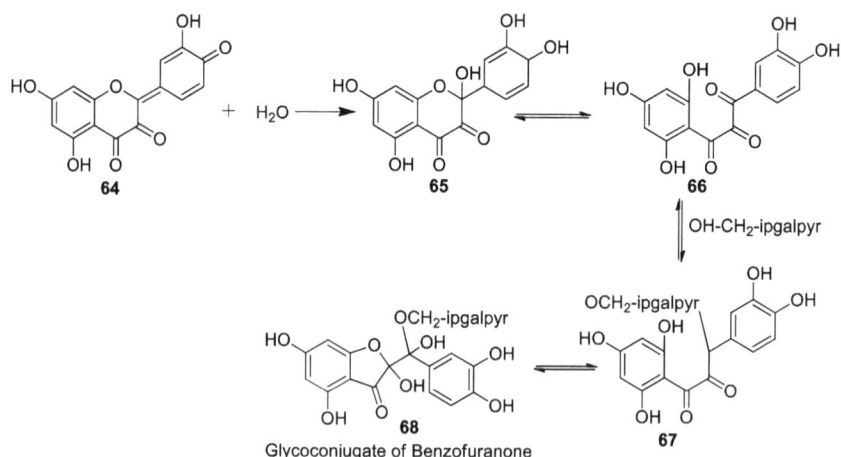

Scheme (14). Series of reactions to form benzofuranone-based glycoconjugate **68**.

Sergey A. Dyshlovoy *et al.* discussed the synthesis of quinone-based glycohybrids. It is shown in the first reaction that tetra-O-acety-
-6-mercaptoglucose **74** in acetone solvent with potassium carbonate could easily condense with halogenoquinones **73a-j**. This produced acetylated conjugates **75 a-j** with moderate to good yields. The acidic β-hydroxyl group in the quinone core prevented tetra-O-acetyl-6-mercaptoglucose from reacting with chloroquinones; hence, these reactions were conducted in a DMSO solution, as shown in Scheme **(16)**. In the second reaction, naphthazarin and juglone derivatives were used to synthesize the acetylated conjugates **76d-f**. Thiols and juglone compounds reacted in ethanol solvent to give 3-substituted compounds [54]. Nevertheless, they found that the primary result of the reaction between 5-acetyljuglone and thiols resulted in the 2-substituted isomer. The 2-monosubstituted product **76d** was primarily synthesized by boiling naphthazarin with excess mercaptoglucose **74**. The next step involved the synthesis of deacetylated conjugates **77a-m** when the appropriate acetylated conjugates were treated with MeONa/MeOH in good to outstanding yields, as shown in Schemes **(17 and 18)** [55]. They assessed the cytotoxic potential for these synthetic compounds in human PC-3 cells, which are resistant to drugs, and in human PNT2 cells, which are not cancerous cells of the prostate. The compounds **75g** and **77g** were assessed in five human prostate cancer cell lines with distinct resistance profiles: PC-3 and DU145 (AR-FL− and AR-V7−, androgen-independent, docetaxel-resistant); 22Rv1 and VCaP (AR-FL+ and AR-V7+, androgen-independent, docetaxel-sensitive); and LNCaP (AR-FL+ and AR-V7−, androgen-dependent, docetaxel-sensitive) [56]. Compound **77g** demonstrated enhanced selectivity toward cancer cells due to its exposed glucose moiety [56].

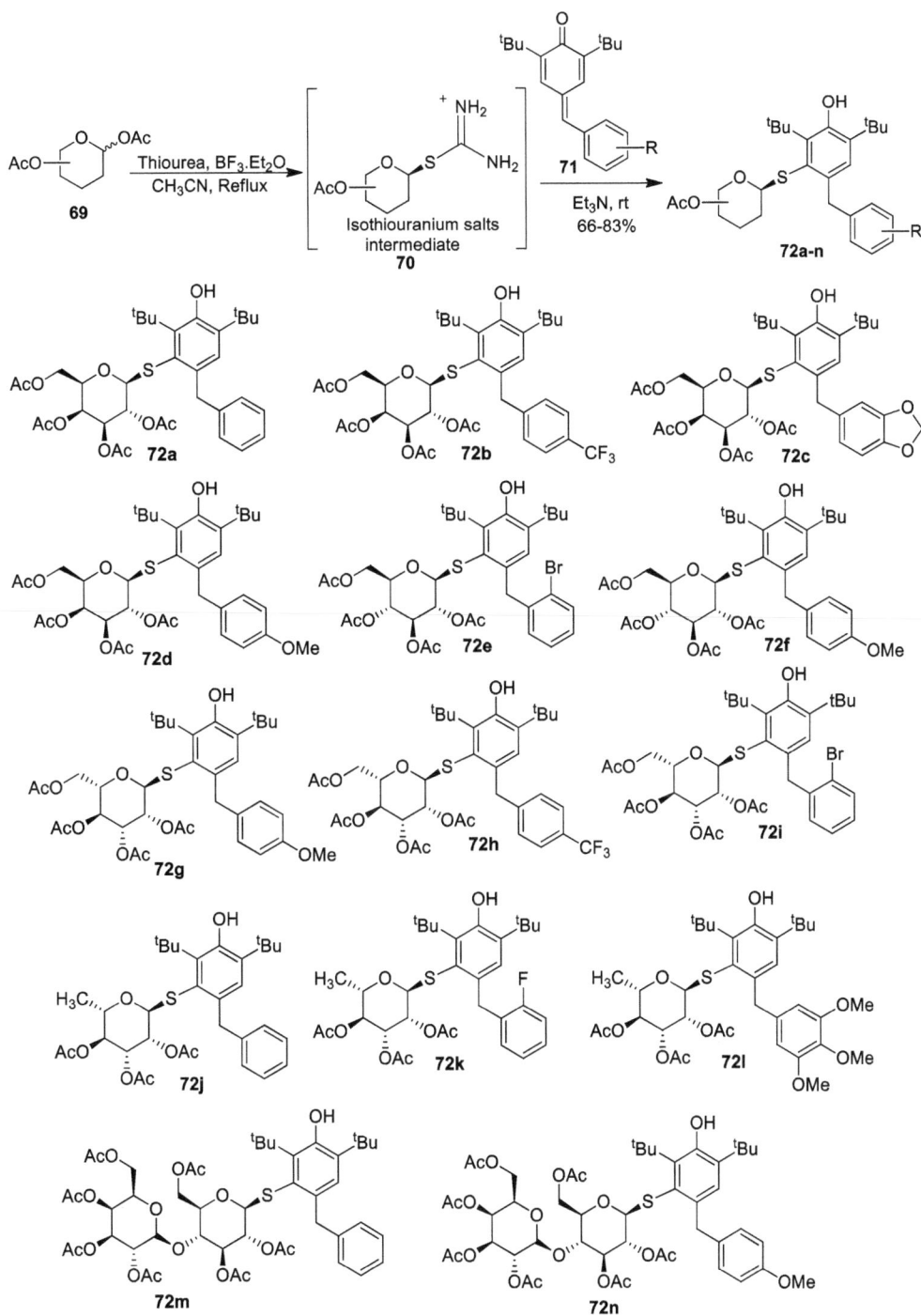

Scheme (15). Synthesis of quinone-derived diarylmethyl thioglycosides **72a-n**.

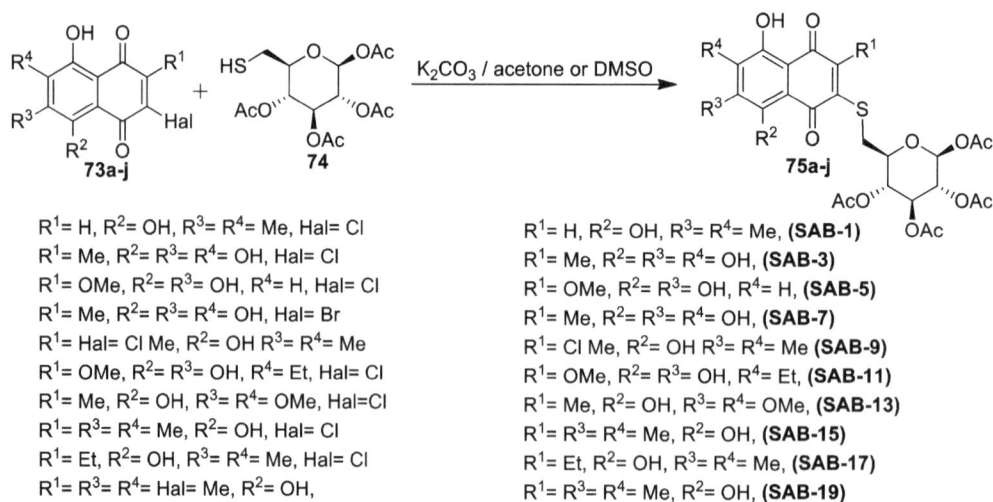

R¹= H, R²= OH, R³= R⁴= Me, Hal= Cl
R¹= Me, R²= R³= R⁴= OH, Hal= Cl
R¹= OMe, R²= R³= OH, R⁴= H, Hal= Cl
R¹= Me, R²= R³= R⁴= OH, Hal= Br
R¹= Hal= Cl Me, R²= OH R³= R⁴= Me
R¹= OMe, R²= R³= OH, R⁴= Et, Hal= Cl
R¹= Me, R²= OH, R³= R⁴= OMe, Hal=Cl
R¹= R³= R⁴= Me, R²= OH, Hal= Cl
R¹= Et, R²= OH, R³= R⁴= Me, Hal= Cl
R¹= R³= R⁴= Hal= Me, R²= OH,

R¹= H, R²= OH, R³= R⁴= Me, **(SAB-1)**
R¹= Me, R²= R³= R⁴= OH, **(SAB-3)**
R¹= OMe, R²= R³= OH, R⁴= H, **(SAB-5)**
R¹= Me, R²= R³= R⁴= OH, **(SAB-7)**
R¹= Cl Me, R²= OH R³= R⁴= Me **(SAB-9)**
R¹= OMe, R²= R³= OH, R⁴= Et, **(SAB-11)**
R¹= Me, R²= OH, R³= R⁴= OMe, **(SAB-13)**
R¹= R³= R⁴= Me, R²= OH, **(SAB-15)**
R¹= Et, R²= OH, R³= R⁴= Me, **(SAB-17)**
R¹= R³= R⁴= Me, R²= OH, **(SAB-19)**

Scheme (16). Synthesis of acetylated compounds **75a-j**.

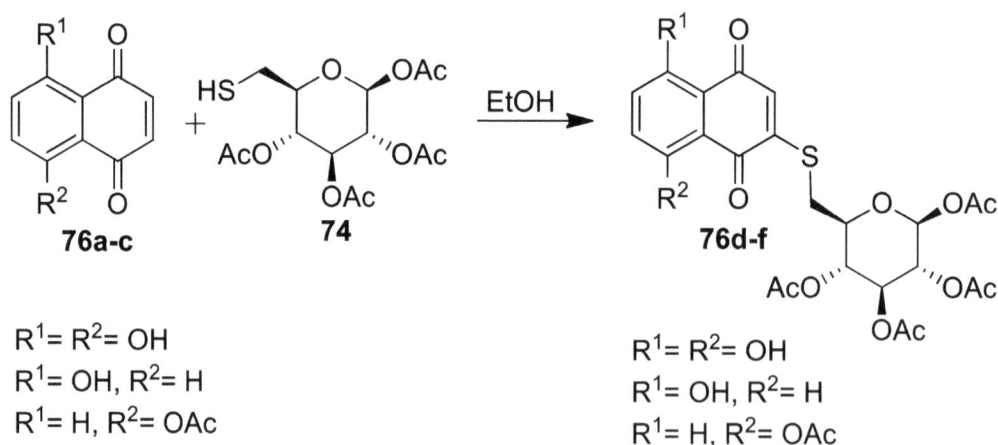

R¹= R²= OH
R¹= OH, R²= H
R¹= H, R²= OAc

R¹= R²= OH
R¹= OH, R²= H
R¹= H, R²= OAc

Scheme (17). Synthesis of acetylated compounds **77a-c**.

K. C. Nicolaou *et al.* synthesized quinone-based glycohybrid Lomaiviticin A **84** from tetracyclic aglycon **78**. When aglycon compound **78** and iodo glycosyl donor compound **79** were coupled with the gold (I) promoter Ph₃PAuNTf₂ [57, 58], the two anomeric products with the intended β-anomer as the predominant isomer produced regioselectivity. Using a radical assisted procedure, this mixture was deiodinated at low temperature (Et₃B, O₂, n-Bu₃SnH, -60 °C) to produce two separable C1 diastereomeric (inconsequential) β-anomers: [(1S)-isomer] and [(1R)-isomer]. Ph3PAuOTf₂ mediated the smooth glycosylation of tertiary alcohols, yielding the intended α-glycosides **80a** and **80b** in good to excellent yield [59]. Then, isomers **80a** and **80b** were exposed to different reaction conditions, and the formation of quinone-based glycohybrid Lomaiviticin A **84** took place in good yield, as shown in Scheme (**19**) [60].

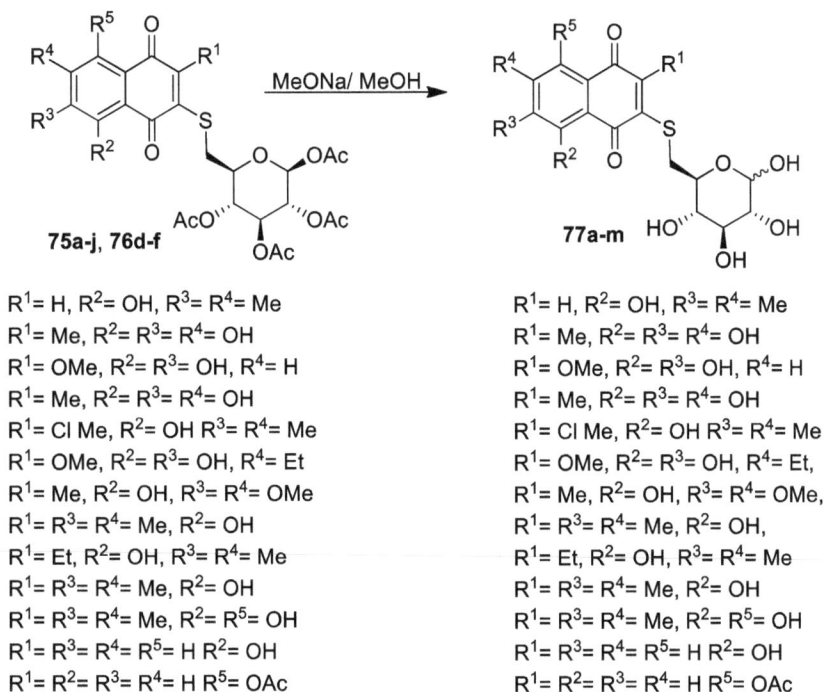

R^1= H, R^2= OH, R^3= R^4= Me
R^1= Me, R^2= R^3= R^4= OH
R^1= OMe, R^2= R^3= OH, R^4= H
R^1= Me, R^2= R^3= R^4= OH
R^1= Cl Me, R^2= OH R^3= R^4= Me
R^1= OMe, R^2= R^3= OH, R^4= Et
R^1= Me, R^2= OH, R^3= R^4= OMe
R^1= R^3= R^4= Me, R^2= OH
R^1= Et, R^2= OH, R^3= R^4= Me
R^1= R^3= R^4= Me, R^2= OH
R^1= R^3= R^4= Me, R^2= R^5= OH
R^1= R^3= R^4= R^5= H R^2= OH
R^1= R^2= R^3= R^4= H R^5= OAc

R^1= H, R^2= OH, R^3= R^4= Me
R^1= Me, R^2= R^3= R^4= OH
R^1= OMe, R^2= R^3= OH, R^4= H
R^1= Me, R^2= R^3= R^4= OH
R^1= Cl Me, R^2= OH R^3= R^4= Me
R^1= OMe, R^2= R^3= OH, R^4= Et,
R^1= Me, R^2= OH, R^3= R^4= OMe,
R^1= R^3= R^4= Me, R^2= OH,
R^1= Et, R^2= OH, R^3= R^4= Me
R^1= R^3= R^4= Me, R^2= OH
R^1= R^3= R^4= Me, R^2= R^5= OH
R^1= R^3= R^4= R^5= H R^2= OH
R^1= R^2= R^3= R^4= H R^5= OAc

Scheme (18). Synthesis of deacetylated compounds **77a-m**.

Sergey Polonik *et al.* synthesized naphthoquinone-based thioglucosides **89a-e** and 2-methoxythiomethylglucosides **92a-e** and **93a-e**. In the first step, synthesis of acetylated thiomethylglucosides **89a-e** took place *via* the reaction of substituted naphthazarins **85a-e** with tetra-O-acetyl-1-mercapto-d-glucose **87a-e** as a thiol component in the presence of paraformaldehyde and formic acid under acetone solvent in good yields. The acetylthioglucosides **89a-e** were readily deacetylated under treatment in MeOH/HCl solution and resulted in quinone-based polar hydrophilic thioglucosides **90a-e** in good yields. The methylation of 2-hydroxy derivatives **89a-e** with diazomethane solution gave the corresponding 2-methoxyderivatives **92a-e** in yields of 85–95%. The subsequent deacetylation 2-methoxyacetylderivatives **91a-e** in MeOH/HCl solution led to a new set of quinone-based polar 2-methoxythiomethylglucosides **93a-e,** as shown in Schemes **20 - 21** [61].

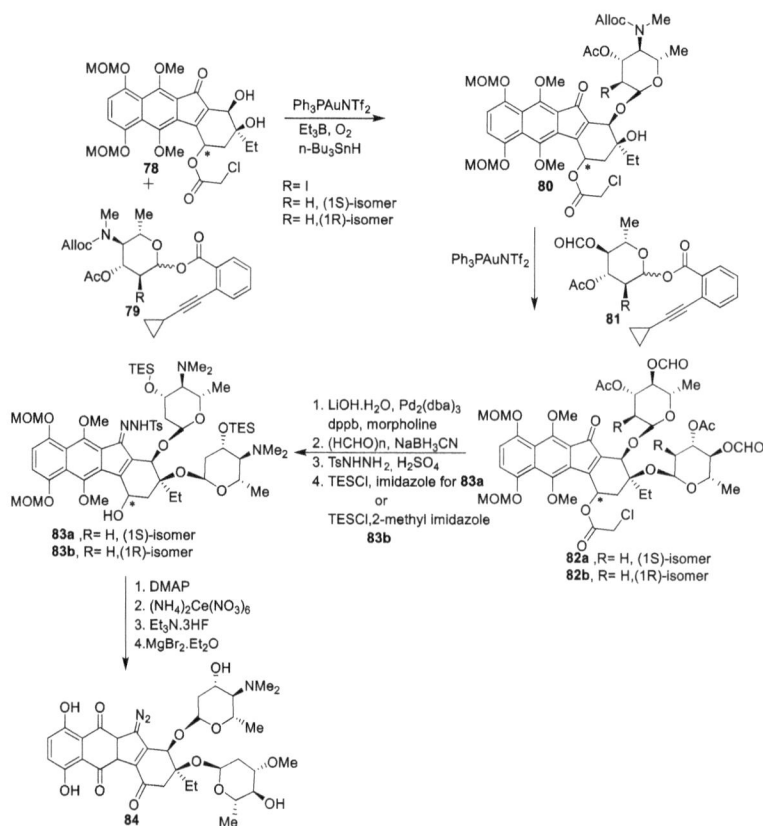

Scheme (19). Synthesis of quinone-based glycohybrid Lomaiviticin A **84**.

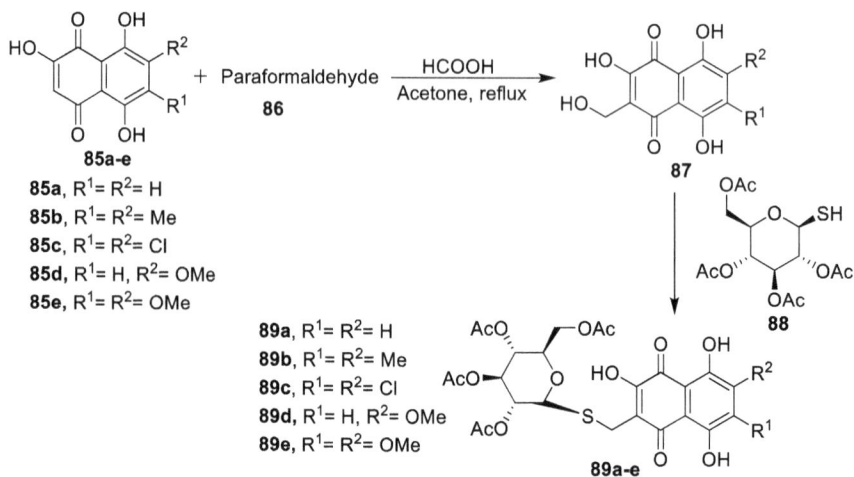

85a-e
85a, R^1= R^2= H
85b, R^1= R^2= Me
85c, R^1= R^2= Cl
85d, R^1= H, R^2= OMe
85e, R^1= R^2= OMe

89a, R^1= R^2= H
89b, R^1= R^2= Me
89c, R^1= R^2= Cl
89d, R^1= H, R^2= OMe
89e, R^1= R^2= OMe

89a-e

Scheme (20). Synthesis of naphthoquinones-based thioglucosides **89a-e**.

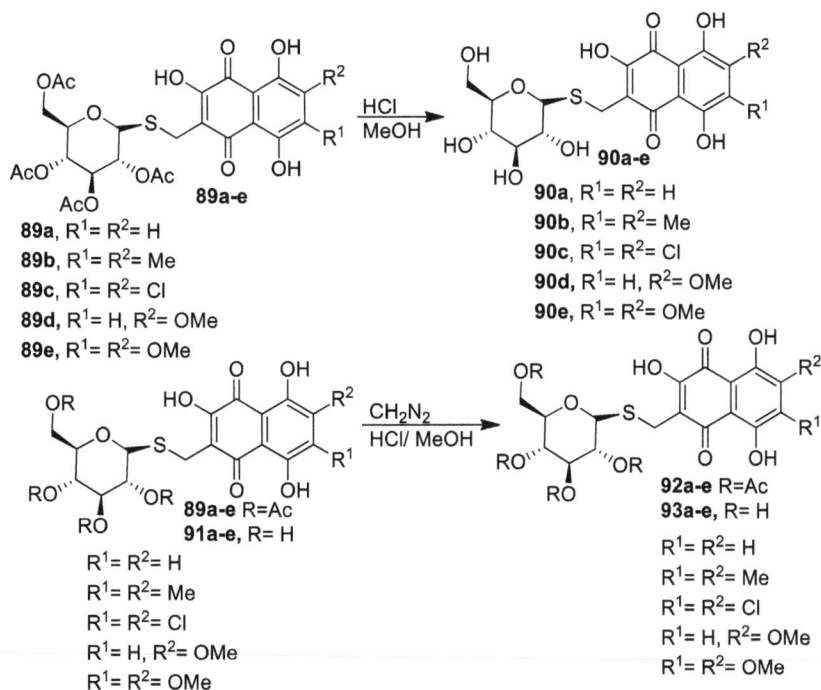

Scheme (21). Synthesis of naphthoquinone-based thioglucosides **92a-e and 93a-e**.

Yuri E. Sabutski *et al.* synthesized tetracyclic quinone–carbohydrate conjugates **97a–d** from substituted chloromethoxynaphthoquinone **94**. In the first step, naphthoquinone acetylglucosides **96a–d** [62] were prepared *via* the condensation reaction of available substituted chloromethoxynaphthoquinone **94** in acetone with per-O-acetyl-1-thioderivatives of D-glucose **88**, D-galactose **95b**, D-xylose **95c**, and L-arabinose **95d**. These naphthoquinone acetylglycoside derivatives, **96a–d**, were readily deacetylated with MeONa/MeOH and immediately converted to the quinone–sugar tetracyclic conjugates **97a–d** in good yields, as shown in Scheme (**22**) [63]. The linear, planar structure and initial sugar stereochemistry were preserved in the tetracyclic quinone–carbohydrate conjugates **97a–d**. These synthesized tetracyclic quinone conjugates **97a-d** were active in vitro against human promyelocytic leukemia HL-60 in 1.0–5.0 μM concentrations, while starting acyclic acetylglycosides were approximately 10–100 times less active.

Rekha Sangwan *et al.* synthesized quinone-based α, α'-diarylmethyl N-glycosides **100a-n**, **102a-f,** and **105a-f** *via* Sc(OTf)$_3$-catalyzed 1,6-conjugate addition of protected and unprotected amino sugars **99a-h** with para-quinone methides (p-QMs) derivatives **98a-i** in acetonitrile solvent at room temperature in good to excellent yields, as shown in Schemes (**23 - 25**). The reactions run easily in the absence of a base and under mild reaction conditions with a wide range of substrates [64].

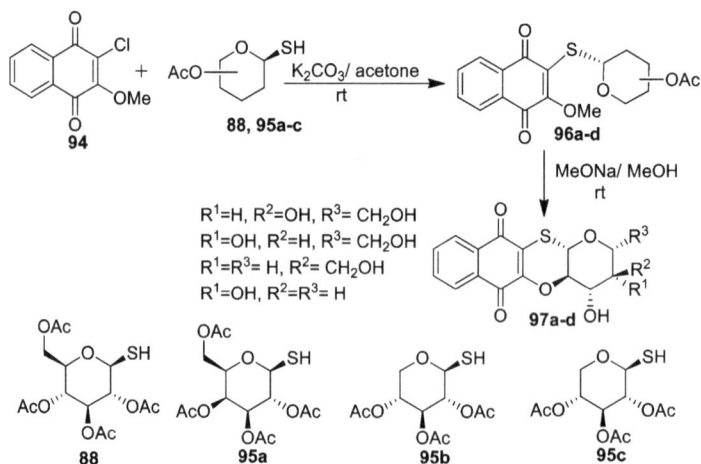

Scheme (22). Synthesis of tetracyclic quinone–carbohydrate conjugates **97a–d**.

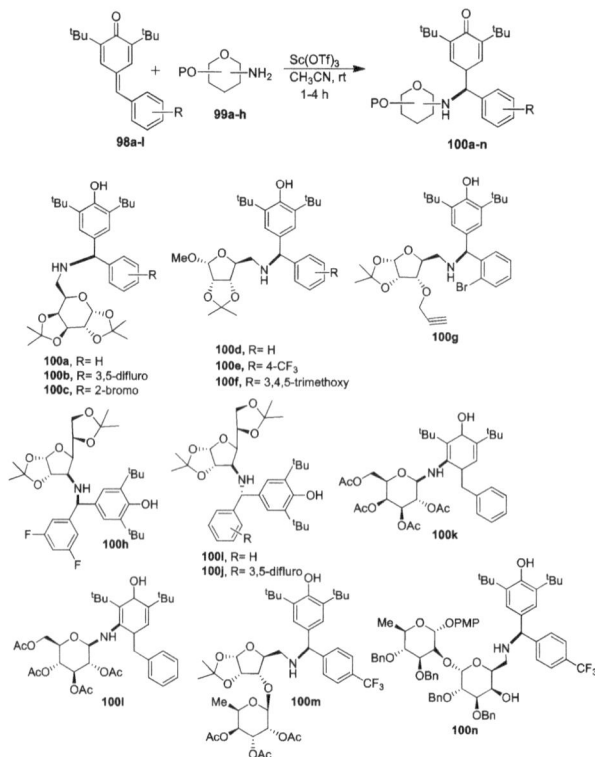

Scheme (23). Synthesis of quinone-based α,α'-diarylmethyl N-glycosides **100a-n**.

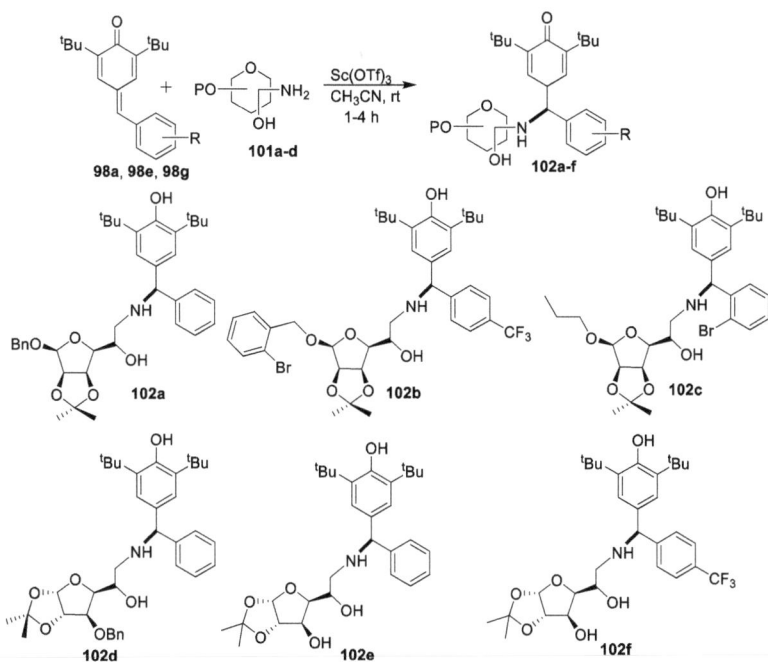

Scheme (24). Synthesis of quinone-based α,α'-diarylmethyl N-glycosides **102a-f**.

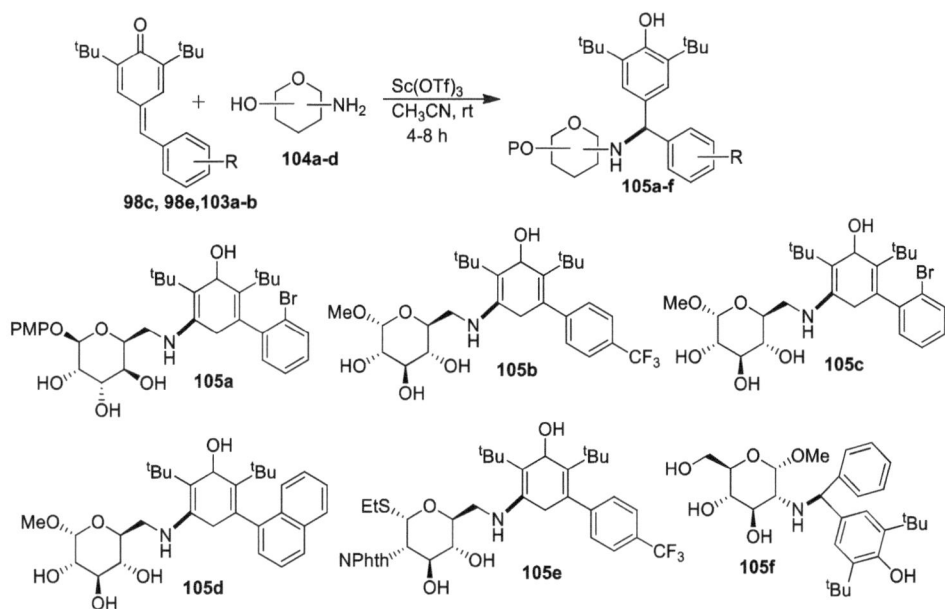

Scheme (25). Synthesis of quinone-based α,α'-diarylmethyl N-glycosides **105a-f**.

Flaviano M. Ottoni *et al* synthesized quinone-based glycohybrids **110a-d** and then assessed the hybrids' cytotoxicity against breast cancer cell lines. Initially, 2--propargyl lawsone **108** was synthesized by reacting lawsone **106** with propargyl bromide **107** in an alkaline medium using potassium carbonate in DMF under reflux conditions. When the propargylated derivative **108** was reacted with the glycosyl azides **109a-d** under [2+3] alkyne-azide cycloaddition reaction conditions using $CuSO_4.5H_2O$, NaAsc in THF/water as solvent at room temperature, the glycosyl triazole derivatives of lawsone were obtained in excellent yields Scheme (**26**). With IC_{50} values less than 10 μM, all compounds exhibited strong anti-SKBR-3 cell line activity. Synthesized from peracetylated D-glucose **110a**, the most promising glycosyl triazole derivative showed improved cytotoxicity against SKBR-3 (IC_{50} = 0.78 μM) and was the most selective (SI > 20) [65].

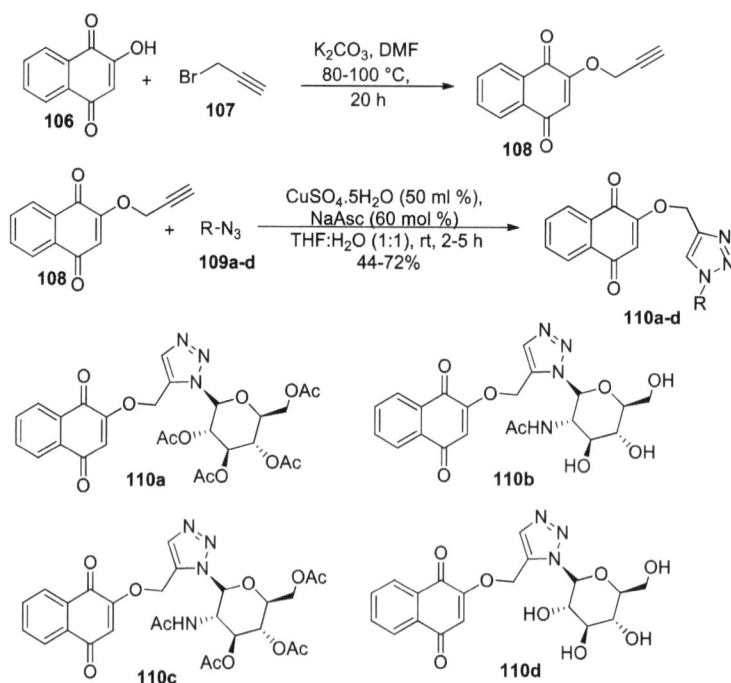

Scheme (26). Synthesis of glycohybrids of lawsone **110a-d**.

Nana Asebi *et al.* synthesized Apios isoflavone glucoside **114** from glycosylated isoflavone **111** [66, 67]. 5-OH was less reactive because of the hydrogen link between it and the carbonyl oxygen at C-4 in **111**. Thus, PvCl was used in the presence of pyridine as a weak base to produce the selective acylation at 2-OH and 4-OH [68]. As a result, the hexa-acylated isoflavone **112** was obtained in good yield. 1,8-diazabicyclo[5.4.0]undec-7-ene (DBU) was used as an organic base to methylate **112** and produce the methyl ether **113** in a moderate amount of yield. By using NaOMe for transesterification, the natural product isoflavone glucoside **114** was obtained in good yield, as shown in Scheme (**27**).

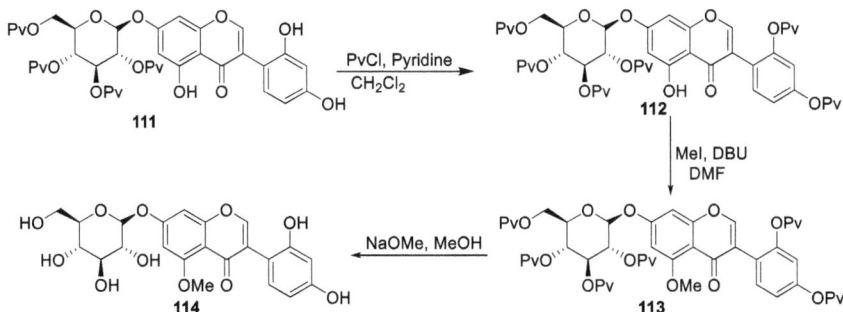

Scheme (27). Synthesis of Apios isoflavone glucoside **114**.

The tyrosinase inhibitory activity of isoflavone glucoside **114** was evaluated using DOPA as a substrate. The IC_{50} of methylated glycoside **114** could not be estimated because its 1 mM solution showed only 24% tyrosinase inhibition. These results suggested that tyrosinase inhibitory effect may be dependent on a hydrogen link between 5-OH and C-4 in the apios isoflavone glucoside **114** [69].

Laura Burchill *et al.* discussed the biosynthesis of Busseihydroquinones D−E **119a**, **122** and Parvinaphthol C **119b** from Busseihydroquinone C **115** meroterpenoid natural products and synthesis of the Busseihydroquinone E Ring System *via* a [4 + 2] cycloaddition reaction.

Busseihydroquinone C **115** undergoes allylic oxidation to furnish the reactive enal **116**, followed by an intramolecular hetero−Diels−Alder reaction with the chromene dienophile *via* an endo transition state, which gives cyclic enol ether **117**. Cyclic enol ether **117**undergoes protonation on its convex face to produce the oxonium ion **118,** and then Busseihydroquinones **119a** and Parvinaphthol C **119b**are synthesized by the nucleophilic addition of MeOH or EtOH (again on the convex face). Also, epoxide **120**is produced by diastereoselective epoxidation of cyclic enol ether **117**, which may be the biosynthetic precursor of busseihydroquinone D **122** on its convex face. Ring opening of the epoxide **120**can then give α-hydroxyaldehyde **121**, followed by stereospecific dehydration to give Busseihydroquinones-D **122,** as shown in Scheme (**28-29**).

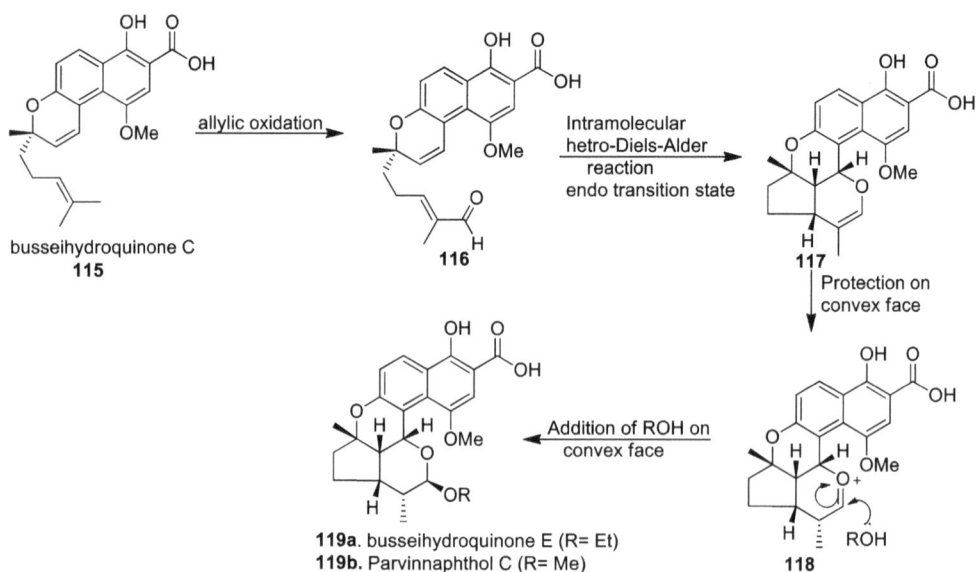

Scheme (28). Synthesis of Busseihydroquinone E **119a** and Parvinaphthol C **119b**.

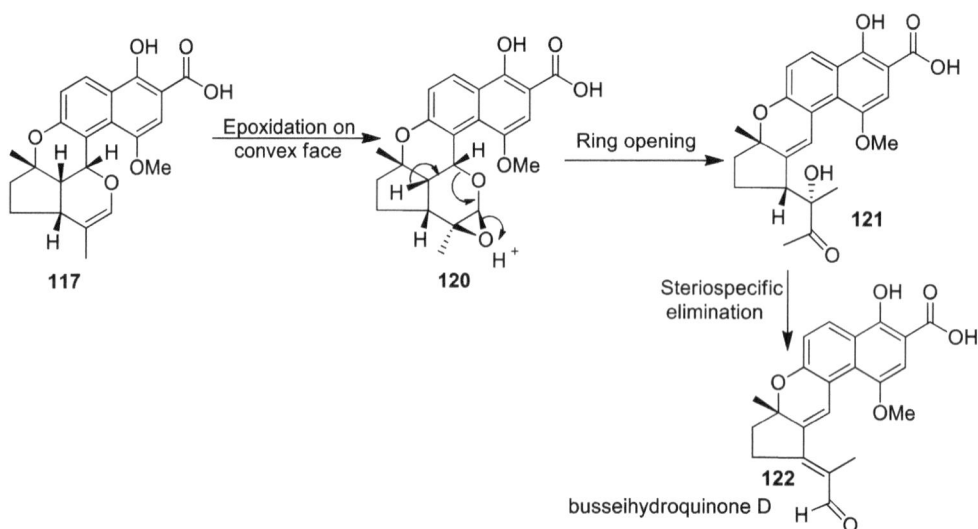

Scheme (29). Synthesis of Busseihydroquinone D **122**.

The synthesis of enal **125** was achieved from Chromene **123**. The oxidation reaction **123** using catalytic SeO_2 and t-BuOOH gave allylic alcohol **124**, which was converted into enal **125** *via* a Swern oxidation. The intended endo Diesels–Alder product **127** was then obtained in 39% yield by heating **125** to 140 °C in xylenes, along with 4% of the exo product **128**. An intramolecular Michael reaction may have produced the o-quinone methide [70 - 72] enolate **126** as a mixture of diastereomers, and then an intramolecular oxo-Michael reaction may have created **127** and **128** in a higher yield when **125** was exposed to a basic condition, as shown in Scheme (**30**) [73].

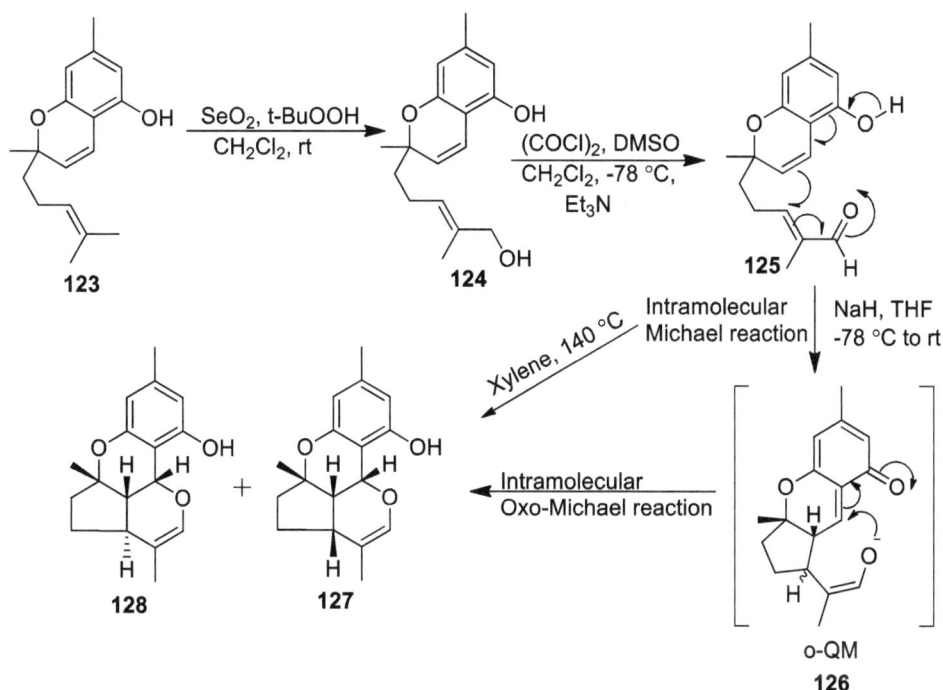

Scheme (30). Synthesis of the Busseihydroquinone **127** and **128**.

Sergey G. Polonik *et al.* synthesized 1,4-naphthoquinone dithioglucoside derivatives **131a-d** *via* the reaction of dichloro naphthoquinones **129a-c** with 1-thioglucose tetra-O-acetyl derivative **88** in basic reaction conditions. Dichloroquinones **129a-c** were readily condensed with thioglucose derivative **88** in CH$_3$CN solution with K$_2$CO$_3$ furnished acetylthioglucoside derivatives **130a-c** in excellent yields. Subsequent saponification of acetyl derivatives **130a-c** under MeONa/MeOH treatment led to the formation of targeted thioglucosides **131a-c** in good yields [74]. Dichloroquinone **129d** with two acidic β-hydroxyl groups in the quinone part did not react with thioglucose **88** under this condition. The presence of two acidic β-hydroxyl groups in the quinone portion of chloroquinone **129d** prevented it from reacting with glucose **88** in these circumstances. It appears that the activity of chlorine atoms to substitution was greatly decreased upon the ionization of quinonoid hydroxyl groups. The desired dithioglucoside **130d** was obtained in good yield when the condensation was carried out in DMSO solution.

Dithioglucoside **130d** was deacetylated in an acidic HCl/MeOH solution to get the desired 1,4-naphthoquinone dithioglucoside derivative **131d,** as shown in Scheme (**31**).

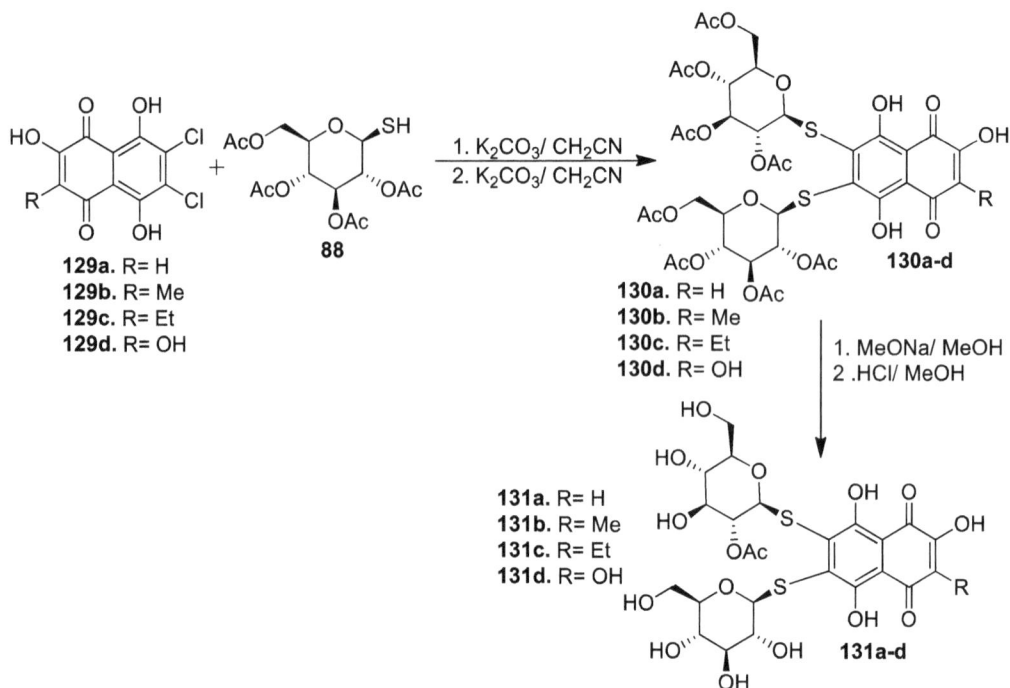

129a. R= H
129b. R= Me
129c. R= Et
129d. R= OH

130a. R= H
130b. R= Me
130c. R= Et
130d. R= OH

1. K$_2$CO$_3$/ CH$_2$CN
2. K$_2$CO$_3$/ CH$_2$CN

1. MeONa/ MeOH
2. HCl/ MeOH

131a. R= H
131b. R= Me
131c. R= Et
131d. R= OH

Scheme (31). Synthesis of 1,4-naphthoquinone dithioglucoside derivatives **131a-d**.

4 hydroxy- and alkyl dithioglucoside derivatives **131a-d** based on natural naphthoquinones were screened for antiradical in 2,2-diphenyl-1-picrylhydrazyl (DPPH) test against echinochrome and ascorbic acid and antiviral activity *in vitro*. Thioglucosides **131a-d** were less active than echinochrome. Thioglucoside **131d** with two β-OH groups showed the highest antiradical properties among the tested compounds [75].

The methylthiazolyl tetrazolium bromide (MTT) assay results were used to compute the 50% cytotoxic concentrations (CC$_{50}$) of all tested compounds. The results showed that the low toxic compounds **131a-d** were formed when 1,4-naphthoquinones were conjugated with thioglucose. These compounds were 1.5 to 2 times less hazardous than the reference compound, echinochrome (P ≤ 0.05). Compound **131c**, which has a lipophilic ethyl substituent, showed the strongest virucidal and strong antiradical activity among the synthesized thioglucosides, comparable to vitamin C.

Rajendra N. Mitra *et al.* synthesized naphthoquinone-based glycohybrids **135a-d** using phthalaldehyde **132** and sugar nitroolfines **133a-d** in the presence of thoazolium bromide carbene **134**, which are activated molecular sieves in dry dichloromethane under inert environment. Sugar-nitrostyrene is slightly mixed with phthalaldehyde 132 to produce useful arylnaphthoquinones **135a-d**, which is the catalyst for the N-heterocycle carbene **134** (NHC)-catalyzed dual Stetter cascade reaction. The authors claim to have used moderate NHC organic catalysis to synthesize optically pure naphthoquinones based on sugar. It was discovered that NHC is an exceptional and potent organocatalyst in this case, which is able to create homoatomic C-C cross-coupling, heteroatomic O-C bonds, and cascade cyclization at room temperature by employing NO_2 as a leaving group, as shown in Scheme (**32**) [76].

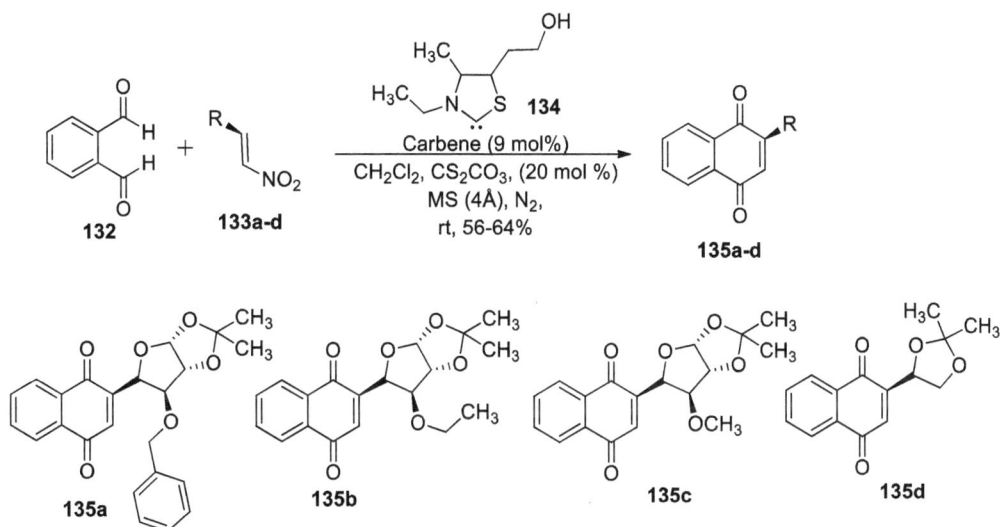

Scheme (32). Naphthoquinone-based glycohybrids **135a-d**.

Ruogu Peng *et al.* synthesized quinone-based glycohybrid, nogalamycin natural product **138**, *via* convergent Hauser annulation. The pivotal Hauser annulation for the anthraquinone core construction was achieved by the fusion of two highly functionalized segments: a cyanophthalide **137** and a tricyclic quinone monoketal **138**. The Hauser annulation between **136** and **137** in the presence of LiOtBu as a base furnished the quinone-based glycohybrid, Nogalamycin **138**, in good yield, as shown in Scheme (**33**) [77].

Sure Siva Prasad *et al.* synthesized a library of iminosugar-isopyrrolonaphthoquinone glycohybrids **140-144**. D-ribose tosylate **139** and 1,4-naphthoquinone **14** reacted in the presence of glycine methyl ester hydrochloride in toluene solvent to produce isopyrrolonaphthoquinone hybrid **140**. The same reaction conditions were used to synthesize glycohybrids **141-144** in moderate to good yields by reacting different iminosugars with the corresponding 1,4-naphthoquinone derivatives, as shown in Scheme (**34**) [78].

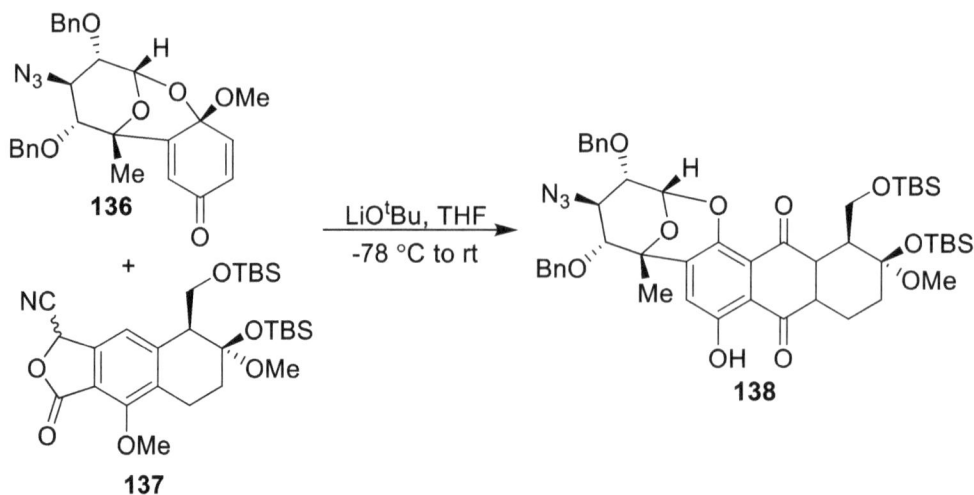

Scheme (33). Synthesis of nogalamycin natural product **138**.

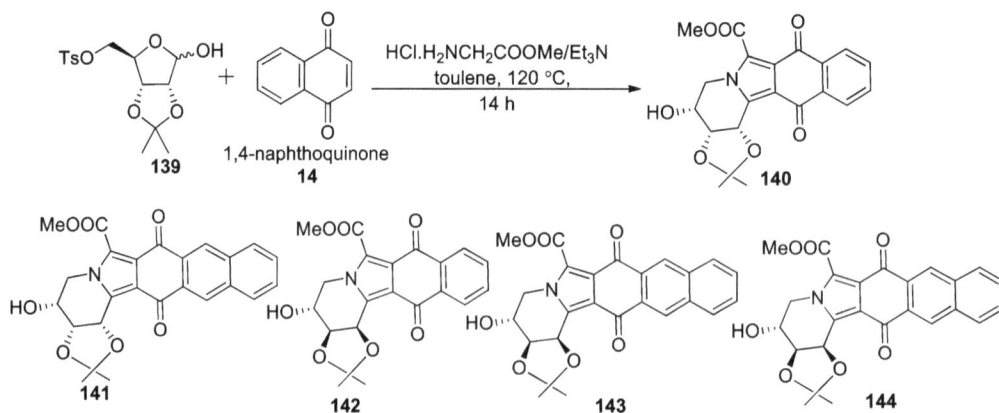

Scheme (34). Iminosugar-isopyrrolonaphthoquinone glycohybrids **140-144**.

Soumen Chakraborty *et al*. synthesized sugar-appended Naphthalenone **152** and C-5 Angucycline glycoside **157** by Hauser Annulation reaction. In the first step, α-lithiated species were generated from ethyl vinyl ether **146**. They were made to react with sugar ketone **145** to furnish intermediate alcohol **147**. It is interesting to note that the required ketone **148** was produced in two steps by the hydrolysis of enol **147** with 1 M HCl. Methylation of α-hydroxy ketone **148** by NaH and MeI provided ketone **149** in good yield. Treatment of alkene **149** with ozone initially furnished molozonide **150**. The ozonide **150**, on treatment with Me$_2$S, resulted in aldehyde **151** in excellent yield. Quinone-based glycohybrid napthalenone **152** was then produced in good yield by intramolecular aldol condensation after keto aldehyde **151** was treated with K^{t}OBu in ^{t}BuOH, as shown in Scheme (**35**).

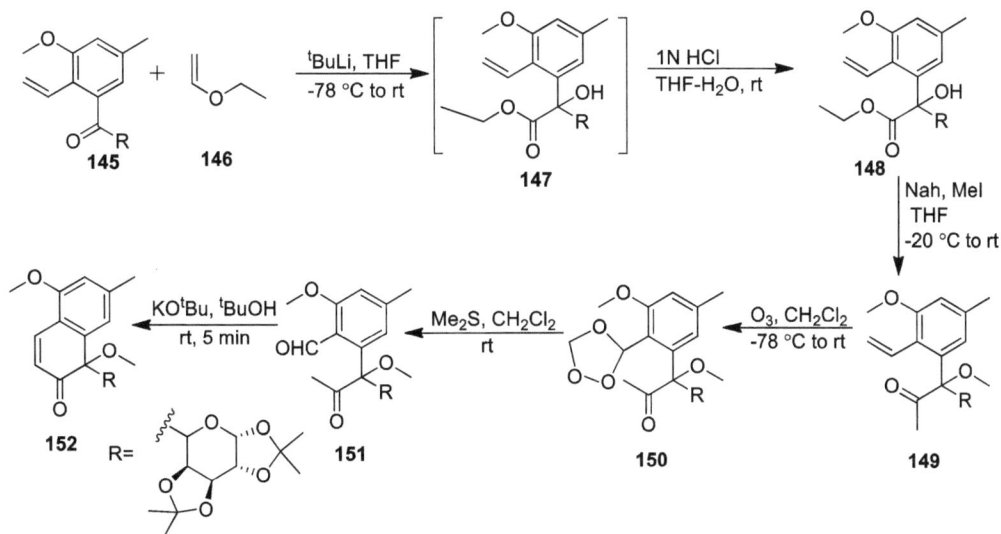

Scheme (35). Synthesis of Sugar-Appended Naphthalenone **152**.

After the synthesis of napthalenone **152,** they subjected it to the Hauser annulation with 7-methoxy-3-cyano-phthalide **153** in the presence of LiO^{t}Bu in THF to furnish annulated product **154**. After standing, airborne oxidation transformed quinol **154** into quinone **155**. Aromatization occurred with the loss of the sugar moiety, giving quinone **156** [79]. The angucycline core of quinone **157**, our intended natural product, was obtained by treating quinol **154** with oxalic acid in a THF and H$_2$O mixture at room temperature, as shown in Scheme (**36**) [80].

Amira A. Ghoneim *et al.* synthesized thioxobenzo[g]pteridine derivatives and 1,4-dihydroquinoxaline derivatives with glycosidic moiety. The ester group of ethyl 3-amino-1,4-dihydroquinoxaline-2-carboxylate **158** [81] reacted with hydrazine hydrate, resulting in the corresponding hydrazide derivative **159**, which was refluxed with CS$_2$ in a solution of 10% KOH to produce the corresponding oxadiazole derivative **160** with good yield. Compound 5-(2-amino--,4-dihydroquinoxalin-3-yl) **160** was glycosylated by reacting it with acetylated glucopyranosyl bromide **161** in the presence of KOH, resulting in glycoside **162**, as shown in Scheme (**37**).

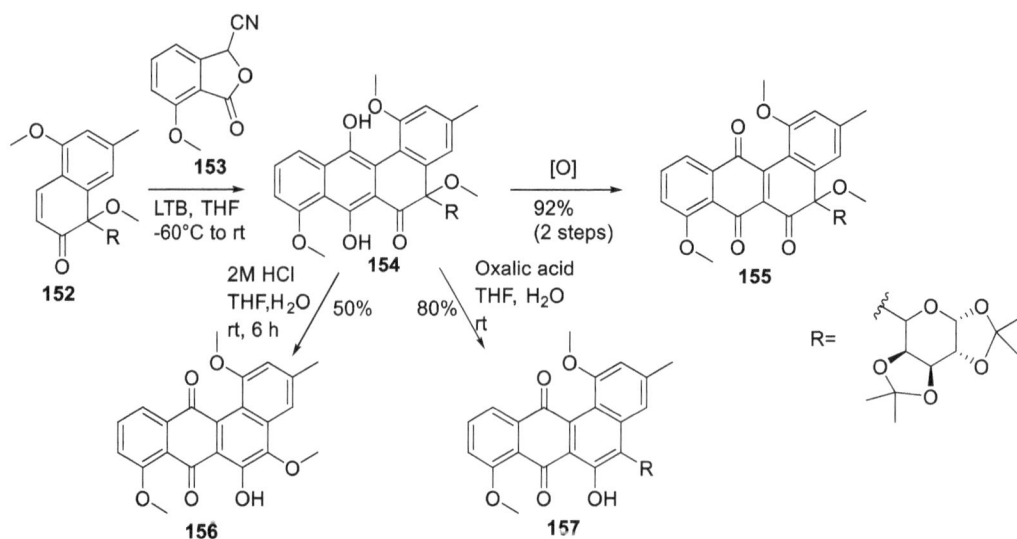

Scheme (36). Synthesis of compound **155-157**.

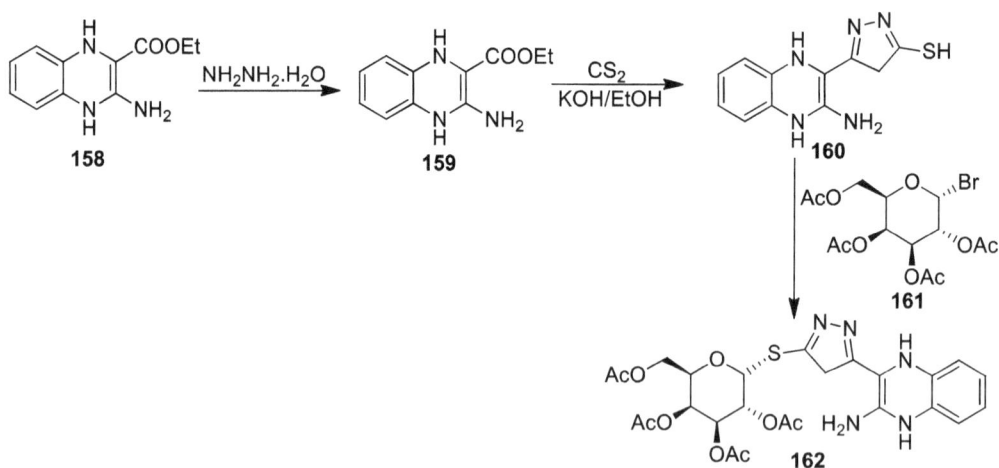

Scheme (37). Synthesis of compounds **160** and **162**.

Benzo[g]pteridine derivatives **163** and **165** react with 2,3,4, 6-tetra-O-α-acetyl glucopyranosyl bromide **161** in aqueous KOH to produce glycosyl derivatives **164** and **166,** as shown in Scheme (**38**). Furthermore, compounds **163** and **165** were methylated by MeI in the presence of KOH, resulting in the creation of 2-(methylthio)benzo[g]pteridine derivatives **168** and **169,** respectively. Compounds **168** and **169** were reacted with hydrazine hydrate in ethanol to afford **170** and **171,** respectively. Additionally, the preparation of Schiff bases **172** and **173** involved heating D-glucose **21** under reflux compounds **170** and **171** in the presence of CH₃COOH acid. Heating hydrazone derivative **172** with acetic anhydride resulted in the synthesis of acetylated glycoside **174,** as shown in Scheme (**39**). The newly synthesized derivatives were docked into the active site of cyclooxygenase-2 (COX-2). This docking study results suggested that the novel compounds may have potent anti-inflammatory activity [82].

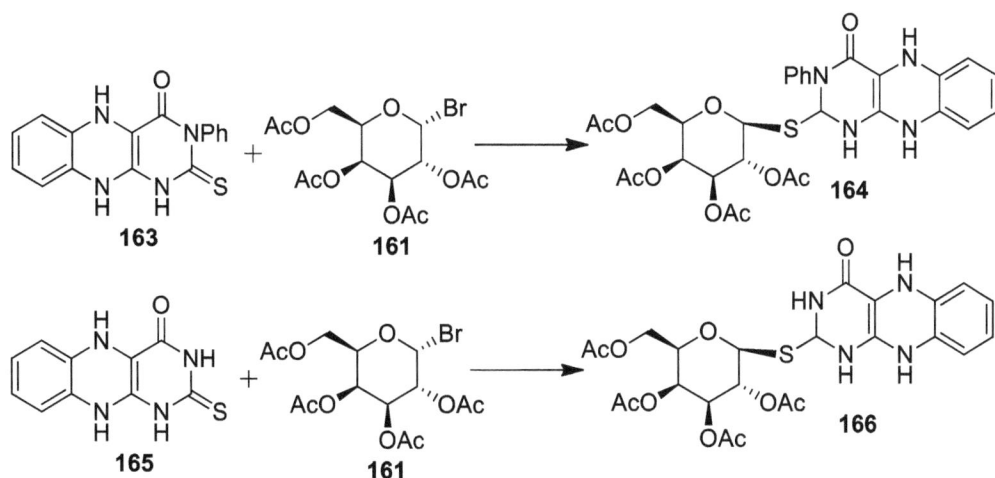

Scheme (38). Thioxobenzo[g]pteridin-derivatives **164** and **166**.

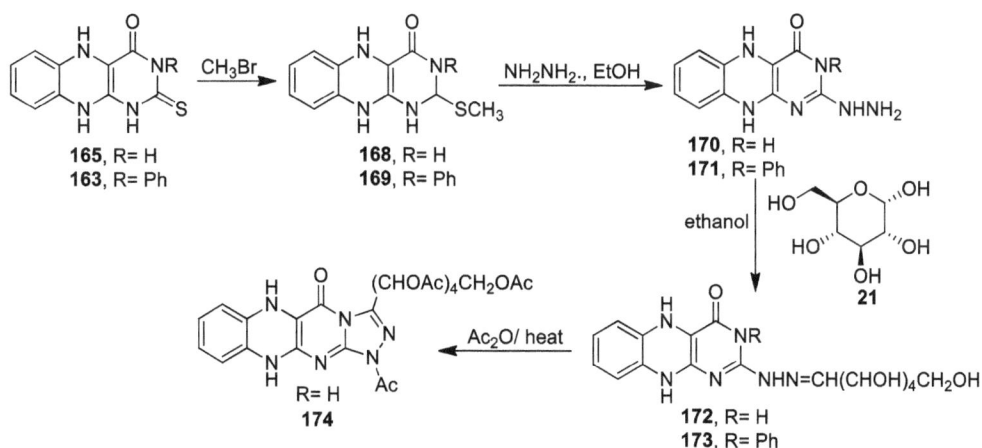

Scheme (39). Synthesis of compounds **172, 173** and **174**.

Wanderson A da Silva *et al.* synthesized quinone-based glycohybrids **178a-c, 179a-c,** and **180a-c** from amino-carbohydrate derivatives **177a–c** [83]. In the first step, treatment of 2,5-dihydroxyacetophenone **173** with methyl-3-aminocrotonate **174** afforded 5,8-dihydroxy-1,3-dimethyl-isoquinoline 4-carboxylate **175**. This was then oxidized to isoquinoline-5,8-dione **176** in good yield *via* MnO$_2$ based oxidation reaction. Compound **176** was subjected to an ultrasound-accelerated

1,4-addition process that led to the formation of new 7-substituted amino-isoquinoline-5,8-quinone derivatives **178a–c**. Compounds **178a–c** reacting with N-halosuccinimides (N-bromosuccinimide [NBS] or N-chlorosuccinimide [NCS]) furnished brominated **179a–c** and chlorinated derivatives **180a–c** in good yields, as shown in Scheme (**40**).

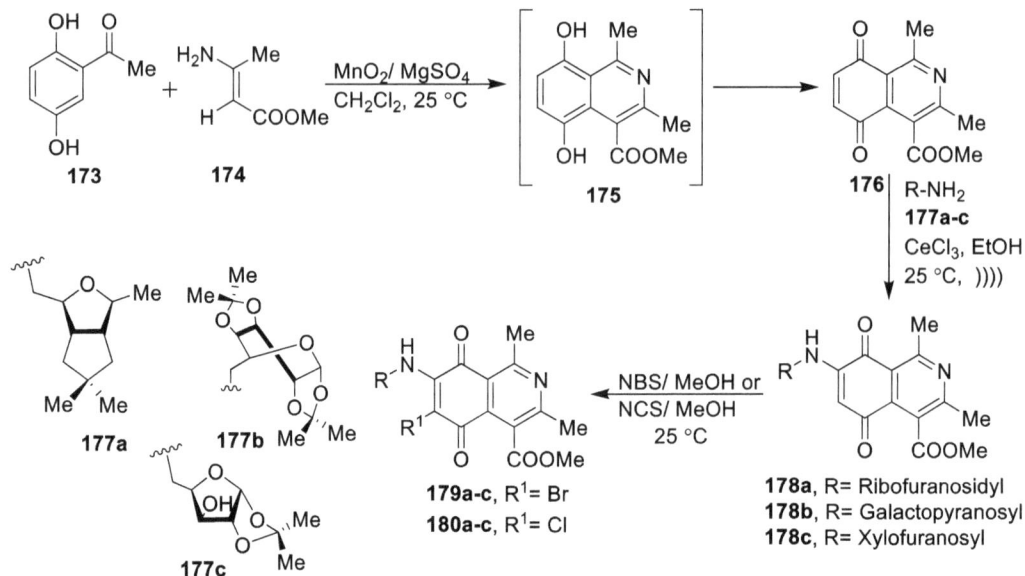

Scheme (40). Synthesis of quinone-based glycohybrids **178a-c**, **179a-c**, and **180a-c**.

These synthesized isoquinoline-5,8-dione compounds were evaluated for *in vitro* antiproliferative activity against normal cell lines (Vero-cells), MDA-MB231 (breast adenocarcinoma), H1299 (pulmonary adenocarcinoma), and DU-145 (prostate carcinoma) human cancer cells lines by MTT reduction assay. Carbohydrate-based quinones may be useful lead molecules in the creation of anticancer medications. The most potent compound of 5,8-dioxo-5-8-dihydroisoquinoline, which has a ribofuranosidyl ring, demonstrated selective action against H1299 cancer cells *in vitro*, with a 1.7-fold increase in activity compared to vinorelbine tartrate, a medication used in clinical settings. The selectivity index of the most active substance approached selectivity index 2, which was higher than that of the reference drug (selectivity index < 1.20) *in vitro* [84].

M. A. Lumba *et al.* described the synthesis of β-galactosidase probes **190**and**191** and quinone alkide **192**. β-galactosidase probes **190** and **191** were synthesized from 2,3,4,6-tetraacetyl-α-D-galactopyranosyl bromide **161**. Phase transfer conditions or Ag$_2$O was used to induce glycosidation with the corresponding nitrophenol that contained carbonyls, resulting in the production of O-linked β-galactosides **181** and **182**. Diethylaminosulfur trifluoride (DAST) was used to directly install difluoromethyl aryl in **185** from **181**. The ketone in **182** was first reduced to a secondary alcohol **183** and then fluorinated using DAST to create the monofluoroethyl aryl in **184**. The nitro groups in **184** and **185** were subsequently reduced to afford anilines **186** and **187**. Propylphosphonic anhydride (T3P) was used to condense the carboxylic acid-functionalized tellurophene with **186** or **187**, yielding **188** and **189** [85]. The acetyl-protected sugars were then deprotected under Zemplén conditions to afford the final β-galactosidase probes **190** and **191** in good yields. The reaction of **190** and **191** with β-galactosidase under hydrolysis formed the quinone alkide **192**, as shown in Scheme (**41**). The inhibitory activity of β-galactosidase probes **190** and **191** against E. coli β-galactosidase was evaluated. They showed that quinone methide was more reactive toward thiols than amines and that the difluoromethyl derivative gave stronger tellurium labeling *in vitro* [86].

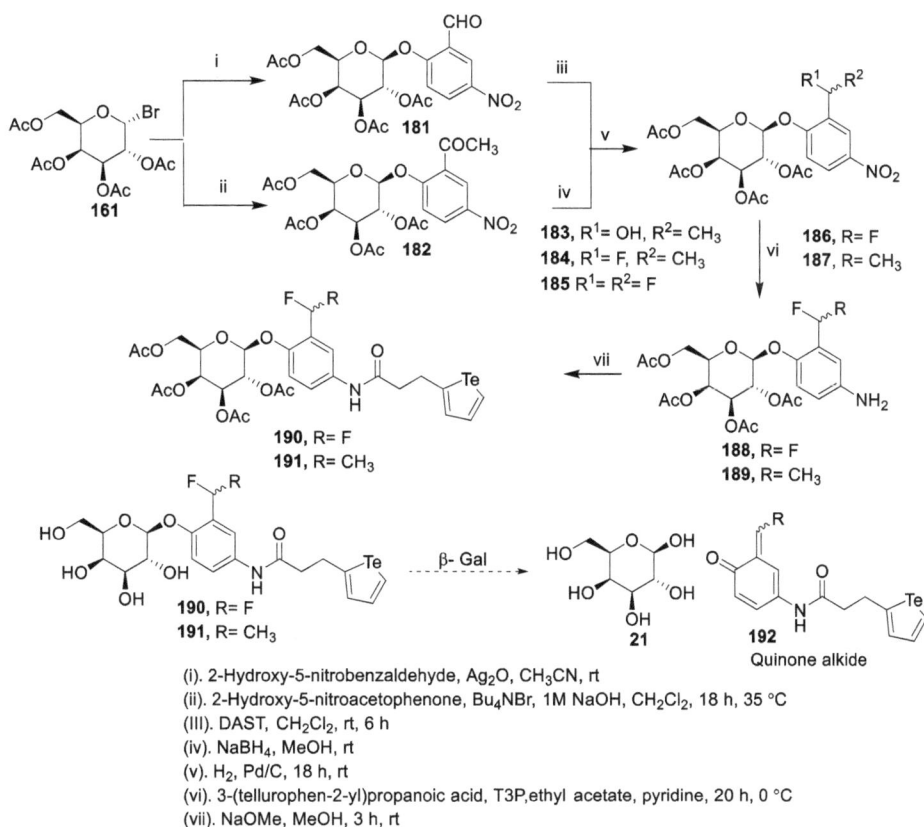

(i). 2-Hydroxy-5-nitrobenzaldehyde, Ag$_2$O, CH$_3$CN, rt
(ii). 2-Hydroxy-5-nitroacetophenone, Bu$_4$NBr, 1M NaOH, CH$_2$Cl$_2$, 18 h, 35 °C
(III). DAST, CH$_2$Cl$_2$, rt, 6 h
(iv). NaBH$_4$, MeOH, rt
(v). H$_2$, Pd/C, 18 h, rt
(vi). 3-(tellurophen-2-yl)propanoic acid, T3P,ethyl acetate, pyridine, 20 h, 0 °C
(vii). NaOMe, MeOH, 3 h, rt

Scheme (41). Synthesis of β-galactosidase probes **190**, **191** and quinone alkide **192**.

CONCLUSION

In this book chapter, we have explored the latest discoveries on the synthesis of diverse quinone-based glycohybrids using a variety of reaction conditions. These reactions include click chemistry, phase transfer catalysis, 6π electrocyclization, Fries-type rearrangement, hydrogenative cycloaddition, intermolecular Diels-Alder reaction, base-catalyzed nucleophilic reactions, [4 + 2] cycloaddition reaction, one-pot iminium-ion based reaction, Bronsted acid catalysis, aldol reaction, *etc*. The triazolyl glycohybrids of quinones showed good to excellent cytotoxicity against anticancer activities against the MCF-7 (breast cancer) cell line, SKBR-3 (IC50 = 0.78 µM), and tumoral cells (SI > 20). Naphthoquinone-based glycohybrids show strong inhibitors of the IRAK1 catalytic site and inhibit P2X7R receptors in murine neuroblastoma cells, indicating their potential as a potent anti-inflammatory, anti-Parkinson disease, anticancer, antiviral, and antiradical agent. Quinone-based glycohybrid sarubicin A exhibited cytotoxicity against cancer cell lines HL-60, SMMC-7721, A-549, MCF-7, and SW480, as well as cytotoxic potential in human PC-3 cells, which are resistant to drugs, and in human PNT2 cells. As a result, numerous well-defined glycohybrids and glycoconjugates were developed quickly to treat a wide range of front-line diseases. We really hope that this book chapter will promote more studies into the synthesis of glycohybrids of physiologically relevant compounds using a greener method, even if several methods for their synthesis have been published. Furthermore, we hope that this chapter will motivate scientists to create innovative inhibitors for the treatment of diverse diseases, hence advancing the creation of new medications.

REFERENCES

[1]   Abraham I, Joshi R, Pardasani P, Pardasani R T. V22N3a02. 2011, 22 (3), 1–37.

[2]   Dandawate PR, Vyas AC, Padhye SB, Singh MW, Baruah JB. Perspectives on medicinal properties of benzoquinone compounds. Mini Rev Med Chem 2010; 10(5): 436-54.
[http://dx.doi.org/10.2174/138955710791330909] [PMID: 20370705]

[3]   Kumagai Y, Shinkai Y, Miura T, Cho AK. The chemical biology of naphthoquinones and its environmental implications. Annu Rev Pharmacol Toxicol 2012; 52(1): 221-47.
[http://dx.doi.org/10.1146/annurev-pharmtox-010611-134517] [PMID: 21942631]

[4]   López López LI, Nery Flores SD, Silva Belmares SY, Sáenz Galindo A. Naphthoquinones: biological properties and synthesis of lawsone and derivates - a structured review. Vitae 2014; 21(3): 248-58.
[http://dx.doi.org/10.17533/udea.vitae.17322]

[5]   Durand R, Zenk MH. Enzymes of the homogentisate ring☐cleavage pathway in cell suspension cultures of higher plants. FEBS Lett 1974; 39(2): 218-20.
[http://dx.doi.org/10.1016/0014-5793(74)80054-2] [PMID: 4152877]

[6]   Babula P, Adam V, Havel L, Kizek R. Noteworthy Secondary Metabolites Naphthoquinones – their Occurrence, Pharmacological Properties and Analysis. Curr Pharm Anal 2009; 5(1): 47-68.
[http://dx.doi.org/10.2174/157341209787314936]

[7]   Grevenstuk T, Coelho N, Gonçalves S, Romano A. *in vitro* propagation of Drosera intermedia in a single step. Biol Plant 2010; 54(2): 391-4.
[http://dx.doi.org/10.1007/s10535-010-0071-6]

[8]   Schettler G. "Lipostabil". BMJ 1960; 1(5186): 1657-8.
[http://dx.doi.org/10.1136/bmj.1.5186.1657-c]

[9]   Ernst-Russell MA, Elix JA, Chai CLL, Willis AC, Hamada N, Nash TH III. Hybocarpone, a novel cytotoxic naphthazarin derivative from mycobiont cultures of the lichen Lecanora hybocarpa. Tetrahedron Lett 1999; 40(34): 6321-4.
[http://dx.doi.org/10.1016/S0040-4039(99)01220-4]

[10]   Guiraud P, Steiman R, Campos-Takaki GM, Seigle-Murandi F, de Buochberg M. Comparison of antibacterial and antifungal activities of lapachol and β-lapachone. Planta Med 1994; 60(4): 373-4.
[http://dx.doi.org/10.1055/s-2006-959504] [PMID: 7938274]

[11]   Tanaka S, Tajima M, Tsukada M, Tabata M. A comparative study on anti-inflammatory activities of the enantiomers, shikonin and alkannin. J Nat Prod 1986; 49(3): 466-9.
[http://dx.doi.org/10.1021/np50045a014] [PMID: 3760886]

[12]   Hinks J, Han EJY, Wang VB, *et al.* Naphthoquinone glycosides for bioelectroanalytical enumeration of the faecal indicator *Escherichia coli.* Microb Biotechnol 2016; 9(6): 746-57.
[http://dx.doi.org/10.1111/1751-7915.12373] [PMID: 27364994]

[13]   Cipolla L, Guerrini M, Nicotra F, Torri G, Vismara E. C-Glucosyl quinones and related spacer-connected C-disaccharide. Chem Commun (Camb) 1997; (17): 1617-8.
[http://dx.doi.org/10.1039/a703559d]

[14]   Vu NQ, Dujardin G, Collet SC, Raiber EA, Guingant AY, Evain M. Synthesis of 5-aza-analogues of angucyclines: manipulation of the 2-deoxy-C-glycoside subunit. Tetrahedron Lett 2005; 46(45): 7669-73.
[http://dx.doi.org/10.1016/j.tetlet.2005.09.053]

[15]   Bringmann G, Zhang G, Hager A, *et al.* Anti-tumoral activities of dioncoquinones B and C and related naphthoquinones gained from total synthesis or isolation from plants. Eur J Med Chem 2011; 46(12): 5778-89.
[http://dx.doi.org/10.1016/j.ejmech.2011.09.012] [PMID: 22019229]

[16]   Dyshlovoy S A, Pelageev D N, Hauschild J, *et al.* Successful Targeting of the Warburg E Ff Ect in Prostate 2019; 11: 1-21.

[17]   de Oliveira MM, Linardi MCF, Sampaio MRP. Effects of quinone derivatives on an experimental tumor. J Pharm Sci 1978; 67(4): 562-3.
[http://dx.doi.org/10.1002/jps.2600670435] [PMID: 641773]

[18]   aLinardi MCF, De Oliveira MM, Sampaio MRP, Sampaio MR. Lapachol derivative active against mouse lymphocytic leukemia P-388. J Med Chem 1975; 18(11): 1159-61.
[http://dx.doi.org/10.1021/jm00245a027] [PMID: 1177264] bSagar R, Singh K, Tyagi R, Mishra VK, Tiwari G. Recent Advances in the Synthesis of Bioactive Glycohybrids *via* Click-Chemistry. SynOpen 2023; 7(3): 322-52.
[http://dx.doi.org/10.1055/a-2130-7319]

[19]   Cute P N. From 2-Hydroxy-1.4~Naphthoquinonest. 1973, 26 (1085), 247–251.

[20]   Shen X, Liang X, He C, *et al.* Structural and pharmacological diversity of 1,4-naphthoquinone glycosides in recent 20 years. Bioorg Chem 2023; 138(June): 106643.
[http://dx.doi.org/10.1016/j.bioorg.2023.106643] [PMID: 37329815]

[21]   Dulo B, Phan K, Githaiga J, Raes K, De Meester S. Natural Quinone Dyes: A Review on Structure, Extraction Techniques, Analysis and Application Potential. Springer Netherlands 2021; Vol. 12.
[http://dx.doi.org/10.1007/s12649-021-01443-9]

[22]   Singh K, Sharma S, Tyagi R, Sagar R. Recent progress in the synthesis of natural product inspired bioactive glycohybrids. Carbohydr Res 2023; 534(July): 108975.
[http://dx.doi.org/10.1016/j.carres.2023.108975] [PMID: 37871479]

[23]   Sagar R, Shankar U, Khanna A, Singh K, Tiwari G. Recent Advances in the Synthetic Developments on the 2-Hydroxy-1,4-Naphthoquinone (Lawsone). SynOpen 2023.
[http://dx.doi.org/10.1055/a-2187-3835] bSharma S, Singh K, Yadav R, Kumar R, Sagar R. Organocatalyzed Synthesis of Anti- tubercular Agents. Curr Organocatal 2023; 10
[http://dx.doi.org/10.2174/2213337210666230901141841]

[24]   aKumari P, Dubey S, Venkatachalapathy S, Narayana C, Gupta A, Sagar R. Synthesis of new triazole linked carbohybrids with ROS-mediated toxicity in breast cancer. New J Chem 2019; 43(47): 18590-600.
[http://dx.doi.org/10.1039/C9NJ03288F] bTyagi R, Singh K, Mishra V K, Sagar R. Recent Advances in Synthesis of Diverse Glycopeptides and Glycohybrids. Synth. Strateg. Carbohydr. Chem. 2024, 523–609.
[http://dx.doi.org/10.1016/B978-0-323-91729-2.00010-0]

[25]   Calvaresi EC, Hergenrother PJ. Glucose conjugation for the specific targeting and treatment of cancer. Chem Sci (Camb) 2013; 4(6): 2319-33.
[http://dx.doi.org/10.1039/c3sc22205e] [PMID: 24077675]

[26]   Shah DK. Pharmacokinetic and pharmacodynamic considerations for the next generation protein therapeutics. J Pharmacokinet Pharmacodyn 2015; 42(5): 553-71.
[http://dx.doi.org/10.1007/s10928-015-9447-8] [PMID: 26373957]

[27]   Tietze LF, Bell HP, Chandrasekhar S. Natural product hybrids as new leads for drug discovery. Angew Chem Int Ed 2003; 42(34): 3996-4028.
[http://dx.doi.org/10.1002/anie.200200553] [PMID: 12973759]

[28]   Claudio Viegas-Junior , Danuello A, da Silva Bolzani V, Barreiro EJ, Fraga CA. Molecular hybridization: a useful tool in the design of new drug prototypes. Curr Med Chem 2007; 14(17): 1829-52.
[http://dx.doi.org/10.2174/092986707781058805] [PMID: 17627520]

[29]   Varki A. Biological roles of oligosaccharides: all of the theories are correct. Glycobiology 1993; 3(2): 97-130.
[http://dx.doi.org/10.1093/glycob/3.2.97] [PMID: 8490246]

[30]   Wilson ZE, Brimble MA. Molecules derived from the extremes of life: a decade later. Nat Prod Rep 2021; 38(1): 24-82.
[http://dx.doi.org/10.1039/D0NP00021C] [PMID: 32672280]

[31]   Li F, He Z, Ye Y. Isocartormin, a novel quinochalcone *C* -glycoside from *Carthamus tinctorius.* Acta Pharm Sin B 2017; 7(4): 527-31.
[http://dx.doi.org/10.1016/j.apsb.2017.04.005] [PMID: 28752041]

[32]   Huynh N O, Krische M J. Enantioselective Transfer Hydrogenative Cycloaddition Unlocks the Total Synthesis of SF2446 B3: An Aglycone of Arenimycin and SF2446 Type II Polyketide Antibiotics. 2023.
[http://dx.doi.org/10.1021/jacs.3c06225]

[33]   Pereyra CE, Dantas RF, Ferreira SB, Gomes LP, Silva- FP Jr. The diverse mechanisms and anticancer potential of naphthoquinones. Cancer Cell Int 2019; 19(1): 207.
[http://dx.doi.org/10.1186/s12935-019-0925-8] [PMID: 31388334]

[34]   Khanna A, Tiwari G, Mishra VK, Singh K, Sagar R. Emerging Trends in Glycoscience Synthesis Efficient Synthesis of Natural Product Inspired Naphthoquinone- Fused Glycohybrids and Their In Silico Docking Studies. Synthesis 2023; 1-10.
[http://dx.doi.org/10.1055/a-2181-9709]

[35]   Chen M, Wang R, Zhao W, *et al.* Isocoumarindole A, a Chlorinated Isocoumarin and Indole Alkaloid Hybrid Metabolite from an Endolichenic Fungus *Aspergillus* sp. Org Lett 2019; 21(5): 1530-3.
[http://dx.doi.org/10.1021/acs.orglett.9b00385] [PMID: 30785290]

[36]   Li J, Wang WX, Chen HP, *et al.* (±)-Xylaridines A and B, Highly Conjugated Alkaloids from the Fungus *Xylaria longipes*. Org Lett 2019; 21(5): 1511-4.
[http://dx.doi.org/10.1021/acs.orglett.9b00312] [PMID: 30767540]

[37]   Miao ZH, Wang H, Yang H, Li Z, Zhen L, Xu CY. Glucose-Derived Carbonaceous Nanospheres for Photoacoustic Imaging and Photothermal Therapy. ACS Appl Mater Interfaces 2016; 8(25): 15904-10.
[http://dx.doi.org/10.1021/acsami.6b03652] [PMID: 27281299]

[38]   Zhang W, Xu W, Wang GY, *et al.* Gelsekoumidines A and B: Two Pairs of Atropisomeric Bisindole Alkaloids from the Roots of *Gelsemium elegans*. Org Lett 2017; 19(19): 5194-7.
[http://dx.doi.org/10.1021/acs.orglett.7b02463] [PMID: 28898085]

[39]   Zhang J, Liu ZW, Ao YL, *et al.* Hunterines A–C, Three Unusual Monoterpenoid Indole Alkaloids from *Hunteria zeylanica*. J Org Chem 2019; 84(22): 14892-7.
[http://dx.doi.org/10.1021/acs.joc.9b01835] [PMID: 31475536]

[40]   Jiao S, Huang H, Wang L, *et al.* Alashanines A–C, Three Quinone-Terpenoid Alkaloids from *Syringa pinnatifolia* with Cytotoxic Potential by Activation of ERK. J Org Chem 2023; 88(11): 7096-103.
[http://dx.doi.org/10.1021/acs.joc.3c00369] [PMID: 37178146]

[41]   Liu H, Lang M, Hazelard D, Compain P. A Fries-Type Rearrangement Strategy for the Construction of Stereodefined Quaternary Pseudoanomeric Centers: An Entry into *C* -Naphthyl Ketosides. J Org Chem 2023; 88(19): 13847-56.
[http://dx.doi.org/10.1021/acs.joc.3c01474] [PMID: 37734008]

[42]   Santos TB, de Moraes LGC, Pacheco PAF, *et al.* Naphthoquinones as a Promising Class of Compounds for Facing the Challenge of Parkinson's Disease. Pharmaceuticals (Basel) 2023; 16(11): 1577.
[http://dx.doi.org/10.3390/ph16111577] [PMID: 38004442]

[43]   Marques LB, Ottoni FM, Pinto MCX, *et al.* Lapachol Acetylglycosylation Enhances Its Cytotoxic and Pro-Apoptotic Activities in HL60 Cells. Toxicol Vitr 2019; 2020: 65.
[http://dx.doi.org/10.1016/j.tiv.2020.104772] [PMID: 31935485]

[44]   Pandey N, Dwivedi P, Jyoti , *et al.* Click Chemistry Inspired Synthesis of Hydroxyanthracene Triazolyl Glycoconjugates. ACS Omega 2022; 7(42): 37112-21.
[http://dx.doi.org/10.1021/acsomega.2c02938] [PMID: 36312433]

[45]   Shimura J, Ando Y, Ohmori K, Suzuki K. Total Synthesis and Structure Assignment of Saptomycin H. Org Lett 2022; 24(7): 1439-43.
[http://dx.doi.org/10.1021/acs.orglett.1c04306] [PMID: 35147030]

[46]   Liu H, Laporte AG, Tardieu D, Hazelard D, Compain P. Formal Glycosylation of Quinones with *exo* - Glycals Enabled by Iron-Mediated Oxidative Radical–Polar Crossover. J Org Chem 2022; 87(19): 13178-94.
[http://dx.doi.org/10.1021/acs.joc.2c01635] [PMID: 36095170]

[47]   Ahuja eg, Janning P, Mentel M, *et al.* PhzA/B catalyzes the formation of the tricycle in phenazine biosynthesis. J Am Chem Soc 2008; 130(50): 17053-61.
[http://dx.doi.org/10.1021/ja806325k] [PMID: 19053436]

[48]   Yu M, Luo J, Luo D, *et al.* Discovery and heterologous production of sarubicins and quinazolinone *C* -glycosides with protecting activity for cardiomyocytes. Org Chem Front 2021; 8(14): 3829-37.
[http://dx.doi.org/10.1039/D1QO00470K]

[49]   Sabutskii YE, Denisenko VA, Popov RS, Polonik SG. The synthesis of thioglucosides substituted 1,4-naphthoquinones and their conversion in oxathiane fused quinone-thioglucoside conjugates. ARKIVOC 2017; 2017(3): 302-15.

[http://dx.doi.org/10.24820/ark.5550190.p010.241]

[50]   Kanaoka Y, Yonemitsu O, Tanizawa K, Ban Y. Chem Pharm Bull 1964, 12, 773–778. NII-Electronic Library Service. Chem Pharm Bull (Tokyo) 1964; 12(7): 773-8.
[http://dx.doi.org/10.1248/cpb.12.773] [PMID: 14206927]

[51]   Pislyagin E, Kozlovskiy S, Menchinskaya E, *et al.* Synthetic 1,4-Naphthoquinones inhibit P2X7 receptors in murine neuroblastoma cells. Bioorg Med Chem 2021; 31(31): 115975.
[http://dx.doi.org/10.1016/j.bmc.2020.115975] [PMID: 33401207]

[52]   Naróg D. Electrochemical study of quercetin in the presence of galactopyranose: Potential application to the electrosynthesis of glycoconjugates of quinone/quinone methide of quercetin. J Electroanal Chem (Lausanne) 2020; 878: 114675.
[http://dx.doi.org/10.1016/j.jelechem.2020.114675]

[53]   Mandal PK, Dubey A. An Efficient One-Pot Protocol for Direct Access to Diarylmethyl Thioglycosides with para-Quinone Methides *via* S-Glycosyl Isothiouronium Salts. Synlett 2020; 31(17): 1713-9.
[http://dx.doi.org/10.1055/s-0040-1707189]

[54]   Thomson RH. Studies in the Juglone Series. III. Addition Reactions. J Org Chem 1951; 16(7): 1082-90.
[http://dx.doi.org/10.1021/jo50001a010]

[55]   Dyshlovoy SA, Pelageev DN, Hauschild J, *et al.* Inspired by Sea Urchins: Warburg Effect Mediated Selectivity of Novel Synthetic Non-Glycoside 1,4-Naphthoquinone-6S-Glucose Conjugates in Prostate Cancer. Mar Drugs 2020; 18(5): 251.
[http://dx.doi.org/10.3390/md18050251] [PMID: 32403427]

[56]   Karimian A, Ahmadi Y, Yousefi B. Multiple functions of p21 in cell cycle, apoptosis and transcriptional regulation after DNA damage. DNA Repair (Amst) 2016; 42: 63-71.
[http://dx.doi.org/10.1016/j.dnarep.2016.04.008] [PMID: 27156098]

[57]   Li Y, Yang X, Liu Y, Zhu C, Yang Y, Yu B. Gold(I)-catalyzed glycosylation with glycosyl ortho-alkynylbenzoates as donors: general scope and application in the synthesis of a cyclic triterpene saponin. Chemistry 2010; 16(6): 1871-82.
[http://dx.doi.org/10.1002/chem.200902548] [PMID: 20039348]

[58]   Zhang Q, Sun J, Zhu Y, Zhang F, Yu B. An efficient approach to the synthesis of nucleosides: gold(I)-catalyzed N-glycosylation of pyrimidines and purines with glycosyl ortho-alkynyl benzoates. Angew Chem Int Ed 2011; 50(21): 4933-6.
[http://dx.doi.org/10.1002/anie.201100514] [PMID: 21500325]

[59]   Li Y, Yang Y, Yu B. An efficient glycosylation protocol with glycosyl ortho-alkynylbenzoates as donors under the catalysis of Ph3PAuOTf. Tetrahedron Lett 2008; 49(22): 3604-8.
[http://dx.doi.org/10.1016/j.tetlet.2008.04.017]

[60]   Nicolaou KC, Chen Q, Li R, Anami Y, Tsuchikama K. Total Synthesis of the Monomeric Unit of Lomaiviticin A. J Am Chem Soc 2020; 142(47): 20201-7.
[http://dx.doi.org/10.1021/jacs.0c10660] [PMID: 33186022]

[61]   Polonik S, Likhatskaya G, Sabutski Y, *et al.* Synthesis, Cytotoxic Activity Evaluation and Quantitative Structure-ActivityAnalysis of Substituted 5,8-Dihydroxy-1,4-naphthoquinones and Their *O*- and *S*-Glycoside Derivatives Tested against Neuro-2a Cancer Cells. Mar Drugs 2020; 18(12): 602.
[http://dx.doi.org/10.3390/md18120602] [PMID: 33260299]

[62]   Polonik SG, Denisenko VA. Synthesis and properties of fused tetracyclic derivatives of 1,4-naphthoquinone thioglycosides. Russ Chem Bull 2009; 58(5): 1062-6.
[http://dx.doi.org/10.1007/s11172-009-0135-y]

[63]   Sabutski YE, Menchinskaya ES, Shevchenko LS, *et al.* Synthesis and Evaluation of Antimicrobial and Cytotoxic Activity of Oxathiine-Fused Quinone-Thioglucoside Conjugates of Substituted 1,4-

Naphthoquinones. Molecules 2020; 25(16): 3577.
[http://dx.doi.org/10.3390/molecules25163577] [PMID: 32781642]

[64] Sangwan R, Dubey A, Tiwari A, Mandal PK. The strategic use of *para* -quinone methides to access synthetically challenging and chemoselective α,α′-diarylmethyl *N* -glycosides from unprotected carbohydrate amines. Org Biomol Chem 2020; 18(7): 1343-8.
[http://dx.doi.org/10.1039/D0OB00039F] [PMID: 32003394]

[65] Ottoni FM, Gomes ER, Pádua RM, Oliveira MC, Silva IT, Alves RJ. Synthesis and cytotoxicity evaluation of glycosidic derivatives of lawsone against breast cancer cell lines. Bioorg Med Chem Lett 2020; 30(2): 126817.
[http://dx.doi.org/10.1016/j.bmcl.2019.126817] [PMID: 31810778]

[66] Ishioka W, Oonuki S, Iwadate T, Nihei K. Resorcinol alkyl glucosides as potent tyrosinase inhibitors. Bioorg Med Chem Lett 2019; 29(2): 313-6.
[http://dx.doi.org/10.1016/j.bmcl.2018.11.029] [PMID: 30470492]

[67] Iwadate T, Nihei K. Chemical synthesis, redox transformation, and identification of sonnerphenolic C, an antioxidant in Acer nikoense. Bioorg Med Chem Lett 2017; 27(8): 1799-802.
[http://dx.doi.org/10.1016/j.bmcl.2017.02.054] [PMID: 28283243]

[68] Mattarei A, Biasutto L, Rastrelli F, *et al*. Regioselective O-derivatization of quercetin *via* ester intermediates. An improved synthesis of rhamnetin and development of a new mitochondriotropic derivative. Molecules 2010; 15(7): 4722-36.
[http://dx.doi.org/10.3390/molecules15074722] [PMID: 20657388]

[69] Asebi N, Nihei K. ichi. Total Synthesis of Apios Isoflavones and Investigation of Their Tyrosinase Inhibitory Activity. Tetrahedron 2019; 75(41): 130589.
[http://dx.doi.org/10.1016/j.tet.2019.130589]

[70] Van De Water RW, Pettus TRR. o-Quinone methides: intermediates underdeveloped and underutilized in organic synthesis. Tetrahedron 2002; 58(27): 5367-405.
[http://dx.doi.org/10.1016/S0040-4020(02)00496-9]

[71] Willis NJ, Bray CD. ortho-Quinone methides in natural product synthesis. Chemistry 2012; 18(30): 9160-73.
[http://dx.doi.org/10.1002/chem.201200619] [PMID: 22707392]

[72] Bai W, David J G, Feng Z, Weaver M G, Wu K, Pettus T R R. The Domestication of Ortho -Quinone Methides. 2014

[73] Burchill L, Pepper HP, Sumby CJ, George JH. *ortho* -Quinone Methide Cyclizations Inspired by the Busseihydroquinone Family of Natural Products. Org Lett 2019; 21(20): 8304-7.
[http://dx.doi.org/10.1021/acs.orglett.9b03060] [PMID: 31593469]

[74] Polonik SG. Synthesis and properties of water-soluble 5,8-dihydroxy-1,4-naphthoquinone thioglucosides structurally related to echinochrome. Russ J Org Chem 2009; 45(10): 1474-80.
[http://dx.doi.org/10.1134/S1070428009100091]

[75] Polonik SG, Krylova NV, Kompanets GG, Iunikhina OV, Sabutski YE. Synthesis and Screening of Anti-HSV-1 Activity of Thioglucoside Derivatives of Natural Polyhydroxy-1,4-Naphthoquinones. Nat Prod Commun 2019; 14(6): 1934578X19860672.
[http://dx.doi.org/10.1177/1934578X19860672]

[76] Mitra RN, Show K, Barman D, Sarkar S, Maiti DK. NHC-Catalyzed Dual Stetter Reaction: A Mild Cascade Annulation for the Syntheses of Naphthoquinones, Isoflavanones, and Sugar-Based Chiral Analogues. J Org Chem 2019; 84(1): 42-52.
[http://dx.doi.org/10.1021/acs.joc.8b01503] [PMID: 30562016]

[77] Peng R, VanNieuwenhze MS. Studies toward the Total Synthesis of Nogalamycin: Construction of the Complete ABCDEF-Ring System *via* a Convergent Hauser Annulation. J Org Chem 2019; 84(2): 760-8.

[http://dx.doi.org/10.1021/acs.joc.8b02602] [PMID: 30584840]

[78]   Prasad SS, Reddy NR, Baskaran S. One-Pot Synthesis of Structurally Diverse Iminosugar-Based Hybrid Molecules. J Org Chem 2018; 83(17): 9604-18.
[http://dx.doi.org/10.1021/acs.joc.8b00748] [PMID: 30101592]

[79]   Hauser FM, Dorsch WA. A new regiospecific preparation of xanthones. Org Lett 2003; 5(20): 3753-4.
[http://dx.doi.org/10.1021/ol0354876] [PMID: 14507222]

[80]   Chakraborty S, Mal D. A Representative Synthetic Route for C5 Angucycline Glycosides: Studies Directed toward the Total Synthesis of Mayamycin. J Org Chem 2018; 83(3): 1328-39.
[http://dx.doi.org/10.1021/acs.joc.7b02833] [PMID: 29231733]

[81]   Dogné JM, Hanson J, Supuran C, Pratico D. Coxibs and cardiovascular side-effects: from light to shadow. Curr Pharm Des 2006; 12(8): 971-5.
[http://dx.doi.org/10.2174/138161206776055949] [PMID: 16533164]

[82]   Ghoneim AA, Ahmed Elkanzi NA, Bakr RB. Synthesis and studies molecular docking of some new thioxobenzo[g]pteridine derivatives and 1,4-dihydroquinoxaline derivatives with glycosidic moiety. J Taibah Univ Sci 2018; 12(6): 774-82.
[http://dx.doi.org/10.1080/16583655.2018.1510163]

[83]   Díaz Pérez P, García-Moreno MI, Ortiz Mellet C, García Fernández JM. Synthesis and Comparative Glycosidase Inhibitory Properties of Reducing Castanospermine Analogues. Eur J Org Chem 2005; 2005(14): 2903-13.
[http://dx.doi.org/10.1002/ejoc.200500071]

[84]   da Silva WA, da Silva LCRP, Campos VR, *et al.* Synthesis and Antitumor Evaluation of Hybrids of 5,8-dioxo-5,8-dihydroisoquinoline-4-carboxylates and Carbohydrates. Future Med Chem 2018; 10(5): 527-40.
[http://dx.doi.org/10.4155/fmc-2017-0173] [PMID: 29424562]

[85]   Park H, Edgar LJ, Lumba MA, Willis LM, Nitz M. Organotellurium scaffolds for mass cytometry reagent development. Org Biomol Chem 2015; 13(25): 7027-33.
[http://dx.doi.org/10.1039/C5OB00593K] [PMID: 26040785]

[86]   Lumba MA, Willis LM, Santra S, *et al.* A β-galactosidase probe for the detection of cellular senescence by mass cytometry. Org Biomol Chem 2017; 15(30): 6388-92.
[http://dx.doi.org/10.1039/C7OB01227F] [PMID: 28726964]

CHAPTER 6

Pharmacodynamics of Quinones and their Derivatives

Ganesh Sonawane[1,*], **Shashikant Bhandari**[2], **Ritu Gilhotra**[3] and **Ashutosh Kumar Dash**[4]

[1] *Divine College of Pharmacy, Satana, Nashik (Maharashtra) India*

[2] *AISSMS College of Pharmacy, Pune (Maharashtra) India*

[3] *School of Pharmacy, Suresh Gyan Vihar University, Jaipur (Rajasthan) India*

[4] *Senior Research Scientist (R&D), Drug Discovery Division, Macleod Pharmaceuticals Ltd, Mumbai, India*

Abstract: Quinones and their derivatives are a diverse group of compounds with significant pharmacological potential rooted in their unique redox properties and ability to interact with various biomolecules. This chapter explores the pharmacodynamics of quinones, highlighting their mechanisms of action, including electron transfer, generation of reactive oxygen species (ROS), and interactions with DNA, proteins, and lipids. These mechanisms underpin their therapeutic applications in oncology, antibacterial and antifungal treatments, antiviral therapies, and other medical areas such as anti-inflammatory and neuroprotective interventions. Despite their promise, the development of quinone-based drugs is challenged by issues of stability, solubility, and toxicity. Advances in drug delivery systems, such as nanoparticles and liposomes, and the creation of novel quinone derivatives are critical to overcoming these obstacles. Moreover, the potential for personalized medicine, leveraging genetic profiling and biomarkers, represents a transformative approach to optimizing quinone therapies. The chapter also addresses the current regulatory and safety considerations in quinone drug development and highlights future research directions, including combination therapies and the use of artificial intelligence in drug discovery. Overall, while challenges remain, ongoing innovations and research efforts are poised to enhance the therapeutic efficacy and safety of quinone-based drugs, unlocking their full potential in modern medicine.

Keywords: Anticancer therapy, Drug delivery systems, Pharmacodynamics, Personalized medicine, Reactive oxygen species, Quinones.

* **Corresponding author Ganesh Sonawane:** Divine College of Pharmacy, Satana, Nashik (Maharashtra) India; E-mail: gbsonawane8@gmail.com

INTRODUCTION

Quinones are a class of organic compounds that are characterized by a fully conjugated cyclic dione structure. Structurally, quinones are derived from aromatic compounds like benzene, naphthalene, or anthracene, where two hydrogen atoms on the ring are replaced by oxygen atoms, creating a system of alternating double bonds. This conjugated system is responsible for the distinctive chemical properties and reactivity of quinones. The general formula for quinones can be represented as $C_6H_4O_2$ for benzoquinones, but this can vary based on the type and complexity of the parent aromatic system [1].

Quinones are known for their ability to participate in redox reactions, which is a key feature underlying their biological and pharmacological activities. The redox cycling of quinones involves the reversible reduction of quinones to hydroquinones (quinols), which can then be reoxidized back to quinones. This redox activity allows quinones to participate in various biochemical processes, including electron transport chains and redox signaling pathways.

The aromaticity of quinones also contributes to their chemical stability and reactivity. The delocalized π-electron system across the conjugated dione structure makes quinones relatively stable compounds yet reactive enough to interact with biological molecules and participate in electron transfer reactions.

Quinones are naturally occurring in many plants, fungi, and bacteria. They are often involved in pigmentation (*e.g.*, anthraquinones in madder root), defense mechanisms (*e.g.*, juglone in walnut trees), and cellular respiration (*e.g.*, ubiquinones in the mitochondrial electron transport chain).

In synthetic chemistry, quinones are typically produced through the oxidation of phenols or anilines. For example, the industrial production of benzoquinone often involves the oxidation of hydroquinone (1,4-dihydroxybenzene) using oxidizing agents like hydrogen peroxide or ferric chloride.

Quinones play crucial roles in various biological processes. One of the most well-known quinones, ubiquinone (coenzyme Q), is vital for the electron transport chain and ATP synthesis in mitochondria. Vitamin K, another important quinone, is essential for blood clotting and bone health. The redox properties of quinones enable them to function as electron carriers in biological systems.

Pharmacologically, quinones and their derivatives exhibit a range of activities, including anticancer, antimicrobial, anti-inflammatory, and antioxidant effects. Their ability to generate reactive oxygen species (ROS) through redox cycling makes them useful in targeting cancer cells, which are often more susceptible to oxidative stress than normal cells [2, 3].

HISTORICAL BACKGROUND AND DISCOVERY

The discovery and study of quinones date back to the early 19th century. The first quinone, benzoquinone, was identified by Carl Wilhelm Scheele in 1786. However, it was not until the 1830s that Friedrich Wohler and Justus von Liebig elucidated the structure of quinones through their pioneering work in organic chemistry. Their research laid the foundation for understanding the chemical properties and reactivity of quinones, leading to the synthesis of numerous quinone derivatives and the exploration of their applications in various fields [4].

SIGNIFICANCE IN PHARMACOLOGY AND MEDICINE

Quinones and their derivatives have significant importance in pharmacology and medicine due to their wide range of biological activities. They exhibit various pharmacodynamic properties, including antimicrobial, anticancer, anti-inflammatory, and antioxidant effects. The biological activity of quinones is primarily attributed to their ability to undergo redox cycling, generating reactive oxygen species (ROS) that can induce oxidative stress and modulate cellular signaling pathways. This unique redox behavior makes quinones promising candidates for therapeutic applications in treating diseases such as cancer, cardiovascular disorders, and neurodegenerative conditions.

Furthermore, quinones are integral components of several vital biochemical processes. For instance, ubiquinone (coenzyme Q) plays a crucial role in the electron transport chain and ATP synthesis in cellular respiration. Similarly, vitamin K, a naphthoquinone derivative, is essential for blood coagulation and bone metabolism. The diverse pharmacological potential and therapeutic applications of quinones underscore their significance in modern medicine and ongoing biomedical research [5].

CHEMICAL STRUCTURE AND CLASSIFICATION

Basic Chemical Structure of Quinones

Quinones are characterized by a fully conjugated cyclic dione structure, typically involving an aromatic ring system where two carbonyl groups (C=O) replace two hydrogen atoms. This conjugation creates a system of alternating double bonds, giving quinones their distinctive reactivity and stability. The simplest quinone, benzoquinone, has the formula $C_6H_4O_2$, with the general structure for quinones being represented as $C_nH2_{n-2}O_2$, where n varies depending on the specific type of quinone.

Types of Quinones

Quinones can be classified into several types (Fig. **1**) based on their parent aromatic system. The simplest forms are benzoquinones, derived from benzene, with para-benzoquinone (p-benzoquinone) having oxygen atoms opposite each other and ortho-benzoquinone (o-benzoquinone) with adjacent oxygen atoms. Naphthoquinones, derived from naphthalene, include 1,4-naphthoquinone (para-naphthoquinone) and 1,2-naphthoquinone (ortho-naphthoquinone). Anthra-quinones, derived from anthracene, are more complex and commonly found in natural pigments and dyes. Additionally, other polycyclic quinones are derived from larger polycyclic aromatic hydrocarbons, adding to the diversity and complexity of this class of compounds.

Benzoquinones: These are the simplest quinones derived from benzene. They include:

- **Para-benzoquinone (p-benzoquinone)**: The oxygen atoms are located opposite each other on the benzene ring, creating a structure conducive to redox reactions.
- **Ortho-benzoquinone (o-benzoquinone)**: The oxygen atoms are adjacent to each other on the benzene ring, which affects its chemical properties and reactivity.

Naphthoquinones: Derived from naphthalene, these quinones have a more extended aromatic system, including:

- **1,4-Naphthoquinone (para-naphthoquinone)**: Similar to p-benzoquinone but with a naphthalene core.
- **1,2-Naphthoquinone (ortho-naphthoquinone)**: Similar to o-benzoquinone but with a naphthalene core.

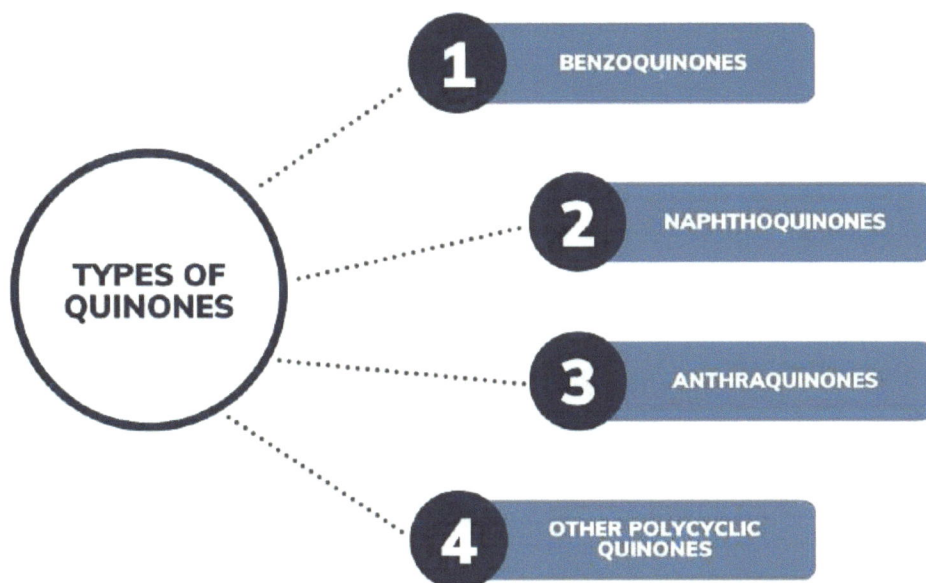

Fig. (1). Types of quinones.

Anthraquinones: Derived from anthracene, these quinones are more complex and widely used in dyes and pigments. The structure consists of three fused benzene rings with two carbonyl groups on adjacent carbon atoms.

Other Polycyclic Quinones: These include quinones derived from larger polycyclic aromatic hydrocarbons (PAHs). They exhibit a variety of structures and chemical properties based on the specific PAH precursor.

Natural *vs.* Synthetic Quinones

Natural Quinones: These quinones occur naturally in plants, fungi, and bacteria. For example, ubiquinone (coenzyme Q) is essential for the mitochondrial electron transport chain, and vitamin K is vital for blood clotting and bone health. Natural quinones often have biological roles due to their redox properties and ability to participate in electron transfer processes.

Synthetic Quinones: These are produced through chemical synthesis for various industrial and pharmaceutical applications. Synthetic methods typically involve the oxidation of phenols or anilines. For example, para-benzoquinone can be synthesized by the oxidation of hydroquinone. Synthetic quinones are used in a wide range of applications, from dyes and pigments to pharmaceuticals [6, 7].

Key Derivatives and their Unique Properties

Quinone derivatives vary widely, and their unique properties are often exploited in different applications (Table **1**):

Table 1. Key Derivatives of Quinone and their Unique Properties

Sr. No.	Quinone derivatives	Unique properties
1	**Ubiquinone (Coenzyme Q10)**	A naturally occurring quinone crucial for ATP synthesis in mitochondria. It acts as an electron carrier in the respiratory chain, highlighting its importance in energy metabolism.
2	**Vitamin K**	A group of structurally similar, fat-soluble vitamins that are essential for the synthesis of proteins involved in blood clotting and bone metabolism.
3	**Plumbagin**	A naturally occurring naphthoquinone with anticancer properties, known for its ability to induce apoptosis in cancer cells through ROS generation.
4	**Mitomycin C**	An anthraquinone derivative used as an anticancer agent. It functions by cross-linking DNA, thereby inhibiting DNA synthesis and function.
5	**Menadione (Vitamin K3)**	A synthetic vitamin K derivative used as a dietary supplement and in various therapeutic applications. It plays a role in oxidative phosphorylation and has anticoagulant properties.

MECHANISMS OF PHARMACODYNAMIC ACTION

Redox Properties and Electron Transfer

Quinones are well-known for their redox properties, which are central to their pharmacodynamic actions. They can easily undergo redox cycling, where they are reduced to hydroquinones (quinols) and then reoxidized back to quinones. This redox cycling involves the transfer of electrons and protons, making quinones effective electron carriers. This property is crucial in biological systems, particularly in processes like the mitochondrial electron transport chain, where ubiquinone (coenzyme Q) plays a vital role in ATP synthesis by shuttling electrons between different complexes.

Generation and Role of Reactive Oxygen Species (ROS)

One of the critical pharmacodynamic actions of quinones is the generation of reactive oxygen species (ROS). During redox cycling, quinones can transfer electrons to molecular oxygen, producing superoxide anions, which are precursors to other ROS, such as hydrogen peroxide and hydroxyl radicals. ROS are highly reactive and can induce oxidative stress within cells, leading to damage to DNA, proteins, and lipids. This property is particularly exploited in anticancer therapies, where elevated ROS levels can selectively induce apoptosis in cancer cells.

Interaction with Biomolecules (DNA, Proteins, Lipids)

Quinones and their derivatives can interact directly with various biomolecules:

DNA: Quinones can cause DNA damage through the formation of adducts and interstrand cross-links or by generating ROS that induce oxidative DNA damage. For example, mitomycin C, an anthraquinone derivative, cross-links DNA, inhibiting replication and transcription, leading to cell death.

Proteins: Quinones can modify proteins by forming covalent adducts with nucleophilic amino acids, affecting protein function. This modification can disrupt normal cellular processes, such as enzyme activity and signal transduction.

Lipids: Quinones can induce lipid peroxidation through ROS generation, leading to cell membrane damage, loss of membrane integrity, and cell death.

Impact on Cellular Pathways

Cellular Respiration and Mitochondrial Function

Quinones, particularly ubiquinone, are essential for mitochondrial function and cellular respiration. Ubiquinone serves as a crucial component of the electron transport chain, facilitating the transfer of electrons from complexes I and II to complex III. This electron transfer is coupled with proton pumping across the mitochondrial membrane, generating a proton gradient that drives ATP synthesis. Disruption of quinone function can impair ATP production, leading to reduced cellular energy levels and affecting cell viability.

Signal Transduction Pathways

Quinones can influence various signal transduction pathways through their redox activity and interaction with cellular components. For instance, they can modulate the activity of kinases and phosphatases, which are crucial for signaling pathways that regulate cell growth, differentiation, and apoptosis. The oxidative stress induced by quinones can activate stress response pathways such as the Nrf2/ARE pathway, which upregulates the expression of antioxidant proteins and detoxifying enzymes to protect cells from oxidative damage.

In cancer therapy, quinones are used to activate pathways leading to apoptosis. For example, the ROS generated by quinones can activate pro-apoptotic signaling cascades, such as the p38 MAPK and JNK pathways, leading to programmed cell death in cancer cells [8, 9].

PHARMACOKINETICS AND METABOLISM

Absorption and Bioavailability

The absorption and bioavailability of quinones vary significantly depending on their chemical structure and physicochemical properties. Generally, quinones are absorbed through passive diffusion due to their lipophilic nature, which allows them to cross cellular membranes. However, their bioavailability can be limited by factors such as poor water solubility and first-pass metabolism in the liver. The extent of absorption can also be influenced by the formulation and administration route. For example, oral administration of quinones like coenzyme Q10 often results in low bioavailability due to its large molecular weight and poor solubility in the gastrointestinal tract.

Distribution in the Body

Tissue and Organ Distribution

After absorption, quinones are distributed throughout the body, with preferential accumulation in tissues with high metabolic activity, such as the liver, kidneys, and heart. The distribution is influenced by the lipophilicity of the quinone, allowing it to integrate into lipid-rich environments like cellular membranes. For instance, ubiquinone is predominantly found in the mitochondria due to its role in the electron transport chain.

Blood-Brain Barrier Penetration

The ability of quinones to penetrate the blood-brain barrier (BBB) is variable. Lipophilic quinones with smaller molecular sizes are more likely to cross the BBB. However, many quinones are modified to enhance their penetration or delivered through nanocarrier systems to improve their efficacy in treating neurological conditions. For example, certain derivatives of naphthoquinones have been studied for their neuroprotective effects due to their ability to cross the BBB and exert antioxidant effects in the brain.

Metabolic Pathways

Quinones undergo extensive metabolism in the liver, involving both Phase I and Phase II reactions.

Phase I Reactions: These primarily involve oxidation, reduction, and hydrolysis. Quinones can be reduced to hydroquinones or undergo oxidation to form more reactive species. Cytochrome P450 enzymes play a significant role in these oxidative transformations.

Phase II Reactions: These involve conjugation reactions where quinones or their metabolites are conjugated with glucuronic acid, sulfate, or glutathione to form more water-soluble compounds, facilitating their excretion. Glutathione conjugation, in particular, helps detoxify quinones by reducing their electrophilicity and reactivity.

Role of Cytochrome P450 Enzymes

Cytochrome P450 enzymes (CYPs) are crucial in the metabolism of quinones. These enzymes catalyze the oxidation of quinones, facilitating their conversion to more water-soluble metabolites. For instance, CYP1A2 and CYP3A4 are involved in the metabolism of various synthetic quinones used in chemotherapy, affecting their pharmacokinetic profiles and therapeutic efficacy.

Excretion Mechanisms

Renal and Hepatic Routes

The primary routes of excretion for quinones are renal (urine) and hepatic (bile/faces). Conjugated metabolites formed during Phase II metabolism are generally more hydrophilic, allowing for efficient renal excretion. Hepatic excretion involves the secretion of these metabolites into the bile, which is then eliminated *via* the feces. The specific route can depend on the quinone's molecular size and polarity.

Half-life and Clearance

The half-life and clearance of quinones depend on their rate of metabolism and excretion. Quinones with rapid metabolism and efficient renal excretion tend to have shorter half-lives. For instance, the half-life of ubiquinone is relatively short due to its rapid utilization in cellular respiration and subsequent metabolism. Clearance rates are also influenced by factors such as age, liver and kidney function, and co-administration of other drugs that may induce or inhibit metabolic enzymes [10, 11].

THERAPEUTIC APPLICATIONS

Quinones are a versatile class of organic compounds known for their diverse therapeutic applications, encompassing anticancer, antibacterial, antifungal, and antiviral activities, among others.

Anticancer Activity

Quinones exhibit potent anticancer activity through several mechanisms:

Generation of Reactive Oxygen Species (ROS): Quinones undergo redox cycling, leading to the generation of ROS, which can induce oxidative stress and apoptosis in cancer cells. Cancer cells often have a higher basal level of oxidative stress, making them more susceptible to additional ROS-induced damage.

DNA Damage and Inhibition of DNA Repair: Quinones can intercalate into DNA and form covalent adducts, leading to DNA strand breaks and cross-links. This DNA damage triggers cell cycle arrest and apoptosis. For example, mitomycin C forms DNA cross-links, preventing replication and transcription.

Inhibition of Topoisomerase: Certain quinones inhibit topoisomerases, enzymes involved in DNA replication and repair. This inhibition prevents DNA unwinding, leading to replication stress and cell death. Doxorubicin, an anthraquinone, inhibits topoisomerase II, causing DNA breaks and apoptosis.

Examples of Quinone-Based Anticancer Drugs

Doxorubicin: An anthracycline antibiotic used in various cancers, including breast cancer, lymphoma, and leukemia. It works by intercalating into DNA and inhibiting topoisomerase II.

Mitomycin C: Used in gastric and pancreatic cancers, mitomycin C cross-links DNA, leading to the inhibition of DNA synthesis and function.

Betulinic Acid: A natural quinone derivative with selective toxicity against melanoma cells, inducing apoptosis through the mitochondrial pathway [12].

Antibacterial and Antifungal Activities

Spectrum of Activity

Quinones exhibit broad-spectrum antibacterial and antifungal activities. They are effective against various Gram-positive and Gram-negative bacteria, as well as several fungal species. Their efficacy depends on the specific quinone derivative and the microorganism's susceptibility.

Mechanisms of Microbial Inhibition

Disruption of Membrane Integrity: Quinones can integrate into microbial cell membranes, disrupting their integrity and leading to cell lysis. For instance, plumbagin disrupts bacterial membranes, leading to leakage of cellular contents and cell death.

Inhibition of Enzymatic Activity: Quinones can inhibit key microbial enzymes involved in energy production and replication. This inhibition can lead to impaired cellular function and death. Naphthoquinones, for example, inhibit bacterial NADH oxidoreductase, disrupting the electron transport chain.

Generation of ROS: Similar to their anticancer mechanism, quinones can induce oxidative stress in microbial cells through ROS generation, leading to oxidative damage and cell death [13, 14].

ANTIVIRAL POTENTIAL

Mechanisms of Antiviral Action

Inhibition of Viral Replication: Quinones can inhibit viral enzymes essential for replication, such as reverse transcriptase in HIV or polymerase in hepatitis viruses. For instance, emodin, a natural anthraquinone, inhibits the 3CL protease of SARS-CoV, impeding viral replication.

Immune Modulation: Quinones can modulate the host immune response, enhancing the body's ability to combat viral infections. By inducing the production of interferons and other cytokines, quinones can enhance antiviral defense mechanisms.

Emerging Applications in Viral Infections

OVID-19: Research is exploring quinones like emodin for their potential to inhibit SARS-CoV-2 replication. Their ability to interfere with viral proteases and polymerases makes them promising candidates for antiviral therapy.

HIV: Quinones like betulinic acid derivatives are being investigated for their potential to inhibit HIV replication and latency reactivation, offering new avenues for treatment [15].

OTHER THERAPEUTIC USES

Anti-inflammatory and Immunomodulatory Effects

Quinones have significant anti-inflammatory and immunomodulatory properties. They can inhibit the production of pro-inflammatory cytokines and enzymes such as COX-2, reducing inflammation. For example, lapachol, a naphthoquinone, reduces inflammation by inhibiting nitric oxide synthase and COX-2 expression.

Potential in Neuroprotection and Cardiovascular Diseases

Neuroprotection: Quinones like coenzyme Q10 have neuroprotective effects due to their role in mitochondrial function and antioxidant properties. Coenzyme Q10 supplementation has been shown to improve mitochondrial function and reduce oxidative damage in neurodegenerative diseases like Parkinson's and Alzheimer's.

Cardiovascular Diseases: Coenzyme Q10 is also beneficial in cardiovascular diseases. It improves mitochondrial function in cardiac cells, enhancing energy production and reducing oxidative stress. Clinical studies have shown that coenzyme Q10 supplementation can improve symptoms of heart failure and reduce the risk of major adverse cardiovascular events [16].

TOXICOLOGY AND SIDE EFFECTS

Quinones can exhibit both acute and chronic toxicity, depending on the dose, duration of exposure, and specific quinone compound.

Acute Toxicity: Acute exposure to high doses of quinones can lead to immediate toxic effects. Symptoms may include nausea, vomiting, diarrhea, and skin irritation. In severe cases, acute toxicity can cause oxidative damage to vital organs, leading to organ failure and death. For example, high doses of para-benzoquinone can cause severe skin and respiratory tract irritation due to its oxidative properties.

Chronic Toxicity: Chronic exposure to lower doses of quinones over an extended period can lead to long-term health effects. These may include carcinogenicity, mutagenicity, and reproductive toxicity. Quinones can cause DNA damage through the formation of DNA adducts and oxidative stress, potentially leading to mutations and cancer. Chronic exposure to naphthoquinones, for instance, has been associated with an increased risk of liver and kidney damage.

Organ-specific Toxicities

Quinones can cause specific toxic effects in various organs:

Hepatotoxicity: Quinones can induce liver damage through oxidative stress and mitochondrial dysfunction. Hepatotoxicity is often characterized by elevated liver enzymes, jaundice, and hepatic necrosis. For example, quinone menadione (vitamin K3) can cause hepatotoxicity through the generation of ROS and depletion of glutathione in hepatocytes.

Nephrotoxicity: Quinones can also affect the kidneys, leading to nephrotoxicity. This is often due to the accumulation of quinone metabolites in renal tissue, causing oxidative damage and inflammation. Chronic exposure to quinones like plumbagin has been shown to cause renal tubular necrosis and interstitial fibrosis.

Cardiotoxicity: Some quinones, particularly anthracyclines like doxorubicin, are known for their cardiotoxic effects. Doxorubicin-induced cardiotoxicity is characterized by cardiomyopathy and congestive heart failure, primarily due to the generation of ROS and oxidative damage to cardiac myocytes [18].

COMMON ADVERSE EFFECTS

Common adverse effects of quinone-based therapies can include:

Gastrointestinal Distress: Nausea, vomiting, diarrhea, and abdominal pain are frequent side effects due to the irritation of the gastrointestinal lining.

Dermatological Reactions: Skin rashes, irritation, and photosensitivity are common, particularly with topical or systemic quinone exposure.

Hematological Effects: Myelosuppression, characterized by reduced bone marrow activity, leading to anemia, leukopenia, and thrombocytopenia, is often seen with chemotherapeutic quinones like mitomycin C.

Neurotoxicity: Peripheral neuropathy, characterized by numbness, tingling, and pain in the extremities, can occur with prolonged exposure to certain quinones.

MITIGATION STRATEGIES

Dose Optimization

Optimizing the dose of quinone-based therapies is crucial to minimize toxicity while maintaining therapeutic efficacy. Strategies include:

Individualized Dosing: Tailoring the dose based on patient-specific factors such as age, weight, liver and kidney function, and genetic polymorphisms in metabolic enzymes can help reduce the risk of toxicity.

Dose Fractionation: Dividing the total dose into smaller, more frequent administrations can help reduce peak plasma levels and associated toxicity.

Use of Protective Agents

Using protective agents alongside quinone therapies can help mitigate adverse effects:

Antioxidants: Co-administration of antioxidants like N-acetylcysteine (NAC) or glutathione can help neutralize ROS and protect against oxidative damage. For example, NAC has been used to reduce the hepatotoxicity of acetaminophen (a quinone-related compound) by replenishing glutathione stores.

Cardioprotective Agents: Agents like dexrazoxane are used to mitigate doxorubicin-induced cardiotoxicity. Dexrazoxane chelates iron, reducing the formation of ROS and protecting cardiac tissue.

Hydration and Diuretics: Adequate hydration and the use of diuretics can help enhance the renal excretion of quinones and their metabolites, reducing nephrotoxicity [19].

CLINICAL STUDIES AND TRIALS

Preclinical Research

In vitro Studies

In vitro studies are the initial phase of preclinical research and involve testing quinones on cell cultures to assess their efficacy and safety. These studies help in understanding the mechanisms of action at a cellular level.

Anticancer Activity: *In vitro* studies have demonstrated that quinones like doxorubicin can effectively induce apoptosis in various cancer cell lines. For example, doxorubicin has been shown to cause cell cycle arrest and apoptosis in breast cancer cells through the generation of ROS and inhibition of topoisomerase II.

Antibacterial and Antifungal Activity: Studies on naphthoquinones have revealed their broad-spectrum antimicrobial properties. For instance, plumbagin has been found to inhibit the growth of Staphylococcus aureus and Candida albicans by disrupting their cell membranes and inducing oxidative stress.

Antiviral Activity:*in vitro* studies on emodin have shown its potential to inhibit the replication of SARS-CoV by blocking the viral 3CL protease, which is essential for viral replication.

Animal Models

Animal models are used to study the pharmacokinetics, pharmacodynamics, efficacy, and toxicity of quinones in a living organism. These studies are crucial for determining the safety profile before proceeding to human trials.

Anticancer Studies: Animal models have been pivotal in studying the efficacy of quinone-based drugs. For instance, doxorubicin has been extensively tested in mouse models of cancer, demonstrating significant tumor regression but also revealing cardiotoxicity, leading to further studies on mitigating these effects.

Toxicological Studies: Animal studies have helped identify the organ-specific toxicities of quinones. For example, studies in rats have shown that high doses of menadione can cause liver and kidney damage due to oxidative stress and mitochondrial dysfunction [20 - 22].

CLINICAL TRIAL PHASES

Phase I: Safety and Dosage

Phase I trials are conducted on a small group of healthy volunteers or patients to evaluate the safety, tolerability, pharmacokinetics, and pharmacodynamics of quinone-based drugs.

Doxorubicin: Phase I trials of doxorubicin involved dose-escalation studies to determine the maximum tolerated dose and identify dose-limiting toxicities. These studies confirmed that cardiotoxicity was a significant adverse effect, necessitating dose adjustments and the development of cardioprotective strategies.

Phase II: Efficacy and Side Effects

Phase II trials involve a larger group of patients and focus on the drug's efficacy and further evaluation of its safety.

Mitomycin C: In phase II trials, mitomycin C was tested in patients with advanced gastric cancer. These studies demonstrated significant antitumor activity but also highlighted adverse effects such as myelosuppression and nephrotoxicity, guiding subsequent dose optimization and supportive care measures.

Phase III: Comparison to Standard Treatments

Phase III trials compare the new quinone-based treatment with standard treatments in a larger population to establish its efficacy, monitor side effects, and collect data to ensure the drug's safety.

Doxorubicin: Phase III trials compared doxorubicin with other chemotherapy regimens in breast cancer patients. These studies established doxorubicin's efficacy in improving survival rates but reinforced the need for monitoring and managing cardiotoxicity.

Phase IV: Post-marketing Surveillance

Phase IV trials are conducted after the drug has been approved for use. They monitor the long-term effectiveness and safety in a larger, real-world population.

Coenzyme Q10: Post-marketing studies on coenzyme Q10, used as a supplement for cardiovascular and neurodegenerative diseases, have continued to evaluate its long-term benefits and safety. These studies have generally confirmed its positive effects on mitochondrial function and minimal adverse effects [23].

Case Studies

Case studies provide detailed accounts of individual patient responses to quinone-based treatments, offering insights into the real-world application and variability in patient outcomes.

Betulinic Acid in Melanoma: A case study reported a patient with metastatic melanoma who showed significant tumor regression after treatment with a betulinic acid derivative. This highlighted the potential for quinone derivatives in targeting specific cancer types and prompted further clinical investigations.

Mitomycin C in Gastric Cancer: Case reports have documented successful tumor reduction and severe adverse effects in patients treated with mitomycin C, illustrating the need for careful patient selection and monitoring during treatment [24].

FUTURE PERSPECTIVES AND CHALLENGES

Current Challenges in Quinone-based Drug Development

Stability and Solubility Issues

One of the primary challenges in the development of quinone-based drugs is their chemical stability and solubility. Quinones are prone to degradation through oxidation and reduction reactions, which can affect their efficacy and shelf life. Additionally, many quinones have poor solubility in aqueous solutions, limiting their bioavailability and therapeutic potential.

Chemical Stability: Quinones can undergo redox cycling, leading to the generation of reactive intermediates that may degrade the active compound. This instability can result in decreased efficacy and a shorter shelf life of the drug. To improve stability, researchers are developing stable prodrugs and utilizing stabilizing excipients in drug formulations. For example, the development of prodrugs can temporarily mask the reactive groups of quinones, reducing their reactivity until they reach the target site in the body.

Solubility: Poor solubility of quinones in aqueous solutions is a significant barrier to their effective use as drugs. Various formulation techniques are being explored to address this issue. These include the use of nanoparticles, liposomes, and micelles. Nanoparticle-based delivery systems can encapsulate quinones, protecting them from degradation and improving their solubility and bioavailability. Liposomes and micelles can similarly enhance the solubility and stability of quinones, ensuring that a higher concentration of the drug reaches the target tissue.

Regulatory and Safety Considerations

The regulatory landscape for quinone-based drugs involves rigorous safety and efficacy evaluations. The potential for toxicity, particularly organ-specific toxicities, poses significant regulatory challenges.

Toxicity: Quinones have potent biological activity, which can lead to adverse effects such as hepatotoxicity, nephrotoxicity, and cardiotoxicity. These toxicities are a major concern for regulatory agencies, which require extensive preclinical and clinical data to ensure that the benefits of quinone-based therapies outweigh the risks. For instance, the cardiotoxicity associated with anthracyclines like doxorubicin has necessitated detailed studies to understand the mechanisms of toxicity and develop strategies to mitigate these effects.

Approval Process: The approval process for quinone-based drugs involves multiple phases of clinical trials to establish safety and efficacy. The complexity of these trials and the need for comprehensive toxicity data can slow down the drug development process. Early collaboration with regulatory agencies can help developers navigate these challenges more effectively, ensuring that the drug development process aligns with regulatory requirements and standards [25].

Innovations and Emerging Research

Novel Quinone Derivatives

Research is ongoing to develop novel quinone derivatives with improved efficacy and reduced toxicity. These efforts include modifying the chemical structure of quinones to enhance their therapeutic properties and minimize adverse effects.

Chemical Modifications: Structural modifications, such as the addition of functional groups, can enhance the selectivity and potency of quinones. For example, the development of second-generation anthracyclines aims to reduce cardiotoxicity while maintaining anticancer efficacy. Modifying the quinone structure can help in targeting specific cancer cells more effectively, reducing damage to healthy cells.

Hybrid Compounds: Combining quinones with other bioactive molecules can produce hybrid compounds with synergistic effects. These hybrids can target multiple pathways simultaneously, potentially leading to improved therapeutic outcomes in cancer and other diseases. For instance, combining quinones with antioxidants or other chemotherapeutic agents can enhance their anticancer effects while reducing oxidative stress and toxicity.

Advances in Drug Delivery Systems

Innovative drug delivery systems are being explored to improve the delivery and efficacy of quinone-based drugs. These systems can enhance solubility, stability, and targeted delivery to specific tissues or cells.

Nanoparticles: Nanoparticle-based delivery systems can encapsulate quinones, protecting them from degradation and improving their solubility and bioavailability. Targeted nanoparticles can also deliver quinones directly to tumor cells, reducing systemic toxicity and enhancing the therapeutic index. For example, nanoparticles can be engineered to release the drug in response to specific stimuli in the tumor microenvironment, ensuring that the drug is released only where it is needed [26].

Liposomes and Micelles: Liposomal and micellar formulations can enhance the stability and solubility of quinones. These carriers can also be functionalized with ligands to target specific receptors on cancer cells, improving the specificity and efficacy of quinone-based therapies. This targeted delivery can help minimize side effects and maximize therapeutic effects by concentrating the drug in the tumor tissue [27].

Potential for Personalized Medicine

The integration of quinone-based therapies into personalized medicine represents a promising future direction. Personalized medicine involves tailoring treatments based on an individual's genetic, phenotypic, and environmental factors to achieve optimal therapeutic outcomes.

Genetic Profiling: Genetic profiling can identify patients who are more likely to respond to quinone-based therapies or those at higher risk of experiencing adverse effects. For example, genetic variations in enzymes involved in quinone metabolism can influence drug efficacy and toxicity. Understanding these genetic differences can guide dose adjustments and treatment choices, improving the safety and effectiveness of quinone-based therapies.

Biomarkers: The identification of biomarkers that predict response to quinone-based treatments can facilitate patient selection and monitoring. Biomarkers of oxidative stress, DNA damage, and cell death pathways can help assess the effectiveness of therapy and adjust treatment regimens accordingly. This approach can lead to more precise and personalized treatment plans, improving outcomes for patients.

Future Trends and Research Directions

The future of quinone-based drug development is likely to be shaped by several emerging trends and research directions:

Combination Therapies: Combining quinone-based drugs with other therapeutic agents, such as immunotherapies, targeted therapies, or conventional chemotherapies, can enhance efficacy and overcome resistance. Combination strategies can also help mitigate toxicity by allowing lower doses of each agent. For example, combining quinones with checkpoint inhibitors in cancer therapy could enhance antitumor immune responses while reducing the dose-related toxicities of each drug.

Artificial Intelligence (AI) and Machine Learning: AI and machine learning can accelerate drug discovery and development by predicting the biological activity and toxicity of new quinone derivatives. These technologies can analyze large datasets to identify promising compounds and optimize drug formulations and delivery systems. AI can also help in designing personalized treatment regimens by integrating patient data, such as genetic profiles and biomarkers.

Epigenetic Modulation: Exploring the role of quinones in epigenetic regulation opens new avenues for therapeutic intervention. Quinones can modulate epigenetic marks, such as DNA methylation and histone modifications, influencing gene expression and cellular behavior. This approach has potential applications in cancer, neurodegenerative diseases, and beyond. For example, quinones could be used to reprogram cancer cells to a less aggressive state or to protect neurons in neurodegenerative diseases [28].

CONCLUSION

The pharmacodynamics of quinones and their derivatives represent a complex interplay of chemical properties, biological interactions, and therapeutic potentials. Quinones, characterized by their redox activity, play significant roles in various cellular processes, including the generation of reactive oxygen species (ROS) and interaction with biomolecules such as DNA, proteins, and lipids. These interactions underpin their diverse pharmacological activities, ranging from anticancer and antimicrobial effects to potential roles in antiviral and anti-inflammatory therapies. However, the development of quinone-based drugs faces substantial challenges, including issues of stability, solubility, and toxicity. Innovations in drug delivery systems, such as nanoparticles and liposomes, along with the development of novel quinone derivatives, hold promise for overcoming these hurdles. Additionally, the integration of quinone-based therapies into personalized medicine, guided by genetic profiling and biomarkers, offers a path toward more effective and safer treatments. As research advances, the potential for quinones to contribute to new therapeutic strategies, especially in combination therapies and through the application of AI in drug development, continues to expand. Despite the challenges, the future of quinone pharmacodynamics looks promising, with ongoing efforts poised to unlock their full therapeutic potential.

REFERENCES

[1]   Dyson PJ, McIndoe JS. Transition Metal Quinone Complexes. Cambridge: Cambridge University Press 2003.

[2]   Thompson DF, Clark RW. Quinone-induced DNA damage and antitumor activity. J Med Chem 1998; 41(19): 3626-41.

[3]   Scheele C W. Manganese oxide and the discovery of benzoquinone. Ann. Chem. 1786.

[4]   Wöhler F, von Liebig J. Untersuchungen über das Chinon. Ann Chem Pharm 1838; 26(1): 241-327.

[5]   Bolton JL, Trush MA, Penning TM, Dryhurst G, Monks TJ. Role of quinones in toxicology. Chem Res Toxicol 2000; 13(3): 135-60.
[http://dx.doi.org/10.1021/tx9902082] [PMID: 10725110]

[6]   Monks TJ, Jones DC. The role of quinones in cellular toxicity. Drug Metab Rev 2002; 34(1-2): 165-83.

[7]   Pawar VN, Mungantiwar AA. Anticancer potential of quinones. J Pharm Pharmacol 2019; 71(3): 315-29.

[8]   Hara H, Matsumoto M. Ubiquinone and mitochondrial health. J Biol Chem 2012; 287(4): 3150-9.

[9]   Shearer MJ. Vitamin K and bone health. Nutr Rev 1997; 55(6): 199-204.

[10]   O'Brien PJ. Molecular mechanisms of quinone cytotoxicity. Chem Biol Interact 1991; 80(1): 1-41.
[http://dx.doi.org/10.1016/0009-2797(91)90029-7] [PMID: 1913977]

[11]   Siegel D, Yan C, Ross D. NAD(P)H oxidoreductase 1 (NQO1) in the sensitivity and resistance to quinones. Biochem Pharmacol 2012; 83(8): 1033-40.
[http://dx.doi.org/10.1016/j.bcp.2011.12.017] [PMID: 22209713]

[12]   Song Y, Hu J, Liu H. The anticancer effect of quinones from medicinal herbs. Pharmacol Res 2014; 90: 102-9.

[13]   Gutierrez RM, Gonzalez AM, Hoyo-Vadillo C. Alkaloids from quinones: A therapeutic perspective. Stud Nat Prod Chem 2010; 37: 149-70.

[14]   Babula P, Mikelova R, Adam V, Kizek R, Havel L, Sladky Z. Noteworthy secondary metabolites naphthoquinones—their occurrence, pharmacological properties and analysis. Curr Pharm Anal 2007;

3(3): 281-94.

[15]   Eswaran S, Adhikari AV, Shetty NS. Quinones as potent antimicrobials: Structural properties, mechanisms of action, and strategies for enhancing their activity. Res Chem Intermed 2009; 35: 269-88.

[16]   Fato R, Bergamini C, Leoni S, Lenaz G, Lenaz G. Mitochondrial production of reactive oxygen species: Role of Complex I and quinone analogues. Biofactors 2008; 32(1-4): 31-9.
       [http://dx.doi.org/10.1002/biof.5520320105] [PMID: 19096098]

[17]   Brabec V, Kasparkova J. Modifications of DNA by platinum complexes: Relation to resistance of tumors to platinum antitumor drugs. Drug Resist Updat 2018; 40: 1-16.
       [PMID: 15894512]

[18]   Minotti G, Menna P, Salvatorelli E, Cairo G, Gianni L. Anthracyclines: molecular advances and pharmacologic developments in antitumor activity and cardiotoxicity. Pharmacol Rev 2004; 56(2): 185-229.
       [http://dx.doi.org/10.1124/pr.56.2.6] [PMID: 15169927]

[19]   Hortobágyi GN. Anthracyclines in the treatment of cancer. An overview. Drugs 1997; 54 (Suppl. 4): 1-7.
       [PMID: 9361955]

[20]   Ishikawa T, Machida H, *et al.* Mitomycin C as a novel therapeutic agent in cancer therapy: Therapeutic potential and mechanisms of action. J Cancer Res Clin Oncol 2018; 144: 1899-908.

[21]   Li T, Liu L, *et al.* Plumbagin induces apoptosis and suppresses metastasis in human pancreatic cancer cells *in vitro* and *in vivo*. Drug Des Devel Ther 2019; 13: 4471-80.

[22]   Thomas JP, Moon TE, *et al.* Menadione for the treatment of drug-resistant infections: A phase I clinical trial. J Clin Pharmacol 2000; 40(9): 1045-50.

[23]   Yamashita T, *et al.* Antiviral potential of quinones in the treatment of viral infections: A clinical perspective. Antiviral Res 2021; 188: 105033.

[24]   Mordente A, Meucci E, Silvestrini A, Martorana GE, Giardina B. Anthracyclines and mitochondria. Adv Exp Med Biol 2009; 652: 14-44.
       [PMID: 22399433]

[25]   Wang L, Zhou GB, Liu P, *et al.* Dissection of mechanisms of Chinese medicinal formula Realgar-*Indigo naturalis* as an effective treatment for promyelocytic leukemia. Proc Natl Acad Sci USA 2008; 105(12): 4826-31.
       [http://dx.doi.org/10.1073/pnas.0712365105] [PMID: 18344322]

[26]   Das PP, Sengupta S, Balram D, *et al.* Recent advancements of nanoparticles for antiviral therapy. Advances in Natural Sciences: Nanoscience and Nanotechnology 2024; 15(4): 043001.

[27]   Shahabipour F, Barati N, Johnston TP, Sahebkar A. Progress in the development of liposomal formulations of doxorubicin: Overcoming the cardiac toxicity. Expert Opin Drug Deliv 2018; 15(5): 499-515.

[28]   Newman DJ, Cragg GM. Natural products as sources of new drugs from 1981 to 2014. J Nat Prod 2016; 79(3): 629-61.
       [http://dx.doi.org/10.1021/acs.jnatprod.5b01055] [PMID: 26852623]

CHAPTER 7

Synthetic and Natural Quinones as Drug Candidates

Santosh Kumar Rath[1,*] and **Ashutosh Kumar Dash**[2]

[1] *School of Pharmaceuticals and Population Health Informatics, Faculty of Pharmacy, DIT University, Dehradun, Uttarakhand-248009, India*

[2] *Senior Research Scientist, Drug Discovery Division, Macleods Pharmaceuticals Ltd, Mumbai, India*

Abstract: Quinones are a group of organic compounds that have a wide range of chemical properties and applications in various fields, such as pharmaceuticals, materials science, and organic synthesis. They are highly versatile and can be modified to produce derivatives with unique properties. This chapter presents a comprehensive and current overview of the chemistry and synthesis of quinones and their derivatives. It serves as an invaluable resource for chemists, researchers, and scientists who are interested in exploring the diverse aspects of this significant class of organic compounds.

Keywords: Mitochondrial activity, Natural naphthoquinones, Oxidative stress, Parkinson's disease, Ubiquinone.

INTRODUCTION

Quinones are a substantial class of naturally occurring intramolecular unsaturated cyclic diketone structures. Synthetically, they can be easily changed into similar structural scaffolds with a wide range of applications. It is well known that they play a crucial function in the biochemistry of living cells [1]. The main structural subtypes of natural quinones are benzoquinone, naphthoquinone, anthraquinone, and phenanthroquinone. Additionally, benzoquinone is further subdivided into o-benzoquinone and p-benzoquinone. However, because of the structural instability of o-benzoquinone, the majority of naturally occurring benzoquinones are derivatives of p-benzoquinone [2]. In addition to these physiological roles, quinones are formed by oxidative metabolism in various xenobiotics. Both a benzoquinoneimine metabolite generated by a cytochrome P450-dependent oxidase reaction and simple p-benzoquinone synthesized from the hydrolysis of

---

[*] **Corresponding author Santosh Kumar Rath:** School of Pharmaceuticals and Population Health Informatics, Faculty of Pharmacy, DIT University, Dehradun, Uttarakhand-248009, India; E-mail: ??

Ashutosh Kumar Dash & Deepak Kumar (Eds.)

the benzoquinoneimine metabolite are responsible for the severe hepatotoxicity that can occur from an overdose of the analgetic paracetamol. Quinones are a unique class of naturally occurring secondary metabolites with anticancercharacteristics. A common anthracycline antibiotic used in clinics to treat cancer is doxorubicin. Its 4-membered ring system comprises aminoglycoside, anthraquinone, and chromophore [3]. It is a first-line chemotherapy for breast cancer and is regarded as one of the most potent cancer medications on the market. Even though anthracycline antibiotics are often used in clinical settings, their usage is restricted due to their major adverse effects on healthy tissues and the emergence of drug resistance in cancer cells. The two most significant side effects of anthracycline chemotherapy are neurotoxicity and cardiotoxicity. As quinone derivatives have a structural resemblance to the anthracycline antibiotics that are already utilized in clinical practice, they may be extremely valuable in terms of their potential anticancer characteristics [4]. Additionally, as quinones are found in natural sources and are secondary metabolites, we should take into account the potential that their natural origin makes them relatively safe. For example, several species within several plant groups include structural similarities of naturally occurring quinones. These include the following: Liliaceae (species of Aloe, *etc.*), Hypericaceae (species of Hypericum, *etc.*), Polygonaceae (species of Rheum, Rumex, Polygonum, *etc.*), Rhamnaceae (species of Rhamnus, *etc.*), Rubiaceae (species of Rubia, Galium, *etc.*), Caeselpinaceae (species of Cassia, *etc.*), Boraginaceae (Alkanna, Arnebia spec., *etc.*), and Julienndaceae (species of Juliens, *etc.*) [5]. Plants belonging to the families Polygonaceae, Rubiaceae, and Leguminosae have been identified as containing anthraquinones. Examples of these species include *Rheum palmatum* L., *Rubia cordifolia* L., *Polygoni multiflori*, *Polygonum cuspidatum*, and *Semen cassiae*. Furthermore, 200 of the approximately 700 distinct anthraquinone derivatives that have been identified are found in plants. The general classification of anthraquinones is into anthraquinone monomers, which are further separated into hydroxy anthraquinones, anthranones and anthranols, and bianthraquinones based on the mother nucleus' structure. Studies have shown that the anthracene nucleus serves as the primary structural component of many anticancer medications and that the activity of this nucleus is significantly influenced by a phenolic hydroxyl group. Anthraquinone monomers like emodin, aloe-emodin, rhein, chrysophanol, and physcion receive more attention. But, hypericin, a bianthraquinone variety, is also well-known for its beneficial pharmacological properties, which include anti-depressant, anti-cancer, and anti-viral properties [6].

NATURAL NAPHTHOQUINONES

Natural naphthoquinones, typically in the form of botanical extracts, have been connected to human existence since prehistoric times, far before they were isolated and identified in the present age. Natural quinones, a diverse class of organic compounds found in plants, fungi, and some marine organisms, have gained enormous attention as potential drug candidates due to their various biological activities. Quinones exhibit various pharmacological properties, including antioxidant, anticancer, antimicrobial, anti-inflammatory, and antiparasitic activities [7]. Furthermore, many quinones, such as the naphthoquinones Plumbagin from *Plumbago rosea* and Juglone from *Juglans nigra*, show growth-inhibitory effects on bacteria or fungus and are employed by plants as defensive compounds [8]. Naphthoquinones, such as Shikonin and Plumbagin, are the primary efficacious molecules in some commonly used medical herbals, particularly those that have antibacterial, insecticidal, antiphlogistic, and wound-healing properties [9]. Thymoquinone (2-isopropyl-5-methylbenzo-1,4-quinone) is a benzoquinone molecule widely distributed in the volatile oil portion of *Nigella sativa* seed [10]. Sargaquinoic acid, a hydroquinone acid isolated from *Sargassum siliquastrum,* has anti-inflammatory properties and impedes macrophages' ability to produce nitric oxide by interfering with LPS-induced signaling. Sargaquinoic acid prevented LPS-stimulated RAW264.7 macrophages from producing NO and from expressing the iNOS protein [11]. The adherence of monocytes to TNF-α-induced adhesion was inhibited by sargaquinoic acid. Additionally, by stopping the proteolytic degradation of inhibitor κB-α, SQA prevented TNF-α-induced nuclear factor kappa B (NF-κB) from translocating into the nucleus. Overall, SQA inhibits the NF-κB pathway in HUVECs to prevent vascular inflammation caused by TNF-α [12]. Throughout their lengthy history of use, naphthoquinones have seen a change in use from their early uses as dyes and decorations to their current use as therapeutic compounds [13]. To date, much research has been done to clarify the pharmacological profile of synthetic and natural naphthoquinones. Naphthoquinones are derivatives of naphthalene with two carbonyl oxygen atoms in their structure. Although there are theoretically multiple naphthoquinone isoforms, 1,4-naphthoquinone is the most stable and well-reported one [14]. Many effective analogs, such as simple modified naphthoquinones like Lawsone, Shikonin, Juglone, Plumbagin, and Menadione, have been found based on this scaffold [15]. Additionally, the chemical space renders naphthoquinones stable ligands for a variety of pathologic targets, and in certain circumstances, naphthoquinones may be the preferred chemotype for the development of novel inhibitors.

NATURAL NAPHTHOQUINONES WITH GREAT IMPORTANCE IN MEDICINAL CHEMISTRY

Natural naphthoquinones have garnered significant interest in medicinal chemistry due to their diverse pharmacological activities and potential therapeutic applications. Here are some natural naphthoquinones that hold great importance in medicinal chemistry:

Ubiquinone (coenzyme Q10): Ubiquinone, commonly known as coenzyme Q10 (CoQ10), is a naturally occurring quinone that plays a crucial role in cellular energy production and acts as a powerful antioxidant [16]. Ubiquinone is a vital component of the electron transport chain and is an antioxidant in the human body. It has been studied for its potential therapeutic applications in treating cardiovascular, neurodegenerative, and mitochondrial disorders [17]. CoQ10 protects cells from oxidative damage by neutralizing free radicals and regenerating other antioxidants like vitamin E [18]. CoQ10 is a lipid-soluble molecule with a quinone ring and a long isoprenoid side chain, which allows it to be highly hydrophobic and embedded within cell membranes [19]. It is an essential component of the mitochondrial electron transport chain, where it facilitates the transfer of electrons from complexes I and II to complex III, aiding in the production of ATP, the primary energy currency of the cell [20]. CoQ10 supplementation has shown benefits in improving symptoms and quality of life in patients with heart failure by enhancing mitochondrial function and reducing oxidative stress. Some studies suggest that CoQ10 may help lower blood pressure, possibly through its antioxidant effects and improvement in endothelial function [21].

Plumbagin is observed in various plant species, such *as Plumbago zeylanica.* It is one of the most studied natural naphthoquinones [22]. It exhibits a wide range of pharmacological properties, including anticancer, antimicrobial, anti-inflammatory, antioxidant, and antiprotozoal activities. Plumbagin has shown promise in preclinical studies for the treatment of various cancers, including breast, lung, prostate, and leukemia [23].

Emodin, derived from plants like *Rheum palmatum* and *Polygonum cuspidatum,* is another natural naphthoquinone with diverse pharmacological activities. It possesses anticancer, anti-inflammatory, antiviral, antibacterial, and antidiabetic properties. Emodin has been investigated for its potential in cancer therapy, particularly against leukemia and solid tumors [24]. Research by Liang *et al.* using the equilibrium dialysis method revealed that emodin has low oral bioavailability in rabbits. Emodin was found to be significantly attached to serum proteins (99.6%) [25]. The distribution of emodin glucuronide/sulfates was seen to be well-established in the kidney and lungs, whereas the liver displayed free emodin following oral administration of *Polygonum cuspidatum* extract (2 and 4 g/kg) in rats. It was observed that the predominant forms of emodin in the kidney and lung were its glucuronides/sulfates, whereas the liver contained a sizable quantity of the drug's free form [26].

Shikonin: Shikonin ((±)-5,8-dihydroxy-2-(1-hydroxy-4-methyl-3-pen-enyl)-1,4-naphthoquinone) is a naturally occurring naphthoquinone found in the roots of *Lithospermum erythrorhizon*. This plant has historically been used to cure a number of illnesses, including measles, burns, carbuncles, macular eruption, and sore throats. Shikonin triggers signaling pathways that control the development of the cytoskeleton, mitochondrial activity, and responses to oxidative stress. This substance builds up in the mitochondria, where it depletes intracellular Ca^{2+} levels and produces reactive oxygen species (ROS). Cell cycle arrest and death are also triggered, and the potential of the mitochondrial membrane and microtubules are deformed. Shikonin may, therefore, be used as a starting point to create new anticancer medications. It exhibits potent anticancer, anti-inflammatory, and antimicrobial activities. It has been studied for its potential in cancer treatment, including leukemia, melanoma, and colorectal cancer [27]. Shikonin also shows promise in the treatment of inflammatory diseases, such as rheumatoid arthritis and inflammatory bowel disease. Natural single naphthoquinone administered intragastrically reduced the malignant symptoms brought on by sodium dextran sulfate. Shikonin or its derivatives significantly increased the inflammatory cytokine interleukin (IL)-10 while lowering the serum levels of pro-inflammatory cytokines. Furthermore, in serum and colonic tissues, the activities of myeloperoxidase (MPO), cyclooxygenase-2 (COX-2), and inducible nitric oxide synthase (iNOS) were inhibited by both SK and alkannin. The disruption of epithelial tight junction (TJ) in colonic tissues caused by DSS was alleviated by SK and its derivatives by blocking the activation of the NF-κB signaling pathway and nucleotide-binding oligomerization domain-like receptors (NLRP3) [28].

Lapachol, derived from various plant species, including *Tabebuia avellanedae* and *Handroanthus impetiginosus*, possesses antitumor, antimicrobial, and anti-inflammatory properties. It is a yellow coloring material found in the grain of some timber trees, has two substituent groups in the quinone ring, and is structurally similar to an amylene hydroxynaphthoquinone. It has been investigated for its potential in cancer therapy, particularly against prostate, breast, and leukemia cancers [29]. The NCI announced that additional cancer research has been terminated due to the failure of Phase I clinical studies to yield a therapeutic result with lapachol without side effects. In three patients, pure lapachol produced total remissions and showed the potential to decrease tumors and lessen the discomfort these tumors caused. It is thought that lapachol's interaction with nucleic acids may cause its anticancer effect. It has been suggested that the naphthoquinone molecule interacts with base pairs in the DNA helix, inhibiting RNA production and DNA replication [30]. Lapachol presumably acts as an antimalarial agent by inhibiting respiratory function against Plasmodium lapohurae. The precise method of action is still up for debate, though. It is postulated that lapachol either directly inhibits an unidentified enzyme between the two cytochromes or inhibits the interaction between cytochromes b and c [31]. Lapachol and its analogs were found to exhibit antipsoriatic effects in an *in vitro* investigation by lowering inflammation and preventing the proliferation of the human keratinocyte cell line HaCaT. The study concluded that lapachol and anthralin both have antipsoriatic activity when it comes to causing harm to the keratinocytes cells' cell membranes [32].

Diosquinone, found in Diospyros species, exhibits antitumor and antimicrobial activities. It has shown cytotoxic effects against various cancer cell lines and has the potential as a lead compound for the development of anticancer drugs [33].

THYMOQUINONE (2-ISOPROPYL-5-METHYL-1,4-BENZOQUINONE), primarily found in the seeds of *Nigella***diosquinone**, *sativa* (black seed), is a benzoquinone derivative with naphthoquinone-like properties. It demonstrates anticancer, anti-inflammatory, antioxidant, and antimicrobial activities. Thymoquinone has been studied for its potential in cancer therapy, particularly against breast, lung, colon, and pancreatic cancers [34]. The anti-inflammatory and antinociceptive properties of thymoquinone, in particular, lend credence to the widely held belief that *N. sativa* is a powerful analgesic and anti-inflammatory. In two stages of the formalin test, animals' paw-licking times were significantly reduced by thymoquinone and its para-benzoquinone counterparts. Thymoquinone may also have antinociceptive effects by blocking the serotonin/5-hydroxytryptamine (5-HT) pathway. It has also been shown that 5-HT and norepinephrine have a function in modulating pain through descending inhibitory pathways [35].

Compounds containing 1,4-naphthoquinone cores have the ability to kill malignant cells by focusing on a variety of biochemical pathways. According to earlier research, 1,4-naphthoquinones can regulate the tumor suppressor protein p53 or specifically block the NAD[P]H-quinone oxidoreductase (NQO1), STAT3, and NF-κB signaling pathways. Additionally, by directly interacting with DNA, these substances can cause DNA damage and the generation of reactive oxygen species (ROS), which in turn can promote the demise of malignant cells [36]. These natural naphthoquinones serve as valuable lead compounds for drug discovery and development. Their diverse pharmacological activities make them attractive candidates for the treatment of various diseases, including cancer, inflammation, infectious diseases, and metabolic disorders. However, further research is needed to elucidate their mechanisms of action, optimize their pharmacokinetic properties, and assess their safety and efficacy in clinical trials.

NEURODEGENERATIVE DISEASES

Parkinson's Disease: Oxidative stress, nigral mitochondrial complex I deficiency, and visual impairment are characteristics of Parkinson's disease (PD) that are also linked to a deficiency in coenzyme Q10 (CoQ10). CoQ10 has been investigated for its potential to slow the progression of Parkinson's disease due to its role in mitochondrial function and protection against oxidative damage. Muller *et al.* conducted a parallel-group, placebo-controlled, double-blind study to ascertain the symptomatic effect of 360 mg of CoQ10 taken orally every day for four weeks on the Farnsworth-Munsell 100 Hue test (FMT), which measures visual function in patients with Parkinson's disease (PD) who are stable and under treatment. When compared to a placebo, CoQ10 supplementation resulted in a considerably ($F_{(1;24)}$ = ¼ 8:48, P = 0:008) improved progress in FMT performance and a significant (P = 0:01) mild symptomatic benefit on PD symptoms. These findings suggest that oral CoQ10 supplementation has a somewhat positive impact on PD patients [37]. A randomized, sham-controlled clinical trial used CoQ10 as an intervention for PD patients' motor impairment. Random-effect models were utilized in the computation of weighted mean differences (WMD). There were eight trials totaling eight hundred ninety-nine subjects. A pooled WMD of 1.02 from a random-effect analysis showed no discernible change in UPDRS part 3 between CoQ10 therapy and placebo (p = 0.54). In the CoQ10 group compared to the placebo group, the effect sizes of UPDRS part 1, part 2, and overall UPDRS scores were comparable (p [0.05). Furthermore, in comparison to the placebo group, CoQ10 was well tolerated. Subgroup analysis revealed that compared to multicenter studies, the impact size of CoQ10 was greater in monocentric studies. According to the results of the current meta-analysis, participants found CoQ10 to be safe and well-tolerated [38].

Alzheimer's Disease: Research is ongoing to determine its effectiveness in reducing the progression of cognitive decline associated with Alzheimer's disease (AD). In a rat model of streptozotocin (STZ)-induced AD, Sheykhhasan *et al.* examined the effects of drug delivery of COQ10 by exosomes produced from adipose-derived stem cells (ADSCs-Exo) on cognition, memory, and neural proliferation. When compared to CoQ10 and Exo groups alone, Exo+CoQ10 dramatically improved STZ-induced memory impairment, as demonstrated by the results of the Morris water maze (MWM) and passive avoidance task. In addition, the STZ-induced rats showed enhanced BDNF expression following Exo+ CoQ10 in contrast to the CoQ10 and Exo groups. When compared to the CoQ10 and Exo groups, Exo+CoQ10 also exhibited the highest cell density and SOX2 gene expression. The results of this study showed that Exo+ COQ10 increased BDNF and SOX2 levels in the hippocampus, which improved cognition and memory deficit in Alzheimer's disease [39]. In the Tg19959 AD-induced mouse model, CoQ10 enhanced the behavioral function while reducing oxidative stress and amyloid pathology. Treatment with CoQ10 reduces brain carbonyl protein levels and acts as an indicator of oxidative stress. After receiving CoQ10 treatment, the hippocampal plaque area and the number decreased, and the Aβ42-specific antibody immunostained the overlaying cortex. CoQ10 supplementation also resulted in a decrease in brain Aβ42 levels. Reduced amounts of β-carboxyterminal fragments of the amyloid-β protein precursor (AβPP) were observed. Notably, mice given CoQ10 demonstrated enhanced cognitive function when tested in the Morris water maze [40]. In an AD-induced rat model, Komaki *et al*. examined the neuroprotective effects of Q10 on Aβ-induced impairment in hippocampus long-term potentiation (LTP), a well-studied model of synaptic plasticity that happens during learning and memory. Q10 was given in three ways: Q10 *via* oral gavage and Q10 + Aβ group; intraventricular PBS injection, Aβ group; and intraventricular Aβ injection, Q10 group. Using oral gavage, Q10 was given once daily for three weeks prior to and three weeks following the Aβ injection. In order to measure the excitatory postsynaptic potential (EPSP) slope and population spike (PS) amplitude in the hippocampus dentate gyrus following the treatment period, *in vivo* electrophysiological recordings were carried out [41]. Ali *et al*. investigated whether Vinpocetine alone or in combination with EGCG, CoQ10, or Vinpocetine (VE) and Se can mitigate aluminum chloride-induced AD in rats, as well as any potential neuroprotective effects and mechanisms of action. Rats were given an intraperitoneal daily dose of $AlCl_3$ (70 mg/kg) for 30 days, either in combination or alone, along with EGCG (10 mg/kg, I.P.), CoQ10 (200 mg/kg, P.O.), VE (100 mg/kg, P.O. & Se (1 mg/kg, P.O.), and Vinpocetine (20 mg/kg, P.O.). The combination of Vinpocetine and EGCG demonstrated the strongest neuroprotection, according to the results. The marked decline in Aβ and ACHE suggested that the brain was protected. The results for BDNF and monoamine levels followed the same pattern [42]

MITOCHONDRIAL DISORDERS

CoQ10 plays a crucial role in mitochondrial function and overall cellular energy production. It is a lipid-soluble molecule found in the mitochondria, the energy-producing organelles in cells. Here are the primary roles and implications of CoQ10 in mitochondrial disorders: CoQ10 is often used as a therapeutic agent in various mitochondrial disorders where defects in mitochondrial function lead to energy deficits in cells. CoQ10 is a vital component of the electron transport chain (ETC), which is responsible for producing ATP (adenosine triphosphate), the primary energy currency of the cell. It functions as an electron carrier, shuttling electrons between complexes I and II to complex III in the *etc*. This process helps generate a proton gradient across the inner mitochondrial membrane, driving ATP synthesis. CoQ10 also acts as an antioxidant, protecting cells from oxidative damage caused by free radicals. This is particularly important in mitochondria, where a high rate of oxidative metabolism occurs, producing reactive oxygen species (ROS) as byproducts. By neutralizing ROS, CoQ10 helps maintain mitochondrial integrity and function. Mitochondrial disorders are a group of conditions caused by dysfunctional mitochondria, often due to mutations in mitochondrial DNA (mtDNA) or nuclear DNA affecting mitochondrial proteins. These disorders can lead to a range of symptoms, including muscle weakness, neurodegenerative diseases, and organ dysfunction. CoQ10 deficiency, whether primary (genetic) or secondary (due to other mitochondrial dysfunctions), can exacerbate these conditions. CoQ10 supplementation shows promise. Its effectiveness depend on the specific mitochondrial disorder, the degree of deficiency, and the formulation used. Further research is ongoing to optimize CoQ10 therapy for individuals with mitochondrial disorders.

MUSCLE HEALTH AND EXERCISE PERFORMANCE

Recent research has highlighted the role of coenzyme Q10 (CoQ10) in muscle health and exercise performance, emphasizing its importance in cellular energy production, antioxidant protection, and overall muscle function. CoQ10 supplementation can improve exercise performance and reduce fatigue, likely due to enhanced mitochondrial energy production and reduced oxidative damage during intense physical activity. Some research indicates that CoQ10 supplementation can enhance aerobic capacity and exercise performance, particularly in endurance athletes. For instance, a study found that CoQ10 supplementation improved time to exhaustion and VO2 max (maximal oxygen uptake) in trained athletes. CoQ10 may help reduce exercise-induced fatigue. In a study involving middle-aged men, CoQ10 supplementation was associated with decreased subjective fatigue levels and improved exercise performance. CoQ10 supplementation has been shown to lower markers of muscle damage, such as creatine kinase (CK) and lactate dehydrogenase (LDH), following strenuous exercise. Athletes taking CoQ10 supplements have reported faster recovery times and less muscle soreness after intense training sessions. A meta-analysis of randomized controlled trials concluded that CoQ10 supplementation could improve exercise performance, particularly in untrained or moderately trained individuals. However, the benefits were less pronounced in highly trained athletes. Research on individuals with chronic conditions, such as fibromyalgia and chronic fatigue syndrome, has shown that CoQ10 supplementation can lead to improvements in muscle function and overall quality of life. Typical dosages used in studies range from 100 to 300 mg per day. Higher doses may be required for therapeutic effects in individuals with significant deficiencies or higher energy demands.

AGING AND SKIN HEALTH

oQ10 is a potent antioxidant that helps reduce oxidative stress, a major contributor to the aging process. By neutralizing free radicals, CoQ10 can protect cells from damage and potentially slow down the aging process. Aging is associated with a decline in mitochondrial function. CoQ10 levels naturally decline with age, contributing to decreased cellular energy and increased oxidative damage. oQ10 supplementation has been shown to improve mitochondrial efficiency and energy production, which can help maintain cellular function and vitality in aging tissues.

CoQ10 has been found to enhance collagen production, which is crucial for maintaining skin elasticity and firmness. Increased collagen levels can reduce the appearance of wrinkles and fine lines. CoQ10 can help protect the skin from UV radiation-induced damage. Studies have shown that topical application of CoQ10 can reduce the depth of wrinkles and prevent oxidative damage caused by UV exposure. It is also used in topical formulations for skin care to reduce wrinkles and improve skin texture. Clinical studies have demonstrated that CoQ10 can reduce the visible signs of aging, such as wrinkles and fine lines. One study found that long-term use of CoQ10-containing creams significantly decreased wrinkle depth and improved skin smoothness. Research on oral CoQ10 supplementation for skin health is also promising. Oral CoQ10 can improve skin's antioxidant defenses and support overall skin health. A study found that oral supplementation with CoQ10 improved skin elasticity and reduced wrinkles after 12 weeks of use. Combining oral and topical CoQ10 treatments may offer synergistic benefits. This dual approach can address both systemic and localized oxidative stress, providing comprehensive support for skin health and anti-aging. CoQ10's primary mechanism is its antioxidant activity, which helps protect the skin from oxidative damage. This is particularly important in the skin, which is exposed to environmental stressors like UV radiation and pollution. Nanoparticles and liposomes are two advanced delivery systems that significantly enhance the bioavailability of CoQ10. Nanoparticles increase the solubility and surface area, improving dissolution and absorption, while liposomes protect CoQ10 from degradation and facilitate direct cellular uptake. Combining these approaches in CoQ10 supplementation offers a promising strategy for maximizing its therapeutic benefits, particularly for conditions requiring high bioavailability.

NATURAL QUINONES AS ANTICANCER AGENTS

A class of naphthofuranequinones was identified from *Tabebuia cassinoides*,

Tabebuia avellanedae, *Crescentia cujete*, and other natural sources. These compounds exhibit several biological characteristics, including antileukemic action and *in vitro* cytotoxicity against KB, K562, and P388 cells. When these quinones were tested against *T. cruzi*, most of them demonstrated an inhibitory effect on the parasite's respiration and the culture's growth [43].

ANTHRACYCLINES

The bacteria *Streptomyces coeruleorubidus* or *Streptomyces peucetius* naturally produce chemotherapy medication daunorubicin [44]. The two most well-known members are doxorubicin and daunorubicin, the latter of which has broad anticancer action against a range of solid malignancies in addition to acute leukemias. The former is mostly active against acute leukemias. Acute myeloid leukemia, acute lymphoblastic leukemia, chronic myelogenous leukemia, and Kaposi's sarcoma are all treated with daunorubicin [45]. The only difference between them on the side chain at position 9 is one hydroxyl group; these variations in clinical activity may come as a surprise. Unfortunately, these medications have drawbacks. The most significant of these is their dose-dependent cumulative cardiomyopathy, which can lead to clinical congestive heart failure even years after therapy ends and is frequently irreversible [46].

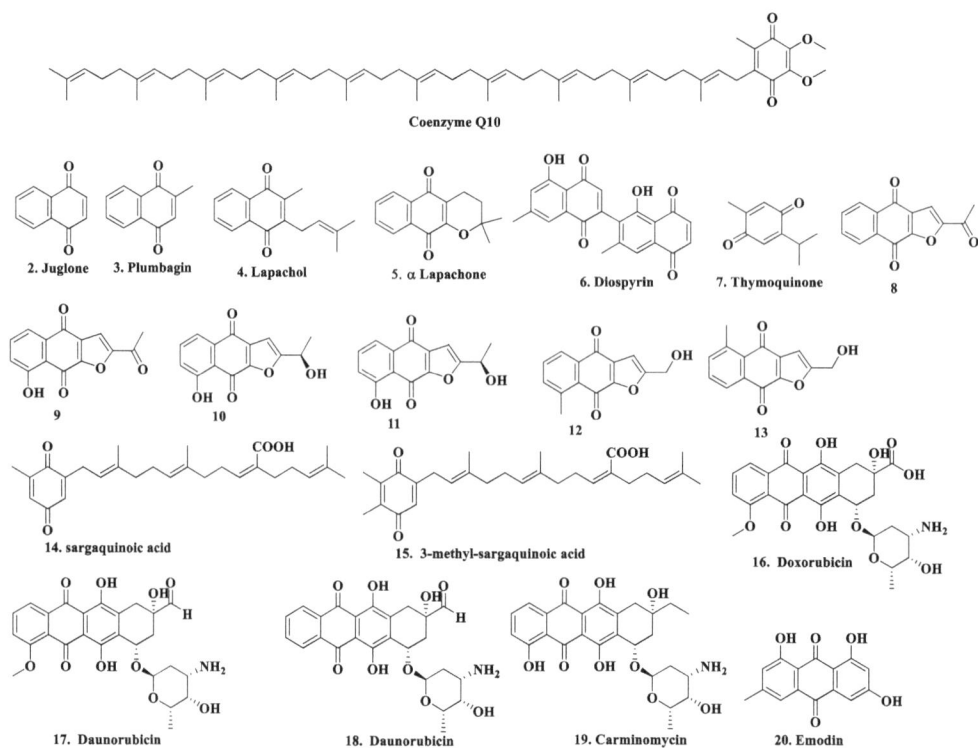

Coenzyme Q10

2. Juglone   3. Plumbagin   4. Lapachol   5. α Lapachone   6. Diospyrin   7. Thymoquinone   8

9   10   11   12   13

14. sargaquinoic acid   15. 3-methyl-sargaquinoic acid   16. Doxorubicin

17. Daunorubicin   18. Daunorubicin   19. Carminomycin   20. Emodin

BIOACTIVITY

Co-enzyme Q10: It acts as a vital component of the electron transport chain and is an antioxidant in the human body. Also, in its potential therapeutic applications in treating cardiovascular, neurodegenerative, and mitochondrial disorders, CoQ10 protects cells from oxidative damage by neutralizing free radicals and regenerating other antioxidants like vitamin E.

Juglone: It shows growth-inhibitory effects on bacteria or fungi and is employed by plants as a defensive compound.

Plumbagin: It has antibacterial, insecticidal, antiphlogistic, wound-healing, anticancer, antimicrobial, anti-inflammatory, antioxidant, and antiprotozoal properties.

Lappaconitine: Itpossesses various biological effects, viz., anticancer, antimalarial, analgesic, antiviral, antiparasitic, antipsoriatic, antioxidant, antimicrobial, antimetastatic, antileishmanial, anti-inflammatory, anti-abscess, anti-trypanosoma cruzi, anti-edemic, fungicidal, acaricidal, bactericidal, pesticidal, termiticidal, molluscicidal, schistosomicidal, insectifugal, and schistosomicidal.

Diospyrin: It possesses various biological effects like antioxidant, hepatoprotective, anti-inflammatory, analgesic, antipyretic, antihypertensive, antidiabetic, neuroprotective, antimicrobial, anti-protozoal, fungicidal, anthelmintic, insecticidal, molluscicidal, cytotoxicity, anti-tumor, multidrug resistance (MDR) reversal, and sedative.

Thymoquinone: Thymoquinone helps in convulsions, depression, memory improvement, nociception, and inflammation.

Sargaquinoic acid: It has anti-inflammatory properties and impedes macrophages' ability to produce nitric oxide by interfering with LPS-induced signaling.

Doxorubicin: Doxorubicin is a potent anticancer drug used in the treatment of various cancers, including breast cancer, leukemia, and lymphoma. It functions by intercalating DNA and inhibiting topoisomerase II, leading to DNA damage and apoptosis.

Emodin: Emodin has been investigated for its potential in cancer therapy, particularly against leukemia and solid tumors.

SYNTHETIC QUINONES AS DRUG CANDIDATES

Synthetic and natural quinones offer a rich source of compounds with diverse pharmacological properties, making them attractive candidates for drug development. Vitamin K_1, a derivative of naphthoquinone, aids in the carboxylation of glutamate to γ−carboxyglutamate and is necessary for blood coagulation [47]. Here is an overview of both synthetic and natural quinones and their potential as drug candidates:

SYNTHETIC QUINONES

1. **Menadione (Vitamin K3)**, primarily known as a synthetic derivative of naphthoquinone, is used as a vitamin supplement. Menadione has also been explored for its potential as an anticancer agent. It exhibits cytotoxic effects on cancer cells and has been studied in combination with other chemotherapy agents [48].
2. **Emitine** is a synthetic quinoline alkaloid. Emetine has historically been used as an anti-protozoal agent for treating amoebiasis. It works by inhibiting protein synthesis in the target organism [49].
3. **Doxorubicin** is a synthetic anthracycline antibiotic derived from the natural compound daunorubicin. Doxorubicin is a potent anticancer drug used in the treatment of various cancers, including breast cancer, leukemia, and lymphoma. It functions by intercalating DNA and inhibiting topoisomerase II, leading to DNA damage and apoptosis [2].
4. **Mitomycin C** is a synthetic anticancer agent. Mitomycin C is derived from Streptomyces bacteria. It works by crosslinking DNA, thereby inhibiting DNA replication and transcription in cancer cells.

Both synthetic and natural quinones offer diverse chemical structures and biological activities, providing ample opportunities for drug discovery and development. However, it is essential to conduct further research to optimize their pharmacokinetic properties, elucidate their mechanisms of action, and assess their safety and efficacy in clinical trials before they can be widely used as pharmaceuticals.

CONCLUSION

In conclusion, quinones, both synthetic and natural, have demonstrated significant potential as drug candidates due to their diverse biological activities. The pharmacological properties of quinones, including their roles as anticancer, antimicrobial, anti-inflammatory, and antioxidant agents, highlight their therapeutic versatility. In the kingdom of plants, anthraquinones are widely distributed, and many of them have exceptional therapeutic benefits and promising future markets. Since research on anthraquinones with a range of biological activities is widely recognized to be of great significance, an overview of related activity aspects undoubtedly helps lay the groundwork for future applications and can potentially serve as an inspiration for future pharmaceutical development. The anticancer properties of anthraquinones are linked to alterations at the C-1, C-2, C-3, and C-6 locations of the anthraquinone ring. Overall, the promising biological activities of quinones underscore their potential as valuable drug candidates. Their diverse biological activities, ranging from anticancer and antimicrobial to anti-inflammatory and antioxidant effects, underscore their therapeutic potential. Natural quinones, derived from various organisms, offer a rich source of bioactive compounds, while synthetic quinones provide opportunities for structural optimization and enhanced pharmacological properties. Despite the promising therapeutic potential of quinones, challenges such as toxicity, side effects, and drug resistance need to be addressed. Future research should focus on developing quinone derivatives with improved safety profiles and efficacy. Additionally, advancements in drug delivery systems can play a crucial role in enhancing the bioavailability and targeted delivery of quinone-based therapies. Ongoing research and development will be crucial in overcoming current limitations and harnessing the full therapeutic potential of both synthetic and natural quinones.

REFERENCES

[1]   Dahlem MA, Nguema Edzang RW, Catto AL. Raimundo J-MJIJoMS Quinones as an efficient molecular scaffold in the antibacterial/antifungal or antitumoral arsenal. 2023, 23 (22):14108

[2]   Zhang L, Zhang G, Xu S. Recent advances of quinones as a privileged structure in drug discovery. 2021, 223:113632.

[3]   Özenver N, Sönmez N. BARAN MY, Uz A, Demirezer LÖJTJoC. Structure-activity relationship of anticancer drug candidate quinones. 2024, 48 (1):152-165.

[4]   Malik EM. Müller CEJMrr. Anthraquinones as pharmacological tools and drugs. 2016, 36 (4):705-748.

[5]   Matysik G, Skalska-Kaminska A. Matysik-Wozniak AJTLCiP, 29Quinone Derivatives. 1998, 825:817.

[6]   Li Y, Jiang J-GJF. Function Health functions and structure–activity relationships of natural anthraquinones from plants. 2018, 9 (12):6063-6080.

[7]   Dahlem MA, Nguema Edzang RW, Catto AL. Raimundo J-MJIJoMS. Quinones as an efficient molecular scaffold in the antibacterial/antifungal or antitumoral arsenal. 2022, 23 (22):14108.

[8]   Widhalm JR, Rhodes DJHR. Biosynthesis and molecular actions of specialized 1, 4-naphthoquinone natural products produced by horticultural plants, 2016.

[9]   Qiu HY, Wang PF, Lin HY, Tang CY, Zhu HL. Yang YHJCb, design d. Naphthoquinones: A continuing source for discovery of therapeutic antineoplastic agents. 2018, 91 (3):681-690.

[10]   Erdoğan Ü, Özmen Ö. Özer MJJoEOBP. Wound Healing, anti-analgesic, and antioxidant activity of Nigella sativa Linn., essential based topical formulations in rat model experimental skin defects. 2023, 26 (1):45-60.

[11]   Croft S, Weiss C. Natural products with antiprotozoal activity.bioassay Methods in Natural Product Research and Drug Development. Springer 1999; pp. 81-99. [http://dx.doi.org/10.1007/978-94-011-4810-8_7]

[12]   Gwon W-G, Lee B, Joung E-J, *et al.* Kim H-RJJoA. Chemistry F Sargaquinoic acid inhibits TNF---induced NF-κB signaling, thereby contributing to decreased monocyte adhesion to human umbilical vein endothelial cells (HUVECs). 2015, 63 (41):9053-9061.

[13]   Qiu HY, Wang PF, Lin HY, Tang CY, Zhu HL. Yang YHJCb, design d. Naphthoquinones: A continuing source for discovery of therapeutic antineoplastic agents. 2018, 91 (3):681-690.

[14]   Riaz MT, Yaqub M, Shafiq Z, *et al.* Synthesis, biological activity and docking calculations of bis-naphthoquinone derivatives from Lawsone. 2021, 114:105069.

[15]   Hook I, Mills C. Sheridan HJSinpc. Bioactive naphthoquinones from higher plants. 2014, 41:119-160.

[16]   Saini RJJoP, Sciences B. Coenzyme Q10: The essential nutrient. 2011, 3 (3):466-467.

[17]   Rodick TC, Seibels DR, Babu JR, *et al.* Potential role of coenzyme Q10 in health and disease conditions. 2018, 1-11.

[18]   Mandelker LJSovm. Oxidative stress, free radicals, and cellular damage. 2011, 1-17.

[19]   Fong CW. Coenzyme Q 10 and Vitamin E synergy, electron transfer, antioxidation in cell membranes, and interaction with cholesterol. Eigenenergy Adelaide South Australia Australia 2023.

[20]   Barcelos IPd, Haas RHJB. CoQ10 and aging.8(2):28, Gonzalez MJ, Miranda-Massari JR Mitochondrial Correction. 2019.

[21]   Nair SV, Baranwal G, Chatterjee M, *et al.* Biswas RJIJoMM. Antimicrobial activity of plumbagin, a naturally occurring naphthoquinone from Plumbago rosea, against Staphylococcus aureus and Candida albicans. 2016, 306 (4):237-248.

[22]   Nair SV, Baranwal G, Chatterjee M, Sachu A, Vasudevan AK, Bose C, Banerji A, Biswas RJIJoMM. Antimicrobial activity of plumbagin, a naturally occurring naphthoquinone from Plumbago rosea, against Staphylococcus aureus and Candida albicans. 2016, 306 (4):237-248.

[24]   Liang J, Hsiu S, Wu P. Chao PJPm. Emodin pharmacokinetics in rabbits. 1995, 61 (05):406-408.

[25]   Lin S-P, Chu P-M, Tsai S-Y, Wu M-H. Hou Y-CJJoe. Pharmacokinetics and tissue distribution of resveratrol, emodin and their metabolites after intake of Polygonum cuspidatum in rats. 2012, 144 (3):671-676.

[26]   Lin S-P, Chu P-M, Tsai S-Y, Wu M-H. Hou Y-CJJoe. Pharmacokinetics and tissue distribution of resveratrol, emodin and their metabolites after intake of Polygonum cuspidatum in rats. 2012, 144 (3):671-676.

[27]   Boulos JC, Rahama M, Hegazy M-EF, Efferth TJCl. Shikonin derivatives for cancer prevention and therapy. 2019, 459:248-267.

[28]   Han H, Sun W, Feng L, *et al.* Differential relieving effects of shikonin and its derivatives on inflammation and mucosal barrier damage caused by ulcerative colitis. 2021, 9:e10675.

[29]   Hussain H, Krohn K, Ahmad VU, Miana GA, Green IRJA. Lapachol: an overview. 2007, 2 (1):145-171.

[30]   Babula P, Adam V, Havel L, Kizek RJCPA. Noteworthy secondary metabolites naphthoquinones-their occurrence, pharmacological properties and analysis. 2009, 5 (1):47-68.

[31]   Fouillaud M, Venkatachalam M, Girard-Valenciennes E, Caro Y. Dufossé LJMd. Anthraquinones and derivatives from marine-derived fungi: Structural diversity and selected biological activities. 2016, 14 (4):64.

[32]   Müller K, Sellmer A. Wiegrebe WJJoNP. Potential antipsoriatic agents: lapacho compounds as potent inhibitors of HaCaT cell growth. 1999, 62 (8):1134-1136.

[33]   Rauf A, Uddin G, Patel S, *et al.* Diospyros, an under-utilized, multi-purpose plant genus: A review. Biomed Pharmacother 2017; 91: 714-30.
[http://dx.doi.org/10.1016/j.biopha.2017.05.012] [PMID: 28499243]

[34]   Asche CJMrimc. Antitumour quinones. 2005, 5 (5):449-467.

[35]   Amin B, Hosseinzadeh HJPm. Black cumin (Nigella sativa) and its active constituent, thymoquinone: an overview on the analgesic and anti-inflammatory effects. 2016; 82 (01/02):8-16.

[36]   Kavaliauskas P, Opazo FS, Acevedo W, *et al.* Synthesis, biological activity, and molecular modelling studies of naphthoquinone derivatives as promising anticancer candidates targeting COX-2. 2022, 15 (5):541.

[37]   Kavaliauskas P, Opazo FS, Acevedo W, *et al.* Synthesis, biological activity, and molecular modelling studies of naphthoquinone derivatives as promising anticancer candidates targeting COX-2. 2022, 15 (5):541.

[38]   Zhu Z-G, Sun M-X, Zhang W-L, Wang W-W, Jin Y-M, Xie C-LJNS. The efficacy and safety of coenzyme Q10 in Parkinson's disease: a meta-analysis of randomized controlled trials. 2017; 38:215-224.

[39]   Sheykhhasan M, Amini R, Asl SS, Saidijam M, Hashemi SM, Najafi RJB. Neuroprotective effects of coenzyme Q10-loaded exosomes obtained from adipose-derived stem cells in a rat model of Alzheimer's disease. 2022; 152:113224.

[40]   Dumont M, Kipiani K, Yu F, *et al.* Beal MFJJoAsd. Coenzyme Q10 decreases amyloid pathology and improves behavior in a transgenic mouse model of Alzheimer's disease. 2011; 27 (1):211-223.

[41]   Qiu HY, Wang PF, Lin HY, Tang CY, Zhu HL. Yang YHJCb, design d. Naphthoquinones: A continuing source for discovery of therapeutic antineoplastic agents. 2018; 91 (3):681-690.

[42]   Ali AA, Khalil MG, Abd El-Latif DM, Okda T, Abdelaziz AI, Kamal MM. Wahid AJaoG, Geriatrics. The influence of vinpocetine alone or in combination with Epigallocatechin-3-gallate, Coenzyme COQ10, Vitamin E and Selenium as a potential neuroprotective combination against aluminium-induced Alzheimer's disease in Wistar Albino Rats. 2022; 98:104557.

[43]   O Salas C, Faúndez M, Morello A, Diego Maya J, A Tapia RJCmc. Natural and synthetic naphthoquinones active against Trypanosoma cruzi: an initial step towards new drugs for Chagas disease. 2011; 18 (1):144-161.

[44]   Hulst MB, Zhang L, van der Heul HU, *et al.* Biotechnology. Metabolic engineering of Streptomyces peucetius for biosynthesis of N, N-dimethylated anthracyclines. 2024; 12:1363803.

[45]   Asche CJMrimc. Antitumour quinones. 2005; 5 (5):449-467.

[46]   Asche CJMrimc (2005) Antitumour quinones. 5 (5):449-467 O Salas C, Faúndez M, Morello A, Diego Maya J, A Tapia RJCmc. Natural and synthetic naphthoquinones active against Trypanosoma cruzi: an initial step towards new drugs for Chagas disease. 2011; 18 (1):144-161.

[47]   Chatterjee K, Mazumder PM. Banerjee SJRBdF. Vitamin K: a Potential Neuroprotective Agent. 2023; 33 (4):676-687.

[48]   Braasch-Turi M, Crans DCJM. Synthesis of naphthoquinone derivatives: menaquinones, lipoquinones and other vitamin K derivatives. 2020; 25 (19):4477.

[49]   Croft S, Weiss C. Natural products with antiprotozoal activity.Bioassay Methods in Natural Product Research and Drug Development. Springer 1999; pp. 81-99.
[http://dx.doi.org/10.1007/978-94-011-4810-8_7]

CHAPTER 8

Understanding Quinones with Reference to Biochemistry

Adil Ali[1], Mohd Hasan Mujahid[1], Ankit Paul[1] and **Tarun Kumar Upadhyay[1,*]**

[1] *Department of Biotechnology, Parul Institute of Applied Sciences and Research and Development Cell, Parul University, Vadodara 391760, Gujarat-India*

Abstract: Quinones are a highly flexible group of organic molecules that are naturally present in a diverse range of organisms, such as plants, algae, bacteria, and fungi. These chemicals are also artificially produced in laboratories for diverse purposes. Quinones possess a distinctive chemical structure that allows them to get involved in redox cycling. This means they can easily switch between oxidized and reduced states, a property that underlies many of their biological and pharmacological functions. They have a crucial function in the electron transport chain in both cellular respiration and photosynthesis. They help transmit electrons, which is essential for energy production in cells. Quinones play a crucial role in cellular signaling pathways and defense mechanisms against oxidative stress due to their capacity to perform redox reactions. Quinones possess a diverse array of pharmacological properties, making them highly valuable in the field of medicine. One of the most important uses of these is in the field of anticancer treatments. Quinone-derived chemicals serve as the foundation for some of the most extensive and potent categories of anticancer medications. Their cytotoxic qualities, which allow them to cause cell death in cancer cells, are utilized in treatments for different types of malignancies. Quinones can be classified into several broad categories, including anthraquinones, benzoquinones, phenanthraquinones, and naphthoquinones. These categories consist of a wide range of molecules that have unique chemical structures and biological properties. These classes constitute the fundamental components of numerous natural and synthetic products utilized across multiple industries.

Keywords: Anticancer properties, Novel drug, Oxidative stress, Pharmacological properties, Quinones, Redox reaction.

INTRODUCTION

Quinones are a group of chemical compounds representing a subclass of the quinoid family characterized by conjugated cyclic dione (–CH= groups converted

---

[*] **Corresponding author Tarun Kumar Upadhyay:** Department of Biotechnology, Parul Institute of Applied Sciences and Research and Development Cell, Parul University, Vadodara 391760, Gujarat-India; E-mail: tarun_bioinfo@yahoo.co.in

Ashutosh Kumar Dash & Deepak Kumar (Eds.)

to $\rightarrow$ –C (=O)– groups) structures and consisting of quinonimines and quinomethanes (Fig. **1**). This chemical group is mostly formed from reactive aromatic compounds like catechols or phenols. Their presence has been determined not only in natural products and biochemicals but also in pharmaceuticals and are requisite compounds having an extensive range of bioactivities [1, 2]. Since quinones represent the group of both naturally existing and synthetically prepared chemicals and are known to exhibit an extensive range of bioactivities such as antitumor, anti-bacterial, anti-cancer, and anticoagulant properties, they are widely applicable for medicinal and industrial purposes [3]. However, DNA is the main target of quinoid antitumor drugs, which contain the structure cyclohexadienedione. It is highly abundant and may be found in endogenous biochemicals, natural products, and environmental pollutants; these agents are alkylating and DNA intercalating agents. Secondly, quinoid chemicals have been demonstrated to target other cellular components, which include heat shock protein (HSP) 90 and telomerase [4, 5]. Examples of some compounds are aziridinylquinones (mitomycin C and Diaziridinyl-benzoquione) [6], naphthoquinones (vitamin K1, phylloquinone) [7], anthracyclines (Daunorubicin, Doxorubicin) [8], aminoquinones (such as streptonigrins), indolequinones (such as mitomycins), and certain vitamins that induce the production of hydrogen peroxide (H_2O_2) in tumor cells *via* redox cycling mechanism and autoxidation reaction to show anticancer activity [9] (Fig. (**2**). The isolation of quinone has been a research topic of global interest in recent times. ^{13}C nuclear magnetic resonance (NMR) spectroscopy is used in the analysis of the intersections of nature-derived quinones. Gathered data from past publications from 2000 to 2022 showed that out of 137 compounds, 70 were newly described [10]. From the biochemistry aspect, the quinones are important reduction-oxidation mediators for numerous electron-transfer chain (ETC) pathways in living systems and, as such, are crucial to countless enzymatic and physiological functional systems such as ubiquinone and plastoquinone and various naturally occurring quinones [11].

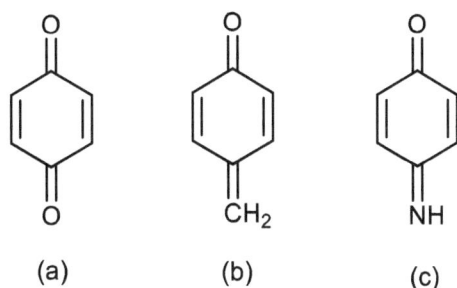

(a)   (b)   (c)

Fig. (1). Simplified structure of quinoids: a) *p*- Benzoquinone b) *p*- Benzoquinone methide c) *p*-Benzoquinone imine.

Mitomycins   Aziridinyl benzoquinone   Doxorubicin

Daunorubicin   Streptonigrins

Vitamin K (Phylloquinone)

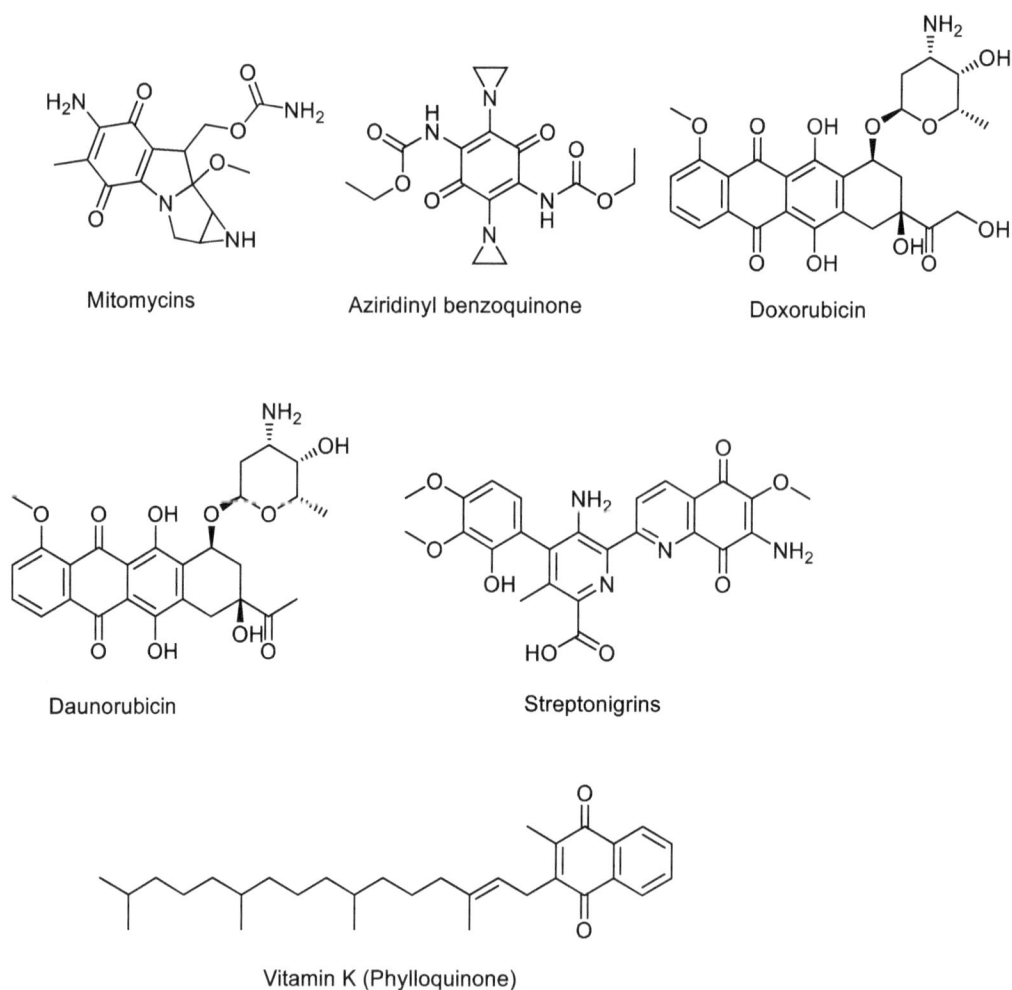

Fig. (2). Diagrammatical illustration of the 2D structure of the different compounds containing quinones moiety.

ISOLATION AND CHARACTERIZATION OF QUINONES

Natural quinones are derived from henna and juglone (walnuts) as well as from various sources such as microorganisms and animals. They are categorized based on the aromatic system in which they are found. The four primary groups of quinones are benzoquinones, naphthoquinones, anthraquinones, and phenanthraquinones, which encompass the majority of known compounds (Table **1**). The subclassification of quinone is shown in Table **2** [10]. Quinone derivatives are often obtained through the process of maceration, percolation, or a mixture of both methods. Before applying these approaches, it is crucial to understand the characteristics of the dissolving solvents (polar or non-polar) to be utilized as they ascertain the solvency of the desired material and impact the effectiveness of the isolation process. According to certain authors, when extracting benzo-quinones ($C_6H_4O_2$), it is preferable to exploit low-polarity solvents, such as dichloromethane, ethyl acetate, and butanol. On the other hand, to obtain naphthoquinones and anthraquinones, it is suggested to aid higher polarity solvents, such as methyl alcohol and ethyl alcohol [12]. The quinone derivative's extraction and distillation can be achieved mainly through conventional chromatographic practices, such as column chromatography, preparatory thin-layer chromatography, and instrumental techniques, including high-pressure liquid chromatography and ultra-high pressure liquid chromatography coupled to mass spectrometry. The compounds can be identified, and their conformations can be determined using 1H and 13C, both unidimensional and bidimensional NMR, as well as infrared (IR) spectroscopic approaches [10]. In general, IR analyses have been shown in spectra that contain both high and low-intensity bands. As a result, benzoquinones can be recognized in the high-intensified bands ranging from 300 to 1650 cm^{-1} and in the low-intensified band at 3200 cm^{-1}. The range of 700 to 1800cm^{-1} has the most potent peaks for naphthoquinones, with a low band at 3200cm^{-1}. On the other hand, anthraquinones display intense peaks in the region of 400cm^{-1}-1810cm^{-1}, with less intensified peaks appearing at about 3300cm^{-1} [12], [10].

Table 1. Categorization of different quinones.

Class	Basic conformation	References
Benzoquinone	1,2-benzoquinone 1,4-benzoquinone	[13]
Naphthoquinone	1,4-naphthoquinone	[14]

Class	Basic conformation	References
Anthraquinone	9,10-anthraquinone	[15]
Phenanthraquinone	Phenanthraquinone	[16]

Table 2. Categorization of quinone sub-classes

Class	Subclass
Benzoquinones	• Monohydroxy benzoquinone • Dihydroxy benzoquinone • Miscellaneous benzoquinones
Naphthoquinones	• Monohydroxy naphthoquinones • Dihydroxy naphthoquinones • Trihydroxy naphthoquinones • Furano naphthoquinones • Piranot Naphthoquinones • Binaphthoquinones
Anthraquinones	• Monohydroxy anthraquinones • Dihydroxy anthraquinone • Trihydroxy anthraquinones • Tetrahydroxy anthraquinones • Furano anthraquinones • Anthraquinone glycosides • Tetrahydro anthraquinone
Phenanthraquinones	Not applicable

BIOSYNTHESIS OF QUINONES

Quinones are compounds formed from the oxidation of phenols. They are distinguished by having two carbonyl groups that are conjugated with a minimum of two double bondings. Quinones are produced in higher-order plants through multiple metabolic processes [17]. The derivatives of hydroxyanthracene can be synthesized from acetyl or malonyl-coenzyme-A units.

Additional approaches involving biosynthesis may employ O-succinyl benzoic acid to synthesize juglone, phylloquinone, and lawsona. Additionally, other naphthoquinones are produced from 4-hydroxybenzoic acid (PHBA). Some quinone compounds, like ubiquinones, have a combination of sources in their biosynthesis. The ring structure is created through the acetate pathway or by the polyketide pathway, while the side chain is derived from the isoprene units [10].

Anthraquinones and other anthraquinone chemicals are largely produced through the malonyl-Coenzyme-A pathway in higher-order plants (Leguminosae families), lichens (Polygonaceae family), and fungi (Ramnaceae family) [18]. In this method, as shown in Fig. (**3**, one unit or one molecule of acetyl-CoA is sequentially combined with 7 molecules or 7 units of the malonyl-CoA to form a long 16-carbon chain compound known as octacetide. Afterward, the octacetide compound undergoes bending and cyclization through condensation reactions between the carbene (C=O) groups and adjacent groups of carbonyls, resulting in the formation of a tricyclic ketone. This intermediary further undergoes analysis to generate the nucleus of the anthrone. Enzymatic dimerization of the nucleus containing anthrone yields diantrones, while the oxidation reaction of the nucleus marks the foundation of anthranols or anthra-quinones [10].

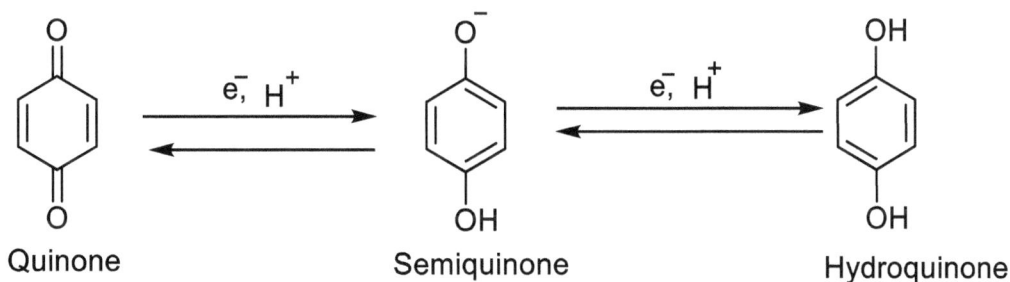

Fig. (3). Malonyl-CoA-mediated anthracene chemical production process. Adopted from Source: Martinez [17].

BENZOQUINONES

Benzoquinones are a specific class of quinones that have a basic chemical formula of $C_6H_4O_2$. There are two primary isomers: 1,4-benzoquinone (often referred to as quinone) and 1,2-benzoquinone (sometimes known as ortho-benzoquinone). The 1,4-isomer is the predominant form and is commonly distinguished by a hexa-membered (6) benzene ringed with 2 opposing carbonyl groups (C=O) instead of two hydrogen atoms. Benzoquinones are characterized by their unique yellow color and intense, pungent odor. They have important functions in biological systems and are crucial in industrial applications. Benzoquinones are naturally occurring compounds that can be retrieved from a variety of plant species and microorganisms. They aid as electron carriers in the processes of cellular respiration and photosynthesis. Ubiquinone, often known as coenzyme Q, plays a vital role as a constituent of the *etc* in mitochondria. Benzoquinones possess antibacterial capabilities, rendering them significant in the field of medical and pharmaceutical research. Benzoquinones are utilized as intermediates in the industrial synthesis of dyes, polymers, and various other compounds. They are also utilized in photography, namely in developing certain photographic processes. The process of creating benzoquinones usually entails the oxidation of hydroquinones and their reduced counterparts, which can be derived from phenolic compounds by several chemical processes. Although benzoquinones have practical applications, they can also pose risks. They possess irritating properties and can induce skin and respiratory complications upon contact. Proper handling of benzoquinones necessitates the implementation of suitable safety measures, such as the utilization of personal protective equipment. Their reactive nature also makes them valuable in organic synthesis, where they participate in various chemical reactions to produce more complex molecules [19].

NAPHTHOQUINONES

Naphthoquinones are a type of chemical compound that has a naphthalene ring with two ketones (C=O) functional groups. The chemical formula of naphthoquinones is $C_{10}H_6O_2$, and they exist in several isomeric forms. Among these forms, 1,4-naphthoquinone, commonly referred to as naphthoquinone, is the most abundant. These chemicals are ubiquitous and can be found in various microorganisms, including bacteria and fungi, and green plants. Naphthoquinones exhibit bright yellow-to-red colors and play a noteworthy function in several bioprocesses. Vitamin K is a widely recognized naphthoquinone that plays a vital role in blood clotting. Vitamin K appears in multiple forms, such as phyllo-quinone (also called Vitamin K1), present in almost all fruits and veggies, and menaquinones (also called Vitamin K2), created by bacteria. Naphthoquinones, such as juglone, found in walnuts, serve as natural pesticides, protecting the plants from herbivores and pathogens. Naphthoquinones possess a diverse array of biological actions, making them highly valuable in the domain of medicinal chemistry [20]. They exhibit antibacterial, antiviral, antifungal, and anticancer characteristics. Their action often involves redox cycling and the production of free reactive oxygen radicals (ROS) that may damage cellular pieces of machinery like DNA, RNA, proteins, peptides, fatty acids, and lipids, resulting in cell death. Naphthoquinones possess strong efficacy against a wide range of infections and cancer cells. Naphthoquinones have industrial applications in addition to their biological importance. They function as precursors for the production of dyes, pigments, and other chemical compounds. Their capacity to engage in redox reactions is utilized in several applications, including their role as electron transfer agents in batteries and other electrical devices. Although naphthoquinones have advantageous applications, they can also be hazardous and necessitate cautious treatment. Exposure to a substance can result in irritation to the skin, eyes, and respiratory system. In large concentrations, such exposure can be hazardous. Hence, it is imperative to implement appropriate safety precautions when handling these substances. In general, naphthoquinones are a flexible and important chemical group with various applications in nature, medicine, and industry [21].

ANTHRAQUINONES

Anthraquinones are a group of chemical compounds that originate from anthracene and have the molecular formula $C_{14}H_8O_2$. These compounds possess a quinone structure connected to an aromatic anthracene ring, forming a unique three-ring system with two carbonyl groups (C=O) located at positions 9 and 10. Anthraquinones are ubiquitous and are especially abundant in diverse living systems. Anthraquinones are found in various plant parts like roots, bark, leafage, and fruits. Notable examples of plants containing anthraquinones include aloe, rhubarb, and senna. These molecules fulfill diverse ecological functions, including preventing herbivores, defending against microbial diseases, and attracting pollinators with their bright colors, which span from yellow to crimson. Anthraquinones are widely recognized for their therapeutic effects. Emodin, chrysophanol, and aloin are key constituents found in both traditional and modern laxatives. They function by inducing peristalsis and enhancing the release of water and electrolytes in the colon, therefore promoting bowel motions. Nevertheless, the overuse of this substance can result in negative consequences, including disturbances in electrolyte levels and the development of dependency. In addition to their laxative qualities, anthraquinones possess heterogenous bioactivities, such as antibacterial, antiviral, anti-inflammatory, and antioncogenic effects [22]. The main cause of these effects is mostly due to their capacity to insert themselves between the DNA strands, hinder enzymes, and generate ROS, resulting in oxidative stress and the demise of infections and cancer cells. Anthraquinones possess notable industrial uses. These substances are employed as dyes and pigments, particularly in the textile sector, because of their durability and bright colors. Alizarin, a well-known anthraquinone dye, was initially obtained from the madder plant and has a historical significance in the dyeing of textiles. Although certain anthraquinones have therapeutic applications, they can also be hazardous and have the potential to cause cancer. Therefore, it is important to handle and regulate their use cautiously, especially in food and medicine. Ongoing research is being conducted to investigate the potential and limitations of these entities, with the goal of utilizing their qualities for therapeutic and industrial purposes while minimizing any associated hazards. Anthraquinones are a very adaptable and important group of molecules that play many roles in nature, medicine, and industry [23].

PHENANTHRAQUINONES

Phenanthraquinones are chemical molecules that have a distinct structure consisting of three rings, with two ketone groups (C=O) usually found on the middle ring. The chemical formula for phenanthraquinones is $C_{14}H_8O_2$. These molecules are less prevalent than other quinones, yet they are of significance due to their distinct chemical characteristics and biological functions. Phenanthraquinones are nature-derived compounds that can be unearthed in a wide range of plant species, fungi, and certain marine creatures. They frequently assume functions in the defensive mechanisms of these organisms, serving as antibacterial and antifungal agents.

Phenanthraquinones in plants and fungi serve to repel diseases and discourage herbivores, thus enhancing their ability to survive and thrive in their natural environment. A significant characteristic of phenanthraquinones is their capacity to engage in redox reactions, which plays a pivotal role in their biological functionality. These chemicals are capable of engaging in electron transfer activities, resulting in the production of ROS. The characteristic of phenanthraquinones to induce cytotoxicity is accredited to their capability to produce ROS, which can instigate detrimental effects on cellular constituents such as DNA, proteins, and lipids, ultimately resulting in the cell's demise. The cytotoxicity of phenanthraquinones is very valuable in anticancer studies, as it allows for the targeted destruction of cancer cells while leaving normal cells unharmed, and some of the biological activities are shown in Fig. (**4**. Phenanthraquinones have anti-inflammatory effects, making them a subject of interest for advancing therapies for inflammatory conditions [24]. Furthermore, researchers are also investigating the potential therapeutic implications of their antibacterial and antiviral activity in combating a variety of infections. Phenanthraquinones are utilized as intermediates in the manufacture of dyes, pigments, and other chemical compounds in manufacturing processes. Due to their stability and bright colors, they are well-suited for applications in the textile industry and other fields that demand robust and vibrant materials. Although phenanthraquinones, like other quinones, possess advantageous properties, they can also be dangerous and require cautious treatment. Exposure to these substances can result in skin, eye, and respiratory irritation, and their cytotoxic qualities indicate that large dosages can be detrimental. Hence, it is imperative to implement appropriate safety precautions when handling phenanthraquinones in both laboratory and industrial environments. Phenanthraquinones are a collection of substances that are both intriguing and have considerable significance in the fields of biology and industry [25].

BIOCHEMICAL PROPERTIES

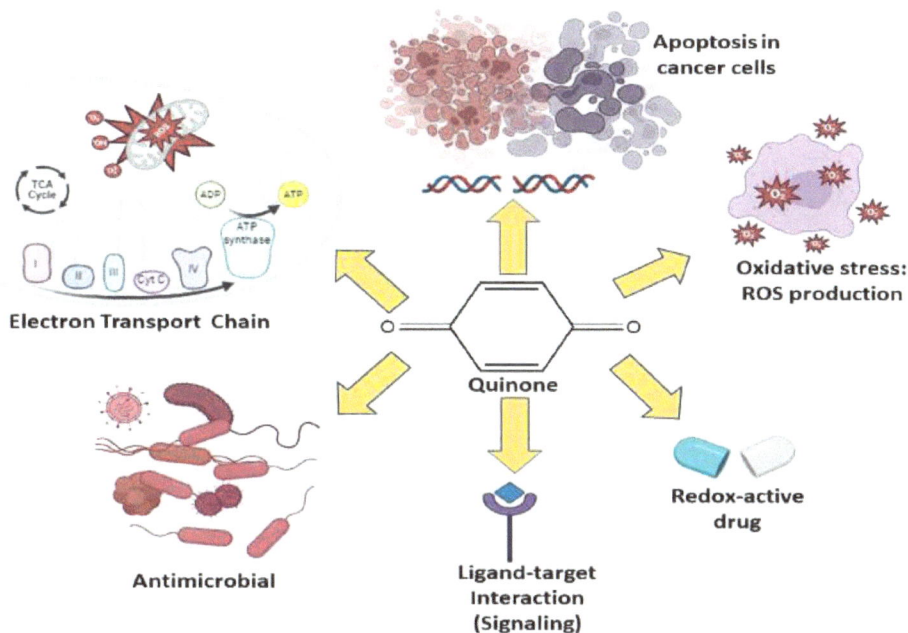

Fig. (4). Schematic illustration of different biological activities of quinones

REDOX REACTION: OXIDATION AND REDUCTION STATES

In practically every organism, quinones are ubiquitous and involved in biological electron (e⁻) transfer processes and play critical roles in these activities. Quinones are very effective chemicals in terms of their capability to undertake reduction-oxidation reactions and can undergo oxidation (loss of e-) or reduction (gain of e-), depending on the circumstances present in their current environment. As a result of this, they are efficient agents for the transport of electrons in a wide range of different processes [26]. Due to the fact that they are redox-characterized, quinones can be found doing almost anything in several biological, chemical, and electronic processes. Electrostatics may play a vital role in the interfaces that might occur between the molecules of quinones [27]. With features such as high energy density, fast charging rates, and stable cycling, these molecules have garnered great interest in energy storage applications, particularly in rechargeable batteries. By generating semiquinone radicals that are persistent through electrochemical processes, quinones have shown that they can act as anticancer agents in the field of cancer research [28]. This highlights the potential therapeutic significance of quinones, which is shown in Fig. (**5.** Quinones include semi-volatile chemicals like 1,2-naphthoquinone and 1,4-benzoquinone, which can occur naturally. It has been recognized that upon reduction, they generate ROS, which can lead to various toxicological effects ranging from cancer to apoptosis [29]. Quinones, including coenzyme Q, are an indispensable component of mitochondria's electron transport chain (ETC), which moves electrons across complexes and generates ATP. Quinones are indispensable constituents of the *etc* because they play a role as electron carriers. This makes them capable of shuttling electrons from dehydrogenases to oxidizing pathways in redox reactions when present [30]. Secondly, quinones participate in the process of formation of reactive oxygen species in mitochondria. They can generate superoxide anions (O^{2-}) directly or act as antioxidants protecting from oxidative damage [31]. Quinones are very important for the effective function of the mitochondrial *etc* of living systems because they are involved in the passage of electrons, synthesis of ATP, and maintenance of redox balance to ensure stability at the cellular level (homeostasis) [32]. Quinone organic cyclic compounds take part in the energy conversion processes, electron transfer, respiration, and photosynthesis. In organic chemistry, 2,3-Dichloro-5,6-dicyano-p-benzoquinone and tetrachloroquinone are two common quinones that often find application as stoichiometric reagents in organic synthesis. Recently, the usage of transition metals or electrochemistry to regenerate oxidized quinones has been developed with catalytic applications. By this example, one sees that the quinone structure impacts reaction processes and the development of catalysis [33].

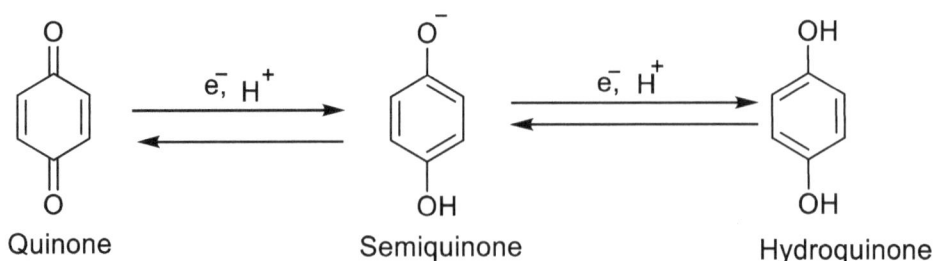

Fig. (5). The simple reversible redox reaction of quinone/hydroquinone redox couple.

QUINONE: A SIGNALING MOLECULES

Quinones are essential signaling molecules in various species, playing vital roles in biological phenomena. For example, a phytoquinone, 2,6-dimethoxy-1-4-benzoquinone (DMBQ), induces the growth of feeding structures and induces genes related to the defense response. This induction is brought about by an influx of cytosolic Ca^{2+} due to leucine-rich-repeat receptor-like kinases [34]. Alkyl quinolones (AQs) are used by microbes, such as *Pseudomonas aeruginosa*, to communicate with one another for interspecies and interkingdom interaction. This interaction plays an equally essential part in both virulence and disease [35]. The Pseudomonas quinolone signal (PQS) has been linked to iron (Fe^{3+}) absorption, the promotion of cell death, and immune regulation. Thus, this new knowledge expands our understanding of the functions of quinones outside of quorum sensing [36]. Chemically, quinones can modify proteins by redox-cycling mechanisms that yield free radicals and through the covalent attachment of quinones to nucleophiles, such as cysteine residues in glutathione (GSH) and proteins. These adducts can cause enzymes to be deactivated, create protein cross-links, and initiate signaling pathways that lead to eventual apoptotic cell demise. Additionally, the oxidation of cysteine residues in Trx also induces the ASK1-mediated p38-MAPK signaling pathway and, as a result, triggers the stimulation of the pathways that induce the death of the cells through apoptosis [37, 38].

PHARMACOLOGICAL ACTIVITY

Numerous researches have been performed on the pharmacological activities of quinones, particularly in the exploration and creation of new drugs [11]. Quinones possess certain inherent characteristics, such as electrophilicity and the capacity for reversible oxido-reduction reactions, which make them highly promising for biological applications [39]. Based on this, analyses of the structural-activity relationship (SAR) of quinones indicate that the greater the polarity of the substituent group in the aromatic system, the greater the corresponding pharmacological activity [40]. The antibacterial potential of quinones and their biological features have been extensively studied. Aloesaponarin showed antibacterial activity against four microorganisms that are resistant to many drugs. Furthermore, it had a higher inhibitory effect when compared against gentamicin. These effects are linked to the existence and arrangement of substituents like carbomethoxy and methyl [10].

It has been important to recognize that the way bacteria resist antibiotics involves the use of enzymes to deactivate the action of antibiotics, allowing changes in the bacterial wall and failure of efflux pump systems. These processes should be studied further to understand how compounds can be effective against bacteria [41]. According to Wang *et al.* [42], the compound 2-methoxy 1,4-naphthoquinone has shown promise in eliminating infections instigated by *Helicobacter pylori*. It is believed to be because of the high reduction-oxidation potential of its hydroquinone form. Quinone derivatives play a significant role in carrying out antiparasitic activities. Naphtho-furanquinone, glycol-quinone, and avice-quinone C showed antiparasitic properties against *Trypanosoma brucei* [43], whereas phenanthra-quinones, burmanin A, B, and C, had such effects on

Leishmania spp [44]. Different biomedical applications are shown in Table **3**. Quinones, such as atovaquone and ubiquinone, have proven potential to suppress the cytochrome bc1 complex of the mitochondrial respiratory chain. This inhibition leads to the lack of mitochondrial functionality in Plasmodium spp. or other protozoan [45]. It is believed that this mechanism of action is possibly the original function of structurally similar quinones.

Table 3. Different quinone compounds with their biomedical applications.

S.No.	Quinone compound	PubChem Id	Source	Structure	Biomedical application	Reference
1.	Alizarin	6293	*Rubia tinctorum*; extracted from the root part.		Towards G⁺: *S. aureus* (MRSA MW2 & MSSA 25923) strains and with *S. epidermidis* (ATCC 14990) showed $\geq$ 70% biofilm inhibition.	[47]
2.	Blattellaquinone	11379050	German cockroaches (*Blattella germanica*), as used to communicate (sex pheromones) with each other, are secreted from the pharyngeal body of insects.		Prominent action in pest control	[48 - 50]
3.	Geldanamycin	5288382	Isolated from the *Streptomyces hygroscopicus*		Antiproliferative action towards MCF-7 (breast carcinoma) cell line (Inhibitory Concentration$_{50}$ =0.03 μM) binding with HsP90.	[51 - 53]
4.	Coenzyme PQQ (pyrroloquinoline quinone)	1024	Isolated from the bacterial sp. *P. aeruginosa*, and *Methylobacterium extorquens*		The antioxidant and anti-inflammatory properties give it promising potential for the treatment of asthma and allergic reactions.	[54 - 56]
5.	Ubiquinones (CoQ10)	119058	Wholegrain cereals, soya beans, meat, fatty fish, nuts, and vegetables like spinach and broccoli are rich in ubiquinone, a vital nutrient.		Useful in clinical diagnostics due to its function in mitochondrial electron transport, trans membranous H⁺ translocation, and antioxidant properties.	[57 - 59]

S.No.	Quinone compound	PubChem Id	Source	Structure	Biomedical application	Reference
6.	Doxorubicin (DXR)	31703	Isolated from *Streptomyces peucetius var. caesius* found in soil.		Chemotherapy drug-induced cell demise occurs through the generation of ROS and DNA-adducted structures that elicit apoptosis and inhibition of topoisomerase II.	[59, 60]
7.	Mitomycin	5746	In *Streptomyces caespitosus*, mitomycin derived from the GlcN (D-glucosamine) and AHBA (N-glycoside composed of a 3-amino-5-hydroxybenzoic acid, $C_7H_7NO_3$) units		Clinically being used as a cancer chemotherapy drug.	[61]
8.	Phylloquinone (Vit. K_1)	5284607	Obtain from green leafy vegetables, vegetable oils, broccoli, spinach, cyanobacteria, green algae, gut microbiota, *etc.*		Required for vascular metabolism, blood coagulation, and bone health.	[7, 62]
9.	Indanthrone	6690	Synthetically produced through dimerization and then cyclization, and oxidation steps.		Indanthrone derivatives have anticancer and anti-inflammatory properties.	[63, 64]
10.	Indan-1,3-dione (isatin)	11815	Synthesis using condensation and decarboxylation method; cyanation and decarboxylation with hydrolysis method.		It stops the action of urease and is used to treat peptic ulcers.	[65, 66]
11.	1,4-Benzoquinone	4650	Two-step Blanc reaction and oxidation from 2,3,4,5-tetramethoxytoluene.		Targeting crucial proteins, drug carrier molecules, and better water solubility	[67, 68]
12.	Lawsone (2-hydroxy-1, 4-naphthoquinone)	6755	Single one-step synthesis includes one-pot synthesis using urea hydrogen peroxide.		Antiplatelet agent; antioxidant, antibacterial, and antifungal properties.	[69 - 71]

S.No.	Quinone compound	PubChem Id	Source	Structure	Biomedical application	Reference
13.	Chloranil (tetrachloro-1,--benzoquinone) (TCBQ)	8371	Tetrachloro-1,4-benzoquinone can be prepared environmentally using tetrachloro-1,4-benzenediol as the raw material and a composite oxidant of sodium chlorite and hydrogen peroxide under certain conditions.		TCBQ can synthesize 1,4-benzoquinone derivatives by various nucleophilic substitution processes; hence, it becomes a good option for drug discovery and medicinal chemistry, apoptosis, intracellular ROS generation, and cytotoxicity against three breast cancer subtypes.	[68, 72]
14.	Juglone (1,4-naphthoquinone)	3806	Metabolite produced in *Juglans nigra*		Antibacterial, sedative, antifungal, antihypertensive, oxidizing, and antiproliferative.	[73]
15.	Naphthoquinones	4227422	Synthesis through one-pot experiment from 2-phenylamino-1-4-naphthoquinones; palladium-catalyzed oxidation of polycyclic naphthalenes to produce fused 1,2-naphthoquinones.		Antioxidant, hypoglycemic potential; cytotoxic.	[74, 75]
16.	Anthraquinones	6780	Oxidation methods have produced electron-deficient aromatic ketones with anthraquinone units, also found in lichens, fungi, and plants.		These chemicals are potential treatments for COVID-19 because of their anti-inflammatory, antioxidant, anticancer, antiviral, and antibacterial activities.	[76 - 78]
17.	2,6-Dimethoxy-1,4-benzoquinone (DMBQ)	68262	DMBQ is found in the juice of *Vitis coignetiae* (mountain grape or Chinese grapes).		Having anti-tumorigenic, anti-inflammatory, and anti-mutagenic components.	[79]

S.No.	Quinone compound	PubChem Id	Source	Structure	Biomedical application	Reference
18.	Plumbagin (PB)	10205	Different families, such as *Ebenaceae, Plumbaginacea*e, and *Droseraceae*, including *Plumbago rosea* and Plumbago zeylanica, PB, are isolated from the roots.		Anti-inflammatory, antioxidant, and anticancer properties.	[80, 81]
19.	Menadione	4055	Synthetically made from 2-methy--1,4-naphthoquinone as a precursor molecule.		Has limited biomedical applications due to potential toxicity.	[82]

Quinones are widely used in clinical practice as a significant class of anticancer drugs [46]. Rhein and aloe-emodin, which are anthraquinone derivatives, strongly suppress the proliferation of HCT or HepG2 cancer cells. This article discusses the bioactivity of quinones, with their capability to suppress the enzyme acetylcholinesterase and their slow aging effects. These properties are summarized in Table **4**.

Table 4. Biological effects of quinones

Compound	Bioactivity	References
Allomicrophyllone	Slow aging	[85]
1,2-dimethoxy-6-methyl-9,10 anthraquinone, (chrysazin)	Anti-malarial activity	[86]
3,4-dihydroxy-1-methoxy anthraquinone-2-carboxaldehyde, (rhein anthrone)	Antimycotic	[87]
6,8-dihydroxy-3-methylanthraquinone, (Ehretiquinone)	Slow aging	[85]
2-hydroxy-3-methylanthraquinone., (Ehretiquinona C)	Slow aging	[85]
2-hydroxy-3-methoxy-9,10-anthraquinone, (Ehretiquinona D)	Slow aging	[85]
3,3'-methylenebis(6-ethyl-4-hydroxy-5-methyl-2H-pyran-2-one), Heliotropinone A	Antimycotic	[87]
Heliotropinone B, (heliespirone B)	Antimycotic	[87]
5-methoxyangenylalkannin	Anti-neoplastic effect	[88]
2-methyl-6-(3-methyl-2 butenyl) benzo-1,4-quinone, (2-methyl-6-geranyl benzoquinone)	Antibacterial activity	[89]
2-methoxy-1,4-naphthoquinone, (MQ)	Antimicrobial and bactericidal activity	[42]

Compound	Bioactivity	References
Morindaparvin E, (6-methoxy-2-cyclohexen-1)	Cell-based toxicity against breast, HeLa cervical, ovarian, and cancer cells	[90]
Morindaparvin F, (Moringin)	Cell-based toxicity against breast, HeLa cervical, ovarian, and cancer cells	[90]
Sterekunthal-A	Anti-malarial activity	[91]
Pyranokuntona A, (pyranoindole)	Anti-malarial activity	[91]
Cynoglosol, (Cynoglossum zeylanicum)	Cell-based toxicity against the HL-60 cancer cell line	[92]
Juglone, (5-hydroxy-1,4-naphthoquinone)	Cell-based toxic	[93]
Glycoquinone, (glucosylthio quinone)	Sleeping sickness	[43]
Aloesaponarin I, (glucosylthio quinone)	Antimicrobial or anti-malarial activity	[94]
Chrysophanol, (chrysophanic acid or Chr)	Suppression of acetylcholinesterase	[95]
Symploquinone A, (cochlioquinone A)	Antimicrobial and bacterial biofilm	[15]
Tectograndone, (tectochrysin)	Antimicrobial	[96]
Physcion, (PSN)	Suppression of acetylcholinesterase	[95]
Xanthopurpurin, (XPP)	Cell-based toxicity against breast cancer cell line	[97]
Rubiadin, (1,3-dihydroxy-2-methyl anthraquinone)	Anti-malarial activity	[98]
Rubiacordone A, (6-acetoxy-1-hydroxy-2-methylanthraquinon--3-O-α-L-rhamnopyranoside)	Anti-malarial activity	[91]
Kniphofiones A, (Kniphofia)	Anti-malarial activity	[99]
Calanquinone A, (5-hydroxy-3,6,7-trimethoxy-1,4-phenanthrenequinone)	Cell-based toxicity against cancer cells of the breast, lung, colon, prostate	[16]

Compound	Bioactivity	References
Calanquinone B, (calothrixin B)	Cell-based toxicity against breast and prostate cancer cell lines	[100]
Calanquinone C, (5-hydroxy-3,6,7-trimethoxy-1,4-phenanthrenequinone)	Cell-based toxicity against breast and prostate cancer cell lines	[100]
Burmanin A, (cinnaburmanin A)	Cell-based toxicity and kala-azar (leishmaniasis) activity	[44]
Burmanin-B	Cell-based toxicity and kala-azar (leishmaniasis) activity	[44]
Burmanin C, (burmannic acid)	Cell-based toxicity and kala-azar (leishmaniasis) activity	[44]
Neodiospyrin, (neosartorin)	Cell-based study suppress effect of 12(S)-HETE	[101]
Prisconnatanone I, (indole fused spiro-1,4-diazocane)	Cell-based toxicity against lung tumor cell	[102]
p-hydroxy methoxy benzobijuglone, (p-hydroxy-3-methoxy acetophenone)	Anti-tumorigenic	[103]
Rhein, (9,10-Dihydro-4,5-dihydroxy-9,10-dioxo-2-anthracenecarboxylic acid)	Cell-based toxicity against HepG2 cancer cell line and HCT	[104]
Helminthosporin	Dual acylcholine acylhydrolase suppression	[95]
Acetylshikonin	Cell-based toxicity against HepG2 cancer cell line and HCT 116	[104]
α-methylbutyrylshikonin, (acetylshikonin)	Antimicrobial and cell-based toxicity activity against the breast carcinoma, MDA-MB 231 cancer cell line	[105]

Compound	Bioactivity	References
Xanthopurpurin, (XPP)	Cell-based toxicity against breast carcinoma cells	[97]

PHARMACOKINETIC PROPERTIES

Pharmacokinetics seeks to explain the complete trajectory of the medication throughout the human body, encompassing crucial stages such as absorption, distribution, metabolism, and elimination. Assessing these criteria is crucial for developing safe and effective pharmaceuticals while requiring the lowest possible concentrations to ensure human well-being [83]. Hence, focusing on pharmacokinetic assessments of substances that have the potential to facilitate the advancement of novel medications is of paramount significance. Quinones attract interest because of their wide range of pharmacological activity (as shown in Table **4**) and their potential for confirmational alteration, rendering them promising candidates for potent or specific medicines [10]. This chemical category possesses distinct benefits: (1) They function as adaptable units to localize dependent functional groups for the purpose of optimizing bond formation; (2) They act as crucial components in pharmaceuticals, facilitating non-covalent interactions to enhance occupancy of binding position in specific drug targets; (3) They additionally contribute to metabolic pathways and biological oxidation processes by acting as redox agents. These qualities enhance and contribute to the therapeutic effects of different diseases [10]. Naphthoquinones and anthraquinones, which are among the primary categories of quinone derivatives, have significant and well-established medical importance. A limited number of isolated compounds of benzoquinones and phenanthraquinones have been reported in the literature. Consequently, there has been a lack of cohort studies focusing on understanding the pharmacokinetic mechanisms of these compounds. Research primarily emphasizes the therapeutic capabilities of naphthoquinones and anthraquinones in treating different types of cancers. These compounds act through many mechanisms, such as promoting cell differentiation, inhibiting processes related to cell death, preventing the spread of cancer cells, and halting the cell cycle [84]. A confirmational-activity link indicates that the confirmational durability and the occurrence of hydroxyl groups at sites C-8 and C-5 in naphthoquinones or at sites C-8 and C-1 in anthraquinones can improve pharmacokinetic and pharmacodynamic activities. Qin devised a technique to assess the pharmacokinetics of anthraquinones, particularly rhein, aloe-emodin, and emodin, through the oral intake of individual nature-based herbal components derived from rhei rhizome or cheng qi-tang in rat blood serum. Using drug disposition variables such as Cmax, AUC, and Tmax, the absorption of all the constituents in the query is enhanced upon delivery in a CCT combination.

Further research has been conducted to enhance the absorption of anthraquinones. Gomes de Carvalho *et al.* [10] showed that emodin cannot be effectively taken orally because it is poorly absorbed, has low bioavailability in living organisms, and is quickly eliminated. Inhibition of glucuronidation metabolism can enhance the pharmacokinetic characteristics.

Acetyl shikonin, a kind of naphthoquinone, is found in various parts of the body, particularly in the colon and stomach. It is not easily absorbed and has a high rate of binding to human plasma proteins. Further pharmacokinetic investigations are required to elucidate its metabolic routes [10].

CONCLUSION

Quinones are important biochemical compounds that play a vital role in various biological processes, specifically in electron transport and redox reactions. They are essential for cellular respiration and photosynthesis as they participate in electron transfer chains. The redox properties of quinones are crucial for their function in biological systems, allowing for the conversion and storage of energy. Quinones are also involved in signaling pathways and defense mechanisms in living organisms. Furthermore, they have been widely researched for their various bioactivities, as demonstrated in this study, including their potential medicinal uses in the treatment of diseases such as malarial parasites and carcinoma. Additionally, quinones have the potential to be used in the synthesis of novel analogs, aiming to create further potent or specific medication and link their activity and structure.

FUTURE PERSPECTIVE

Future research on quinones is poised to explore their potential in therapeutic applications, mainly in treating mitochondrial dysfunction and disorders associated with oxidative stress. Advancements in biotechnology and synthetic biology can produce quinone-based pharmaceuticals and antioxidants. Quinones can interact with various proteins, which can lead to non-specific signaling. This can make it difficult to achieve a specific cellular response. Moreover, further elucidation of quinone biosynthesis pathways may reveal novel targets for antibiotic and anticancer therapies. Additionally, the application of quinones in bioengineering and renewable energy, such as bio-inspired solar cells and bioelectronic devices, represents a promising area for sustainable technological innovations.

ACKNOWLEDGMENT

The authors are thankful to Geetika Madan Patel, Vice President & Medical Director, as well as the R&D team of the Research and Development Cell, Parul University, Vadodara, for providing the facility and motivation to carry out multidisciplinary collaborative publication.

REFERENCES

[1] Bolton J. Quinone Methide Bioactivation Pathway: Contribution to Toxicity and/or Cytoprotection? Curr Org Chem 2014; 18(1): 61-9.
[http://dx.doi.org/10.2174/1385272818011401211230046] [PMID: 25346613]

[2] Sokolova K V, Podpletnia O A, Konovalova S O, Avdeenko A P. KomarovskaPorokhnyavets, O. Z, Lubenets, V. I, Kovalenko, S. I. N-Arylsulfonyl-2-Aroylamino-1,4- Quinone Imines and Their Hydrogenated Analogues: Prediction of Toxicity and Prospects for Use as Diuretics. Медичні перспективи = Medicni perspektivi (Medical perspectives) 2023; No. 2, 20–28.

[3] Lin M, Han P, Li Y, Wang W, Lai D, Zhou L. Quinoa Secondary Metabolites and Their Biological Activities or Functions. Molecules 2019; 24(13): 2512.
[http://dx.doi.org/10.3390/molecules24132512] [PMID: 31324047]

[4] Rendic S, Guengerich FP. Contributions of human enzymes in carcinogen metabolism. Chem Res Toxicol 2012; 25(7): 1316-83.
[http://dx.doi.org/10.1021/tx300132k] [PMID: 22531028]

[5] Faizan S, Mohammed Abdo Mohsen M, Amarakanth C, *et al.* Quinone scaffolds as potential therapeutic anticancer agents: Chemistry, mechanism of Actions, Structure-Activity relationships and future perspectives. Results Chem 2024; 7: 101432.
[http://dx.doi.org/10.1016/j.rechem.2024.101432]

[6] Winski SL, Hargreaves RH, Butler J, Ross D. A new screening system for NAD(P)H:quinone oxidoreductase (NQO1)-directed antitumor quinones: identification of a new aziridinylbenzoquinone, RH1, as a NQO1-directed antitumor agent. Clin Cancer Res 1998; 4(12): 3083-8.
[PMID: 9865924]

[7] Basset GJ, Latimer S, Fatihi A, Soubeyrand E, Block A. Phylloquinone (Vitamin K1): Occurrence, Biosynthesis and Functions. Mini Rev Med Chem 2017; 17(12): 1028-38.
[http://dx.doi.org/10.2174/1389557516666160623082714] [PMID: 27337968]

[8] Soni I, Kumari A, Jayaprakash GK, Naik P, Rajendrachari S. Evaluation of the role of ionic liquid as a modifier for carbon paste electrodes in the detection of anthracyclines and purine-pyrimidine-based anticancer agents. Mater Res Express 2024; 11(1): 012005.
[http://dx.doi.org/10.1088/2053-1591/ad1bff]

[9] Ali T, Li D, Ponnamperumage TNF, *et al.* Generation of Hydrogen Peroxide in Cancer Cells: Advancing Therapeutic Approaches for Cancer Treatment. Preprints 2024.
[http://dx.doi.org/10.20944/preprints202405.0194.v1]

[10] Gomes de Carvalho NK, Wellisson da Silva Mendes J, Martins da Costa JG. Quinones: Biosynthesis, Characterization of ^{13}C Spectroscopical Data and Pharmacological Activities. Chem Biodivers 2023; 20(12): e202301365.
[http://dx.doi.org/10.1002/cbdv.202301365] [PMID: 37926679]

[11] Zhang L, Zhang G, Xu S, Song Y. Recent advances of quinones as a privileged structure in drug discovery. Eur J Med Chem 2021; 223: 113632.
[http://dx.doi.org/10.1016/j.ejmech.2021.113632] [PMID: 34153576]

[12] Dulo B, Phan K, Githaiga J, Raes K, De Meester S. Natural Quinone Dyes: A Review on Structure,

Extraction Techniques, Analysis and Application Potential. Waste Biomass Valoriz 2021; 12(12): 6339-74.
[http://dx.doi.org/10.1007/s12649-021-01443-9]

[13]   Barreto A, Santiago V, Freire R, *et al.* Magnetic nanosystem for cancer therapy using oncocalyxone a, an antitomour secondary metabolite isolated from a Brazilian plant. Int J Mol Sci 2013; 14(9): 18269-83.
[http://dx.doi.org/10.3390/ijms140918269] [PMID: 24013376]

[14]   Prawat U, Chaimanee S, Butsuri A, Salae AW, Tuntiwachwuttikul P. Bioactive styryllactones, two new naphthoquinones and one new styryllactone, and other constituents from *Goniothalamus scortechinii.* Phytochem Lett 2012; 5(3): 529-34.
[http://dx.doi.org/10.1016/j.phytol.2012.05.007]

[15]   Farooq U, Khan S, Naz S, *et al.* Three new anthraquinone derivatives isolated from *Symplocos racemosa* and their antibiofilm activity. Chin J Nat Med 2017; 15(12): 944-9.
[http://dx.doi.org/10.1016/S1875-5364(18)30011-6] [PMID: 29329652]

[16]   Lee CL, Nakagawa-Goto K, Yu D, *et al.* Cytotoxic calanquinone A from *Calanthe arisanensis* and its first total synthesis. Bioorg Med Chem Lett 2008; 18(15): 4275-7.
[http://dx.doi.org/10.1016/j.bmcl.2008.06.099] [PMID: 18640035]

[17]   Martínez A M. Quinonas y compuestos relacionados.

[18]   Schripsema J, Ramos-Valdivia A, Verpoorte R. Robustaquinones, novel anthraquinones from an elicited Cinchona robusta suspension culture. Phytochemistry 1999; 51(1): 55-60.
[http://dx.doi.org/10.1016/S0031-9422(98)00470-1]

[19]   Dandawate PR, Vyas AC, Padhye SB, Singh MW, Baruah JB. Perspectives on medicinal properties of benzoquinone compounds. Mini Rev Med Chem 2010; 10(5): 436-54.
[http://dx.doi.org/10.2174/138955710791330909] [PMID: 20370705]

[20]   Ventura Pinto A, Lisboa de Castro S. The trypanocidal activity of naphthoquinones: a review. Molecules 2009; 14(11): 4570-90.
[http://dx.doi.org/10.3390/molecules14114570] [PMID: 19924086]

[21]   Kumagai Y, Shinkai Y, Miura T, Cho A K. The Chemical Biology of Naphthoquinones and Its Environmental Implications. Annual Review of Pharmacology and Toxicology 2012; 52: 221-47.
[http://dx.doi.org/10.1146/annurev-pharmtox-010611-134517]

[22]   Rahman MM, Islam MR, Akash S, *et al.* Naphthoquinones and derivatives as potential anticancer agents: An updated review. Chem Biol Interact 2022; 368: 110198.
[http://dx.doi.org/10.1016/j.cbi.2022.110198] [PMID: 36179774]

[23]   Wellington KW, Understanding K. Understanding cancer and the anticancer activities of naphthoquinones – a review. RSC Advances 2015; 5(26): 20309-38.
[http://dx.doi.org/10.1039/C4RA13547D]

[24]   Steck E A, Day A R. Reactions of Phenanthraquinone and Retenequinone with Aldehydes and Ammonium Acetate in Acetic Acid Solution1. ACS Publications.
[http://dx.doi.org/10.1021/ja01243a043]

[25]   Zhang ZJ, Zhang XQ, Ye WC, Wang Y, Che CT, Zhao SX. A new 1,4-phenanthraquinone from Menispermum dauricum. Nat Prod Res 2004; 18(4): 301-4.
[http://dx.doi.org/10.1080/14786410310001620592] [PMID: 15214480]

[26]   Prince RC, Dutton PL, Gunner MR. The aprotic electrochemistry of quinones. Biochim Biophys Acta Bioenerg 2022; 1863(6): 148558.
[http://dx.doi.org/10.1016/j.bbabio.2022.148558] [PMID: 35413248]

[27]   Pingale SS, Ware AP, Gadre SR. Unveiling electrostatic portraits of quinones in reduction and protonation states. J Chem Sci 2018; 130(5): 50.
[http://dx.doi.org/10.1007/s12039-018-1450-3]

[28] Krayz GT, Bittner S, Dhiman A, Becker JY. Electrochemistry of Quinones with Respect to their Role in Biomedical Chemistry. Chem Rec 2021; 21(9): 2332-43.
[http://dx.doi.org/10.1002/tcr.202100069] [PMID: 34107155]

[29] Sousa ET, Lopes WA, de Andrade JB. Fontes, formação, reatividade e determinação de quinonas na atmosfera. Quim Nova 2016; 39: 486-95.
[http://dx.doi.org/10.5935/0100-4042.20160034]

[30] Zhao RZ, Jiang S, Zhang L, Yu ZB. Mitochondrial electron transport chain, ROS generation and uncoupling (Review). Int J Mol Med 2019; 44(1): 3-15.
[http://dx.doi.org/10.3892/ijmm.2019.4188] [PMID: 31115493]

[31] Wang F, Stahl SS. Electrochemical Oxidation of Organic Molecules at Lower Overpotential: Accessing Broader Functional Group Compatibility with Electron–Proton Transfer Mediators. Acc Chem Res 2020; 53(3): 561-74.
[http://dx.doi.org/10.1021/acs.accounts.9b00544] [PMID: 32049487]

[32] Sarewicz M, Osyczka A. Electronic connection between the quinone and cytochrome C redox pools and its role in regulation of mitochondrial electron transport and redox signaling. Physiol Rev 2015; 95(1): 219-43.
[http://dx.doi.org/10.1152/physrev.00006.2014] [PMID: 25540143]

[33] Wendlandt AE, Stahl SS. Quinone☐Catalyzed Selective Oxidation of Organic Molecules. Angew Chem Int Ed 2015; 54(49): 14638-58.
[http://dx.doi.org/10.1002/anie.201505017] [PMID: 26530485]

[34] Laohavisit A, Wakatake T, Ishihama N, *et al.* Quinone perception in plants *via* leucine-rich-repeat receptor-like kinases. Nature 2020; 587(7832): 92-7.
[http://dx.doi.org/10.1038/s41586-020-2655-4] [PMID: 32879491]

[35] Reen F J, McGlacken G P, O'Gara F. The Expanding Horizon of Alkyl Quinolone Signalling and Communication in Polycellular Interactomes 2018.
[http://dx.doi.org/10.1093/femsle/fny076]

[36] Lin J, Cheng J, Wang Y, Shen X. The *Pseudomonas* Quinolone Signal (PQS): Not Just for Quorum Sensing Anymore. Front Cell Infect Microbiol 2018; 8: 230.
[http://dx.doi.org/10.3389/fcimb.2018.00230] [PMID: 30023354]

[37] Shu N, Hägglund P, Cai H, Hawkins CL, Davies MJ. Modification of Cys residues in human thioredoxin-1 by *p*-benzoquinone causes inhibition of its catalytic activity and activation of the ASK1/p38-MAPK signalling pathway. Redox Biol 2020; 29: 101400.
[http://dx.doi.org/10.1016/j.redox.2019.101400] [PMID: 31926625]

[38] Chen SH, Li CW. Detection and Characterization of Catechol Quinone-Derived Protein Adducts Using Biomolecular Mass Spectrometry. Front Chem 2019; 7: 571.
[http://dx.doi.org/10.3389/fchem.2019.00571] [PMID: 31497592]

[39] El-Najjar N, Gali-Muhtasib H, Ketola RA, Vuorela P, Urtti A, Vuorela H. The chemical and biological activities of quinones: overview and implications in analytical detection. Phytochem Rev 2011; 10(3): 353-70.
[http://dx.doi.org/10.1007/s11101-011-9209-1]

[40] Li Y, Jiang JG. Health functions and structure–activity relationships of natural anthraquinones from plants. Food Funct 2018; 9(12): 6063-80.
[http://dx.doi.org/10.1039/C8FO01569D] [PMID: 30484455]

[41] Garneau-Tsodikova S, Labby KJ. Mechanisms of resistance to aminoglycoside antibiotics: overview and perspectives. MedChemComm 2016; 7(1): 11-27.
[http://dx.doi.org/10.1039/C5MD00344J] [PMID: 26877861]

[42] Garneau-Tsodikova, S, J. Labby, K. Mechanisms of Resistance to Aminoglycoside Antibiotics: Overview and Perspectives. MedChemComm 2016; 7 (1), 11–27. Available from:

https://www.proquest.com/openview/537513ba94b4f808f783ff7c8d70b142/1?pq-origsite=gscholar&c bl=2037463

[43] Mazlan NW, Clements C, Edrada-Ebel R. Targeted Isolation of Anti-Trypanosomal Naphthofuran-Quinone Compounds from the Mangrove Plant *Avicennia lanata.* Mar Drugs 2020; 18(12): 661.
[http://dx.doi.org/10.3390/md18120661] [PMID: 33371387]

[44] Mori-Yasumoto K, Izumoto R, Fuchino H, *et al.* Leishmanicidal activities and cytotoxicities of bisnaphthoquinone analogues and naphthol derivatives from Burman *Diospyros burmanica.* Bioorg Med Chem 2012; 20(17): 5215-9.
[http://dx.doi.org/10.1016/j.bmc.2012.06.055] [PMID: 22858297]

[45] Patel OPS, Beteck RM, Legoabe LJ. Antimalarial application of quinones: A recent update. Eur J Med Chem 2021; 210: 113084.
[http://dx.doi.org/10.1016/j.ejmech.2020.113084] [PMID: 33333397]

[46] Nonell S, Bresolí Obach R, Agut Bonsfills M, *et al.* On the Mechanism of Candida Tropicalis Biofilm Reduction by the Combined Action of Naturally-Occurring Anthraquinones and Blue Light RECERCAT. Dipòsit de la Recerca de Catalunya 2017.
[http://dx.doi.org/10.1371/journal.pone.0181517]

[47] Abou Elmaaty T, Sayed-Ahmed K, Magdi M, Elsisi H. An eco-friendly method of extracting alizarin from Rubia tinctorum roots under supercritical carbon dioxide and its application to wool dyeing. Sci Rep 2023; 13(1): 30.
[http://dx.doi.org/10.1038/s41598-022-27110-0] [PMID: 36593257]

[48] Wada-Katsumata A, Schal C. Antennal grooming facilitates courtship performance in a group-living insect, the German cockroach Blattella germanica. Sci Rep 2019; 9(1): 2942.
[http://dx.doi.org/10.1038/s41598-019-39868-x] [PMID: 30814635]

[49] Liang S, Zhang Y, Li J, Yao S. Phytochemical Profiling, Isolation, and Pharmacological Applications of Bioactive Compounds from Insects of the Family Blattidae Together with Related Drug Development. Molecules 2022; 27(24): 8882.
[http://dx.doi.org/10.3390/molecules27248882] [PMID: 36558015]

[50] Mishra SS, Shroff S, Sahu JK, Naik PP, Baitharu I. Insect Pheromones and Its Applications in Management of Pest Population.Natural Materials and Products from Insects: Chemistry and Applications. Cham: Springer International Publishing 2020; pp. 121-36.
[http://dx.doi.org/10.1007/978-3-030-36610-0_8]

[51] Turbyville TJ, Wijeratne EMK, Liu MX, *et al.* Search for Hsp90 inhibitors with potential anticancer activity: isolation and SAR studies of radicicol and monocillin I from two plant-associated fungi of the Sonoran desert. J Nat Prod 2006; 69(2): 178-84.
[http://dx.doi.org/10.1021/np058095b] [PMID: 16499313]

[52] Ibrahim SRM, Mohamed SGA, Altyar AE, Mohamed GA. Natural Products of the Fungal Genus Humicola: Diversity, Biological Activity, and Industrial Importance. Curr Microbiol 2021; 78(7): 2488-509.
[http://dx.doi.org/10.1007/s00284-021-02533-6] [PMID: 34003333]

[53] Zhang H, Sun GZ, Li X, Pan HY, Zhang YS. A new geldanamycin analogue from Streptomyces hygroscopicus. Molecules 2010; 15(3): 1161-7.
[http://dx.doi.org/10.3390/molecules15031161] [PMID: 20335971]

[54] Pyrroloquinoline quinone (PQQ): Role in Plant-Microbe Interactions | SpringerLink. Available from: https://link.springer.com/chapter/10.1007/978-981-13-5862-3_9 (accessed 2024-05-29).

[55] Carpagnano GE, Resta O, Foschino-Barbaro MP, *et al.* Exhaled Interleukine-6 and 8-isoprostane in chronic obstructive pulmonary disease: effect of carbocysteine lysine salt monohydrate (SCMC-Lys). Eur J Pharmacol 2004; 505(1-3): 169-75.
[http://dx.doi.org/10.1016/j.ejphar.2004.10.007] [PMID: 15556150]

[56]   Good NM, Vu HN, Suriano CJ, Subuyuj GA, Skovran E, Martinez-Gomez NC. Pyrroloquinoline Quinone Ethanol Dehydrogenase in Methylobacterium extorquens AM1 Extends Lanthanide-Dependent Metabolism to Multicarbon Substrates. J Bacteriol 2016; 198(22): 3109-18.
[http://dx.doi.org/10.1128/JB.00478-16] [PMID: 27573017]

[57]   Timofeeva EO, Gorbunova EV, Chertov AN. Fluorescence Analysis of Ubiquinone and Its Application in Quality Control of Medical Supplies. 2017.
[http://dx.doi.org/10.1117/12.2252879]

[58]   Shaikh S. Sources and Health Benefits of Functional Food Components.Current Topics in Functional Food. IntechOpen 2022.
[http://dx.doi.org/10.5772/intechopen.104091]

[59]   Hutchinson CR, Colombo AL. Genetic engineering of doxorubicin production in Streptomyces peucetius : a review. J Ind Microbiol Biotechnol 1999; 23(1): 647-52.
[http://dx.doi.org/10.1038/sj.jim.2900673] [PMID: 10455495]

[60]   Lee J, Choi MK, Song IS. Recent Advances in Doxorubicin Formulation to Enhance Pharmacokinetics and Tumor Targeting. Pharmaceuticals (Basel) 2023; 16(6): 802.
[http://dx.doi.org/10.3390/ph16060802] [PMID: 37375753]

[61]   Wang S, Cheng Y, Wang X, Yang Q, Liu W. Tracing of Acyl Carrier Protein-channeled Mitomycin Intermediates in *Streptomyces caespitosus* Facilitates Characterization of the Biosynthetic Steps for AHBA–GlcN Formation and Processing. J Am Chem Soc 2022; 144(32): 14945-56.
[http://dx.doi.org/10.1021/jacs.2c06969] [PMID: 35943208]

[62]   Vambhurkar G, Amulya E, Sikder A, *et al.* Nanomedicine based potentially transformative strategies for colon targeting of peptides: State-of-the-art. Colloids Surf B Biointerfaces 2022; 219: 112816.
[http://dx.doi.org/10.1016/j.colsurfb.2022.112816] [PMID: 36108367]

[63]   Khattab T, Rehan M. A review on synthesis of nitrogen-containing heterocyclic dyes for textile fibers - Part 1: Five and six-membered heterocycles. Egypt J Chem 2018; 0(0): 0.
[http://dx.doi.org/10.21608/ejchem.2018.4130.1362]

[64]   Pluskota R, Koba M. Indandione and Its Derivatives - Chemical Compounds with High Biological Potential. Mini Rev Med Chem 2018; 18(15): 1321-30.
[http://dx.doi.org/10.2174/1389557518666180330101809] [PMID: 29600759]

[65]   Singh K. Applications of Indan-1,3-Dione in Heterocyclic Synthesis. Curr Org Synth 2016; 13(3): 385-407.
[http://dx.doi.org/10.2174/1570179412666150817222851]

[66]   Bano B, Kanwal , Khan KM, *et al.* Benzylidine indane-1,3-diones: As novel urease inhibitors; synthesis, *in vitro*, and in silico studies. Bioorg Chem 2018; 81: 658-71.
[http://dx.doi.org/10.1016/j.bioorg.2018.09.030] [PMID: 30253339]

[67]   Shuveksh P S, Ahmed K, Padhye S, Schobert R, Biersack B. Chemical and Biological Aspects of the Natural 1,4-Benzoquinone Embelin and its (semi-)Synthetic Derivatives.
[http://dx.doi.org/10.2174/0929867324666170116125731]

[68]   Qiu YF, Lu B, Yan YY, Luo WY, Gao ZQ, Wang J. A convenient synthesis of 1,4-benzoquinones. J Chem Res 2019; 43(3-4): 124-6.
[http://dx.doi.org/10.1177/1747519819841806]

[69]   Sivakumar D, Thanusu J, Kanagarajan V, Nagarajan S, Manikandan H, Gopalakrishnan M. One-pot Synthesis of 2-Hydroxy-1,4-Naphthoquinone (Lawsone).
[http://dx.doi.org/10.2174/1570179416666190111155328]

[70]   Monroy-Cárdenas M, Méndez D, Trostchansky A, Martínez-Cifuentes M, Araya-Maturana R, Fuentes E. Synthesis and Biological Evaluation of Thio-Derivatives of 2-Hydroxy-1,4-Naphthoquinone (Lawsone) as Novel Antiplatelet Agents. Front Chem 2020; 8: 533.
[http://dx.doi.org/10.3389/fchem.2020.00533] [PMID: 32850615]

[71]   Ríos D, Valderrama JA, Cautin M, *et al.* New 2-Acetyl-3-aminophenyl-1,4-naphthoquinones: Synthesis and *in vitro* Antiproliferative Activities on Breast and Prostate Human Cancer Cells. Oxid Med Cell Longev 2020; 2020: 1-11.
[http://dx.doi.org/10.1155/2020/8939716] [PMID: 33101594]

[72]   Ling B, Gao B, Yang J. Evaluating the Effects of Tetrachloro-1,4-benzoquinone, an Active Metabolite of Pentachlorophenol, on the Growth of Human Breast Cancer Cells. J Toxicol 2016; 2016: 1-8.
[http://dx.doi.org/10.1155/2016/8253726] [PMID: 26981120]

[73]   Dos S Moreira C, Santos TB, Freitas RHCN, Pacheco PAF, da Rocha DR. Juglone: A Versatile Natural Platform for Obtaining New Bioactive Compounds. Curr Top Med Chem 2021; 21(22): 2018-45.
[http://dx.doi.org/10.2174/1568026621666210804121054] [PMID: 34348624]

[74]   Ribeiro RCB, Ferreira PG, Borges AA, Forezi LSM, da Silva FC, Ferreira VF. 1,2-Naphthoquinone-4-sulfonic acid salts in organic synthesis. Beilstein J Org Chem 2022; 18(1): 53-69.
[http://dx.doi.org/10.3762/bjoc.18.5] [PMID: 35047082]

[75]   Razaque R, Raza AR, Irshad M, *et al.* Synthesis and evaluation of 2-phenylamino-1-4-naphthoquinones derivatives as potential hypoglycaemic agents. Braz J Biol 2024; 84: e254234.
[http://dx.doi.org/10.1590/1519-6984.254234] [PMID: 35293531]

[76]   Zhai H, Wang C, Li J, *et al.* Novel anthraquinone derivatives trigger endoplasmic reticulum stress response and induce apoptosis. Future Med Chem 2023; 15(2): 129-45.
[http://dx.doi.org/10.4155/fmc-2022-0217] [PMID: 36799271]

[77]   Abdullah, Hussain, Y. Chapter 7 - Anthraquinones and SARS-CoV-2. In Application of Natural Products in SARS-CoV-2; Niaz, K., Ed.; Academic Press, 2023; pp 171–184.
[http://dx.doi.org/10.1016/B978-0-323-95047-3.00006-X]

[78]   Shafiq N, Zareen G, Arshad U, *et al.* A Mini Review on the Chemical and Bio-Medicinal Aspects along with Energy Storage Applications of Anthraquinone and its Analogues. Mini Rev Org Chem 2024; 21(2): 134-50.
[http://dx.doi.org/10.2174/1570193X19666220512141411]

[79]   Kamiya T, Tanimoto Y, Fujii N, *et al.* 2,6-Dimethoxy-1,4-benzoquinone, isolation and identification of anti-carcinogenic, anti-mutagenic and anti-inflammatory component from the juice of *Vitis coignetiae.* Food Chem Toxicol 2018; 122: 172-80.
[http://dx.doi.org/10.1016/j.fct.2018.10.028] [PMID: 30316843]

[80]   Bothiraja C, Joshi PP, Dama GY, Pawar AP. Rapid method for isolation of plumbagin, an alternative medicine from roots of *Plumbago zeylanica.* Eur J Integr Med 2011; 3(1): 39-42.
[http://dx.doi.org/10.1016/j.eujim.2011.02.008]

[81]   Shukla B, Saxena S, Usmani S, Kushwaha P. Phytochemistry and pharmacological studies of Plumbago zeylanica L.: a medicinal plant review. Clinical Phytoscience 2021; 7(1): 34.
[http://dx.doi.org/10.1186/s40816-021-00271-7]

[82]   Available from: Indianjournals.Com/Ijor.Aspx?Target=ijor:Ajrc&volume=5&issue=9&article= 021https://www.indianjournals.com/ijor.aspx?target=ijor:ajrc&volume=5&issue=9&article=021

[83]   Prateeksha , Yusuf MA, Singh BN, *et al.* Chrysophanol: A Natural Anthraquinone with Multifaceted Biotherapeutic Potential. Biomolecules 2019; 9(2): 68.
[http://dx.doi.org/10.3390/biom9020068] [PMID: 30781696]

[84]   Chen Q, He H, Xiong L, Li P, Li P. A novel GC–MS method for determination of chrysophanol in rat plasma and tissues: Application to the pharmacokinetics, tissue distribution and plasma protein binding studies. J Chromatogr B Analyt Technol Biomed Life Sci 2014; 973: 76-83.
[http://dx.doi.org/10.1016/j.jchromb.2014.10.011] [PMID: 25464098]

[85]   Farooq U, Pan Y, Disasa D, Qi J. Novel Anti-Aging Benzoquinone Derivatives from *Onosma bracteatum* Wall. Molecules 2019; 24(7): 1428.

[http://dx.doi.org/10.3390/molecules24071428] [PMID: 30978970]

[86]   Osman CP, Ismail NH, Ahmad R, Ahmat N, Awang K, Jaafar FM. Anthraquinones with antiplasmodial activity from the roots of Rennellia elliptica Korth. (Rubiaceae). Molecules 2010; 15(10): 7218-26.
[http://dx.doi.org/10.3390/molecules15107218] [PMID: 20966871]

[87]   Singh DN, Verma N, Raghuwanshi S, Shukla PK, Kulshreshtha DK. Antifungal anthraquinones from *Saprosma fragrans*. Bioorg Med Chem Lett 2006; 16(17): 4512-4.
[http://dx.doi.org/10.1016/j.bmcl.2006.06.027] [PMID: 16824761]

[88]   Tung NH, Du GJ, Yuan CS, Shoyama Y, Wang CZ. Isolation and chemopreventive evaluation of novel naphthoquinone compounds from Alkanna tinctoria. Anticancer Drugs 2013; 24(10): 1058-68.
[http://dx.doi.org/10.1097/CAD.0000000000000017] [PMID: 24025561]

[89]   Drewes SE, Khan F, van Vuuren SF, Viljoen AM. Simple 1,4-benzoquinones with antibacterial activity from stems and leaves of *Gunnera perpensa*. Phytochemistry 2005; 66(15): 1812-6.
[http://dx.doi.org/10.1016/j.phytochem.2005.05.024] [PMID: 16019043]

[90]   Kang J, Zhang P, Gao Z, *et al.* Naphthohydroquinones, naphthoquinones, anthraquinones, and a naphthohydroquinone dimer isolated from the aerial parts of *Morinda parvifolia* and their cytotoxic effects through up-regulation of p53. Phytochemistry 2016; 130: 144-51.
[http://dx.doi.org/10.1016/j.phytochem.2016.04.001] [PMID: 27298278]

[91]   Onegi B, Kraft C, Köhler I, *et al.* Antiplasmodial activity of naphthoquinones and one anthraquinone from *Stereospermum kunthianum*. Phytochemistry 2002; 60(1): 39-44.
[http://dx.doi.org/10.1016/S0031-9422(02)00072-9] [PMID: 11985850]

[92]   Jeziorek M, Damianakos H, Kawiak A, *et al.* Bioactive rinderol and cynoglosol isolated from *Cynoglossum columnae* Ten. *in vitro* root culture. Ind Crops Prod 2019; 137: 446-52.
[http://dx.doi.org/10.1016/j.indcrop.2019.04.046]

[93]   Zhou Y, Yang B, Jiang Y, *et al.* Studies on Cytotoxic Activity against HepG-2 Cells of Naphthoquinones from Green Walnut Husks of Juglans mandshurica Maxim. Molecules 2015; 20(9): 15572-88.
[http://dx.doi.org/10.3390/molecules200915572] [PMID: 26343618]

[94]   Abdissa N, Gohlke S, Frese M, Sewald N. Cytotoxic Compounds from Aloe megalacantha. Molecules 2017; 22(7): 1136.
[http://dx.doi.org/10.3390/molecules22071136] [PMID: 28686200]

[95]   Augustin N, Nuthakki VK, Abdullaha M, Hassan QP, Gandhi SG, Bharate SB. Discovery of Helminthosporin, an Anthraquinone Isolated from *Rumex abyssinicus* Jacq as a Dual Cholinesterase Inhibitor. ACS Omega 2020; 5(3): 1616-24.
[http://dx.doi.org/10.1021/acsomega.9b03693] [PMID: 32010836]

[96]   Bitchagno GTM, Sama Fonkeng L, Kopa TK, *et al.* Antibacterial activity of ethanolic extract and compounds from fruits of Tectona grandis (Verbenaceae). BMC Complement Altern Med 2015; 15(1): 265.
[http://dx.doi.org/10.1186/s12906-015-0790-5] [PMID: 26245866]

[97]   Bajpai VK, Alam MB, Quan KT, *et al.* Cytotoxic properties of the anthraquinone derivatives isolated from the roots of Rubia philippinensis. BMC Complement Altern Med 2018; 18(1): 200.
[http://dx.doi.org/10.1186/s12906-018-2253-2] [PMID: 29970094]

[98]   Endale M, Ekberg A, Alao J, *et al.* Anthraquinones of the roots of Pentas micrantha. Molecules 2012; 18(1): 311-21.
[http://dx.doi.org/10.3390/molecules18010311] [PMID: 23271468]

[99]   Dai Y, Harinantenaina L, Bowman JD, *et al.* Isolation of antiplasmodial anthraquinones from *Kniphofia ensifolia*, and synthesis and structure–activity relationships of related compounds. Bioorg Med Chem 2014; 22(1): 269-76.

[http://dx.doi.org/10.1016/j.bmc.2013.11.032] [PMID: 24326280]

[100] Lee CL, Chang FR, Yen MH, *et al.* Cytotoxic phenanthrenequinones and 9,10-dihydrophenanthrenes from Calanthe arisanensis. J Nat Prod 2009; 72(2): 210-3.
[http://dx.doi.org/10.1021/np800622a] [PMID: 19193043]

[101] Wube AA, Streit B, Gibbons S, Asres K, Bucar F. *in vitro* 12(*S*)-HETE inhibitory activities of naphthoquinones isolated from the root bark of *Euclea racemosa* ssp. *schimperi.* J Ethnopharmacol 2005; 102(2): 191-6.
[http://dx.doi.org/10.1016/j.jep.2005.06.009] [PMID: 16019177]

[102] Wang C, Ding X, Feng SX, *et al.* Seven New Tetrahydroanthraquinones from the Root of Prismatomeris connata and Their Cytotoxicity against Lung Tumor Cell Growth. Molecules 2015; 20(12): 22565-77.
[http://dx.doi.org/10.3390/molecules201219856] [PMID: 26694340]

[103] Li ZB, Wang JY, Jiang B, Zhang XL, An LJ, Bao YM. Benzobijuglone, a novel cytotoxic compound from *Juglans mandshurica*, induced apoptosis in HeLa cervical cancer cells. Phytomedicine 2007; 14(12): 846-52.
[http://dx.doi.org/10.1016/j.phymed.2007.09.004] [PMID: 17959366]

[104] Cui XR, Tsukada M, Suzuki N, *et al.* Comparison of the cytotoxic activities of naturally occurring hydroxyanthraquinones and hydroxynaphthoquinones. Eur J Med Chem 2008; 43(6): 1206-15.
[http://dx.doi.org/10.1016/j.ejmech.2007.08.009] [PMID: 17949858]

[105] (Vukic, M. D.; Vukovic, N. L.; Djelic, G. T.; Popovic, S. Lj.; Zaric, M. M.; Baskic, D. D.; Krstic, G. B.; Tesevic, V. V.; Kacaniova, M. M. Antibacterial and Cytotoxic Activities of Naphthoquinone Pigments from *Onosma Visianii* Clem. EXCLI J 2017; 16: 73-88.
[http://dx.doi.org/10.17179/excli2016-762]

CHAPTER 9

Quinone Compounds in Medicine: A Biological Perspective

Rajendra Dighe[1], Ashutosh Kumar Dash[2], Shashikant Bhandari[3] and Ritu Gilhotra[4,*]

[1] *KBHSS Trust's, Institute of Pharmacy, Malegaon, Maharashtra, India*

[2] *Senior Research Scientist (R&D), Drug Discovery Division, Macleods Pharmaceuticals Ltd, India*

[3] *AISSMS College of Pharmacy, Pune, Maharashtra, India*

[4] *Gyan Vihar School of Pharmacy, Suresh Gyan Vihar University, Jaipur, Rajasthan, India*

Abstract: Quinone compounds are versatile molecules with significant biological importance and have therapeutic potential in medicine. This chapter provides a comprehensive overview of quinones, beginning with their definition, historical background, and chemical structure. It explores their diverse roles in biological systems, including their involvement in cellular respiration, enzymatic reactions as co-factors, and their function as endogenous compounds. Mechanistically, quinones employ their effects through redox properties, electron transfer processes, and interactions with cellular components such as proteins, lipids, and DNA. Therapeutically, quinones are pragmatic for their anti-cancer, antimicrobial, anti-inflammatory, and antioxidant properties. Key drugs like doxorubicin and mitomycin C exemplify their efficacy in cancer treatment, while other quinones serve as antimicrobial agents against bacteria, fungi, and viruses. Challenges in drug development, including toxicity and stability issues, are addressed alongside strategies to mitigate these concerns. Case studies and clinical trial data underscore the clinical relevance of quinone-based therapies. Looking forward, future research opportunities include exploring novel quinone derivatives, integrating quinones in combination therapies, and advancing drug delivery systems to enhance their efficacy and safety profiles. The chapter concludes by emphasizing the significant role of quinone compounds in modern medicine and outlining potential breakthroughs that may further expand their therapeutic applications.

Keywords: Anthraquinones, Benzoquinones, Doxorubicin, Mitomycin, Naphthoquinones, Quinones, Reactive oxygen species, Vitamin K, Ubiquinone.

* **Corresponding author Ritu Gilhotra:** Gyan Vihar School of Pharmacy, Suresh Gyan Vihar University, Jaipur, Rajasthan, India; E-mail: drritugilhotra@gmail.com

Ashutosh Kumar Dash & Deepak Kumar (Eds.)

INTRODUCTION

Quinones are a class of organic compounds characterized by a fully conjugated cyclic di-one structure. The most common quinones include benzoquinones, naphthoquinones, and anthraquinones [1]. Quinones are derived from aromatic compounds through the oxidation of hydroquinones. Their chemical structure typically includes a six-membered aromatic ring with two ketone substitutions, leading to their highly reactive nature due to the presence of electron-deficient carbonyl groups [2].

Quinones possess a basic structure of $C_6H_4O_2$ in the case of benzoquinones, extending to more complex forms such as naphthoquinones ($C_{10}H_6O_2$) and anthraquinones ($C_{14}H_8O_2$). The electron-deficient nature of the carbonyl groups makes quinones highly reactive and capable of participating in various redox reactions [3]. Quinones are typically yellow to red crystalline substances, exhibiting a distinctive coloration due to their conjugated system [4]. They have relatively low melting points and are soluble in organic solvents but exhibit limited solubility in water [5].

Quinones readily undergo reversible redox reactions, cycling between quinone and hydroquinone forms. This redox capability underpins many of their biological activities, including roles in electron transport and enzymatic reactions [6]. The redox properties are influenced by substituents on the aromatic ring, which can either donate or withdraw electrons, thus modifying the quinone's reactivity [7].

Quinones are ubiquitous in nature, playing vital roles in biological processes. For instance, ubiquinones (coenzyme Q) are essential for cellular respiration in the mitochondrial electron transport chain. They act as electron carriers and are involved in the synthesis of ATP, showcasing their importance in energy metabolism [8].

Naturally occurring quinones are found in a variety of plants, fungi, and bacteria. They are involved in pigmentation, such as in the case of lawsone (henna) and juglone (black walnut). Synthetically, quinones can be produced through various chemical reactions, including the oxidation of aromatic precursors and the cyclization of appropriate intermediates. The reactivity of quinones makes them suitable for a variety of applications, including medicinal chemistry. Their derivatives are used in anti-cancer, anti-microbial, and anti-inflammatory drugs due to their ability to generate reactive oxygen species and interact with biological macromolecules [9].

HISTORICAL BACKGROUND AND DISCOVERY IN MEDICINE

Early uses and Discovery

The medicinal use of quinone compounds dates back to ancient times, even before their chemical nature was understood. Natural quinones, especially those found in plants, have been used in traditional medicine for their therapeutic properties. One of the earliest known uses of a quinone compound is henna, derived from the plant Lawsonia inermis, which contains lawsone, a naphthoquinone. Henna has been used for millennia for its dyeing properties and potential medicinal benefits, including antimicrobial and anti-inflammatory effects [10].

19th Century: Isolation and Chemical Characterization

The 19th century marked significant advancements in the chemical isolation and characterization of quinones. In 1838, Pierre Joseph Pelletier and Joseph Bienaimé Caventou isolated the first quinone, quinone itself (benzoquinone), from the oxidation of quinic acid. This discovery laid the groundwork for understanding the chemical structure and reactivity of quinones.

Following this, in the late 1800s, notable chemists such as Friedrich Wöhler and August Kekulé contributed to the elucidation of the structures of various quinones. Wöhler, known for his synthesis of urea, also worked on the synthesis and study of benzoquinone. Kekulé's structural theories further advanced the understanding of aromatic compounds, including quinones [10].

20th Century: Biomedical Discoveries

The 20th century saw significant breakthroughs in the biological and medicinal applications of quinones. In the 1930s, research into the role of quinones in cellular respiration led to the discovery of ubiquinone (coenzyme Q10) by Frederick L. Crane and colleagues in 1957. Ubiquinone's crucial role in the mitochondrial electron transport chain and ATP synthesis underscored the biological importance of quinones [11].

Simultaneously, the anti-cancer properties of quinone compounds began to be explored. The anthracycline antibiotic doxorubicin, derived from the bacterium Streptomyces peucetius, was discovered in the 1960s and became a cornerstone in chemotherapy for various cancers. Its mechanism, involving DNA intercalation and the generation of reactive oxygen species, highlighted the potential of quinones in cancer treatment [12].

MODERN APPLICATIONS AND RESEARCH

In recent decades, the medicinal use of quinones has expanded significantly. Advances in synthetic chemistry have enabled the development of numerous quinone-based drugs with improved efficacy and reduced toxicity. For example, the discovery and development of atovaquone, an anti-malarial drug, in the 1990s provided an effective treatment for resistant strains of Plasmodium falciparum [13].

Current research continues to explore new therapeutic applications of quinones. The redox properties of quinones are being harnessed in novel drug delivery systems and in the design of drugs targeting oxidative stress-related diseases, including neurodegenerative disorders and cardiovascular diseases. Additionally, the role of quinones in modulating immune responses is an emerging field with potential implications for treating inflammatory and autoimmune conditions [14].

OVERVIEW OF THE BIOLOGICAL IMPORTANCE OF QUINONES

Quinones are integral to numerous biological processes due to their unique chemical properties, particularly their redox activity. These compounds are involved in electron transport, enzymatic reactions, cellular signaling, and protection against oxidative stress. The key biological importance of quinones is illustrated in Fig. (**1**).

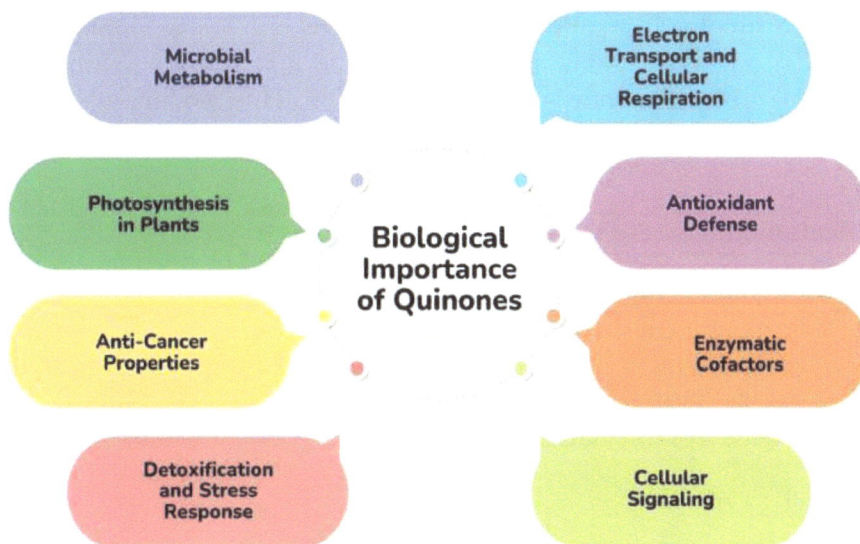

Fig. (1). Biological Importance of Quinones.

Electron Transport and Cellular Respiration

Quinones play a crucial role in cellular energy production. Ubiquinone, also known as coenzyme Q10, is a prime example. It is a vital component of the mitochondrial electron transport chain, where it functions as an electron carrier. Ubiquinone accepts electrons from complexes I and II and transfers them to complex III, facilitating the generation of ATP through oxidative phosphorylation.

Antioxidant Defense

Quinones, particularly ubiquinone, are significant antioxidants. They protect cells from oxidative damage by neutralizing reactive oxygen species (ROS). The reduced form of ubiquinone, ubiquinol, is particularly effective in scavenging free radicals and preventing lipid peroxidation in cell membranes.

Enzymatic Cofactors

Quinones act as cofactors for various enzymes. For instance, vitamin K, a type of naphthoquinone, is essential for the activity of enzymes involved in the carboxylation of glutamate residues in certain proteins, which is crucial for blood clotting. Without vitamin K, these proteins cannot bind calcium, leading to impaired blood coagulation.

Cellular Signaling

Quinones are involved in cellular signaling pathways. For example, menadione (vitamin K3) and other quinones can modulate signal transduction pathways related to cell growth, apoptosis, and inflammation. This modulation often occurs through the generation of ROS, which act as secondary messengers in signaling cascades.

Detoxification and Stress Response

Quinones are implicated in the cellular detoxification process. Enzymes such as NAD(P)H oxidoreductase 1 (NQO1) reduce quinones to hydroquinones, which are less reactive and can be excreted from the body more easily. This detoxification pathway is crucial for protecting cells from quinone-induced oxidative stress and potential toxicity.

Anti-Cancer Properties

Quinones are widely studied for their anti-cancer properties. Many quinone-based drugs, such as doxorubicin and mitomycin C, exert their effects by intercalating into DNA, generating ROS, and inducing apoptosis in cancer cells. The redox cycling of quinones in cancer cells leads to the selective generation of cytotoxic ROS, which can kill rapidly dividing cells while sparing normal cells.

Photosynthesis in Plants

In plants, quinones like plastoquinone play a crucial role in photosynthesis. Plastoquinone functions in the electron transport chain within the thylakoid membranes of chloroplasts. It transfers electrons from photosystem II to the cytochrome b6f complex, which is essential for the synthesis of ATP and NADPH, the energy molecules required for carbon fixation in the Calvin cycle.

Microbial Metabolism

Quinones are also important in microbial metabolism. Bacteria, such as those in the genus Pseudomonas, use quinones like ubiquinone and menaquinone in their electron transport chains to generate energy under both aerobic and anaerobic conditions. These quinones help in maintaining cellular redox balance and energy production in diverse environmental conditions [15, 16].

CHEMICAL STRUCTURE AND CLASSIFICATION

Quinones are a class of organic compounds that are characterized by a fully conjugated cyclic dione structure. They are important in various biological and industrial processes. Quinones have the general formula $C_6H_4O_2$, consisting of a six-membered benzene ring with two ketone substitutions.

Types of Quinones

Quinones are classified based on the parent hydrocarbon structure from which they are derived. The primary types include benzoquinones, naphthoquinones, and anthraquinones, each differing in the complexity and arrangement of their ring structures.

Benzoquinones

Benzoquinones (Fig. **2**) are the simplest quinones derived from benzene with the general formula $C_6H_4O_2$. They have a six-membered aromatic ring with two ketone groups. The most common types of benzoquinones are para-benzoquinones and ortho-benzoquinones, named based on the relative positions of the carbonyl (C=O) groups on the benzene ring.

1,4-Benzoquinone (Para-benzoquinone): This is the most common form, with ketone groups at the 1 and 4 positions. 1,4-Benzoquinone (Fig. **3**) is a yellow crystalline solid, commonly used in organic synthesis and as an oxidizing agent.

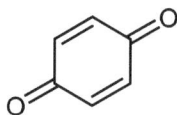

Fig. (2). Structure of Benzoquinone.

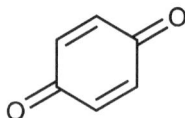

Fig. (3). Structure of 1,4-Benzoquinone.

1,2-Benzoquinone (Ortho-benzoquinone): Less common, with ketone groups at the 1 and 2 positions. 1,2-Benzoquinone (Fig. **4**) is typically found in certain biochemical pathways [17].

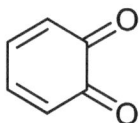

Fig. (4). Structure of 1,2-Benzoquinone.

2,5-Dihydroxy-1,4-benzoquinone: The carbonyl groups are at the 1 and 4 positions, with hydroxyl groups at the 2 and 5 positions. This compound is also known as quinizarin, used in dye manufacture and as a pH indicator.

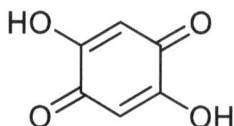

Fig. (5). Structure of 2,5-Dihydroxy-1,4-benzoquinone.

Tetrahydroxy-1,4-benzoquinone: The carbonyl groups are at the 1 and 4 positions, with hydroxyl groups at the 2, 3, 5, and 6 positions. This highly hydroxylated compound is used in various chemical applications and as a precursor in synthesis.

NAPHTHOQUINONES

Naphthoquinones (Fig. **7**) are derived from naphthalene and have two benzene rings fused together with two ketone groups. The most prevalent types of naphthoquinones are para-naphthoquinones and ortho-naphthoquinones, which are classified according to the positions of the carbonyl (C=O) groups on the naphthalene ring.

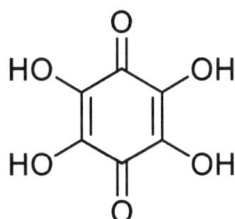

Fig. (6). Structure of Tetrahydroxy-1,4-benzoquinone.

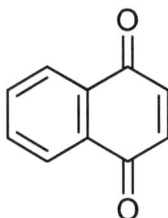

Fig. (7). Structure of Naphthoquinone.

1,4-Naphthoquinone (Para-napthoquinone): The ketone groups are at the 1 and 4 positions on the naphthalene ring. The simplest naphthoquinone is used in the production of vitamin K and certain dyes.

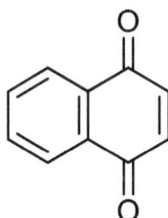

Fig. (8). Structure of 1,4-Naphthoquinone.

1,2-Naphthoquinone (Ortho-napthoquinone): The carbonyl groups are positioned at the 1 and 2 positions of the benzene ring. It is less common than 1,4-benzoquinone and is typically more reactive due to the proximity of the carbonyl groups.

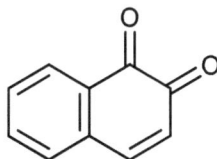

Fig. (9). Structure of 1,2-Naphthoquinone.

Lawsone (2-Hydroxy-1,4-Naphthoquinone): Lawsone (Fig. **10**) contains a hydroxyl group at the 2 position. It is found in the henna plant, used as a dye and in traditional medicines [18, 19].

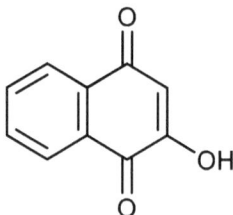

Fig. (10). Structure of Lawsone.

Juglone (5-Hydroxy-1,4-Naphthoquinone): A hydroxyl group at position 5 and carbonyl groups at the 1st and 4th positions. Found in walnut trees; has allelopathic properties and used in biological research.

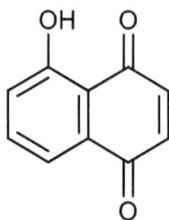

Fig. (11). Structure of 5-Hydroxy-1,4-naphthoquinone.

Vitamin K Derivatives: Substituted naphthoquinones with additional functional groups, such as phytyl side chains. Vitamin K is essential for blood clotting and bone health.

ANTHRAQUINONES

Anthraquinones (Fig. **12**) are derived from anthracene and consist of three fused benzene rings with two ketone groups. The basic structure includes ketone groups on the central ring. The parent compound is used as an intermediate in the dye industry and as a precursor for various pharmaceuticals. Alzarin, quinizarin and 1,4-Diaminoanthraquinone are some examples of antraquinone.

Alizarin: Alizarin (Fig. **13**) is derived from anthraquinone with hydroxyl groups. A natural dye originally obtained from the madder plant [20].

Quinizarin: Quinizarin (Fig. **14**), also known as 1,4-dihydroxyanthraquinone, is a derivative of anthraquinone with the chemical formula $C_{14}H_8O_4$. It is an important synthetic dye and intermediate used in various industrial applications.

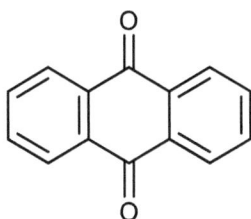

Fig. (12). Structure of Anthraquinone.

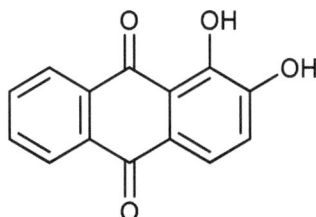

Fig. (13). Structure of Alizarin.

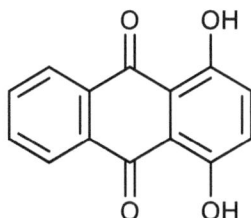

Fig. (14). Structure of Quinizarin.

1,4-Diaminoanthraquinone: 1,4-Diaminoanthraquinone (Fig. **15**), also known as disperse orange 11, is a synthetic organic compound derived from anthraquinone. It has notable applications in the dye industry.

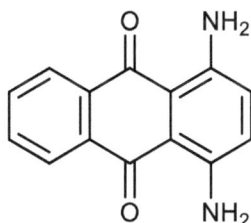

Fig. (15). Structure of 1,4-Diaminoanthraquinone.

KEY CHEMICAL PROPERTIES INFLUENCING BIOLOGICAL ACTIVITY

Quinones are known for their significant biological activities, which are largely influenced by their unique chemical properties. Fig. (**16**) shows some key chemical properties of quinones that influence their biological activity.

REDOX ACTIVITY

Quinones can undergo reversible redox reactions, cycling between oxidized (quinone) and reduced (hydroquinone) forms. This redox cycling is crucial for their role in biological systems, such as in cellular respiration and photosynthesis. Quinones can accept and donate electrons, making them integral to electron transport chains in mitochondria and chloroplasts. For instance, ubiquinone (coenzyme Q) plays a vital role in the mitochondrial electron transport chain [21].

REACTIVE OXYGEN SPECIES (ROS) GENERATION

Quinones can generate reactive oxygen species (ROS) through redox cycling, leading to oxidative stress. This property is leveraged in anticancer therapies but can also result in cytotoxicity. Quinones like doxorubicin generate ROS that damage cellular components, leading to cell death. This mechanism is used to target cancer cells but can also cause side effects due to damage to healthy cells [22].

ALKYLATION ABILITY

Quinones can act as electrophiles, reacting with nucleophilic sites in biological macromolecules. This alkylation can modify DNA, proteins, and other cellular components, affecting their function. Quinones can form covalent bonds with DNA and proteins, leading to mutations, enzyme inhibition, and other modifications that impact cell function and viability [23].

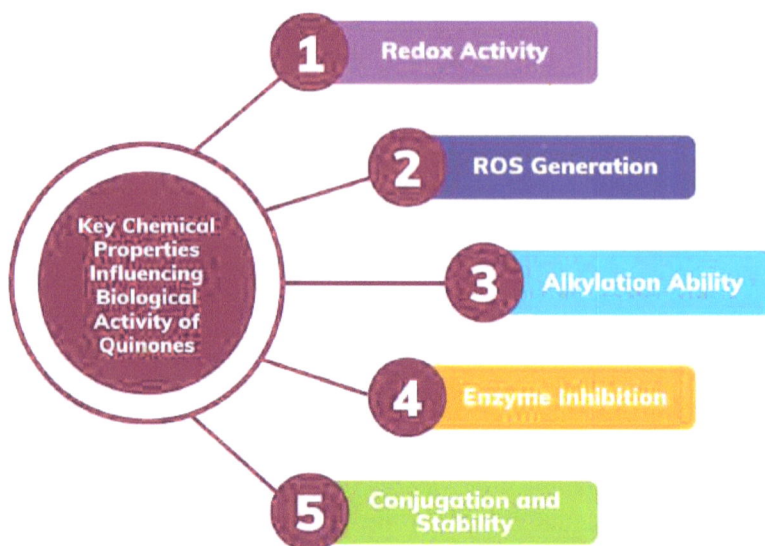

Fig. (16). Key Chemical Properties Influencing Biological Activity of Quinones.

ENZYME INHIBITION

Quinones can inhibit various enzymes by binding to their active sites or modifying essential amino acid residues. This inhibition can disrupt metabolic pathways and cellular functions. Compounds like plumbagin and juglone inhibit enzymes involved in cellular proliferation and survival, contributing to their antimicrobial and anticancer properties [24].

CONJUGATION AND STABILITY

The conjugated system of quinones contributes to their stability and reactivity. The extended π-system allows for interactions with various biomolecules, affecting their distribution and persistence in biological systems. The conjugated double bonds in quinones facilitate their interactions with cellular components, influencing their bioavailability and activity [25].

MECHANISMS OF ACTION

The detailed exploration of the mechanisms of action of quinones, covering their redox properties, electron transfer, radical formation, interaction with cellular components, and enzymatic pathways, is as follows.

REDOX PROPERTIES OF QUINONES

Quinones exhibit significant biological activity largely due to their redox properties, which involve the ability to undergo reversible redox reactions. Here is an overview of the redox properties of quinones and their biological implications, supported by references:

REDUCTION-OXIDATION (REDOX) CYCLING

Quinones can cycle between a quinone (oxidized) and a hydroquinone (reduced) form by accepting and donating electrons. This redox cycling is crucial for their role in various biological processes, including electron transport chains and cellular signaling pathways.

ELECTRON ACCEPTORS IN BIOLOGICAL SYSTEMS

Quinones serve as electron carriers in biological systems, participating in electron transport chains (ETC) in mitochondria and chloroplasts. For instance, ubiquinone (coenzyme Q) plays a vital role in ATP synthesis through its involvement in the mitochondrial *etc.*

PRODUCTION OF REACTIVE OXYGEN SPECIES (ROS)

During their redox cycling, quinones can generate reactive oxygen species (ROS), such as superoxide anion and hydrogen peroxide. This property is essential in their antimicrobial and cytotoxic effects but can also contribute to oxidative stress and cellular damage [26].

ELECTRON TRANSFER AND RADICAL FORMATION

Electron transfer and radical formation are fundamental aspects of quinone chemistry that underpin their diverse biological activities. Quinones can form radicals during their redox reactions, including semiquinone radicals and reactive oxygen species. Semiquinone radicals formed during quinone redox cycling can initiate chain reactions and modify cellular molecules, leading to oxidative stress and damage.

ELECTRON TRANSFER MECHANISMS

Quinone Reduction and Oxidation

Quinones undergo reversible redox reactions where they alternate between a quinone (oxidized) and a hydroquinone (reduced) form by accepting or donating electrons.

Example: Ubiquinone (coenzyme Q) in the mitochondrial electron transport chain accepts electrons from complex I and II and donates them to complex III, playing a crucial role in ATP synthesis.

Electron Acceptors in Biological Systems

Quinones act as electron carriers in various biological processes, including cellular respiration and photosynthesis.

Example: Plastoquinone in photosystem II of plants and algae accepts electrons from photosystem II and transfers them to the cytochrome b6f complex during photosynthesis.

RADICAL FORMATION AND ROS GENERATION

Production OF Reactive Oxygen Species (Ros)

During redox cycling, quinones can undergo incomplete reduction processes, leading to the formation of reactive oxygen species (ROS) such as superoxide anion and hydrogen peroxide. ROS can cause oxidative damage to cellular components, including lipids, proteins, and DNA, contributing to aging, inflammation, and various diseases.

Radical Formation

Quinones can also form radicals during their redox cycling, which can initiate chain reactions or react with other molecules, altering their structure and function.

Example: Semiquinone radicals formed during the reduction of quinones are highly reactive and can contribute to oxidative stress in cells [27].

INTERACTION WITH CELLULAR COMPONENTS

Quinones can interact with various cellular components, including proteins, lipids, and DNA, through covalent and non-covalent interactions. These interactions can significantly impact cellular function and health.

Proteins: Quinones can modify proteins by forming adducts or oxidizing critical amino acid residues, influencing enzyme activity and protein function.

Lipids: Quinones can oxidize membrane lipids, disrupting cellular membranes and affecting cell integrity and function.

DNA: Quinones can form DNA adducts, leading to mutations and potentially contributing to carcinogenesis and genotoxicity.

Enzymatic Pathways Involving Quinones

Quinones interact with specific enzymatic pathways, including those involving quinone reductases and other redox enzymes.

Quinone Reductases (QRs): These enzymes catalyze the reduction of quinones to hydroquinones, playing a role in detoxification and cellular defense against oxidative stress.

Biological Significance: QRs are crucial in maintaining redox balance and protecting cells from quinone-induced toxicity [28, 29].

QUINONES IN BIOLOGICAL SYSTEMS

Quinones are a class of organic compounds characterized by a fully conjugated cyclic dione structure. They play vital roles in various biological processes, particularly in cellular respiration and enzymatic reactions.

ROLE OF QUINONES IN CELLULAR RESPIRATION

Quinones are crucial in the electron transport chain (ETC), a series of complexes located in the inner mitochondrial membrane responsible for oxidative phosphorylation. One key quinone in this process is ubiquinone (coenzyme Q10).

Ubiquinone (Fig. **17**) is lipid-soluble and can move freely within the inner mitochondrial membrane. It serves as an electron carrier, transferring electrons between Complex I (NADH oxidoreductase) and Complex II (succinate oxidoreductase) to Complex III (cytochrome bc1 complex). During this process, ubiquinone is reduced to ubiquinol (QH2), which then donates electrons to Complex III, facilitating the creation of a proton gradient used to produce ATP.

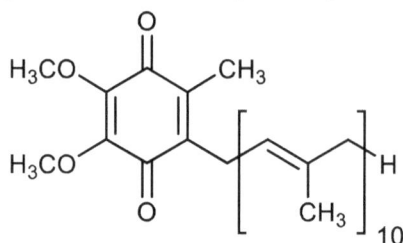

Fig. (17). Structure of Ubiquinone.

QUINONES AS CO-FACTORS IN ENZYMATIC REACTIONS

Quinones also act as essential cofactors in various enzymatic reactions, helping enzymes catalyze redox reactions.

Vitamin K: One well-known quinone is vitamin K (Fig. **18**), which functions as a cofactor for the enzyme γ-glutamyl carboxylase. This enzyme is critical in the carboxylation of glutamate residues on proteins required for blood clotting. Vitamin K undergoes a redox cycle, converting to its epoxide form and then being recycled back to its quinone form to continue the process.

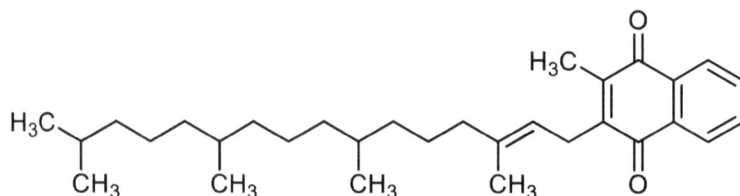

Fig. (18). Structure of Vitamin K.

Pyrroloquinoline Quinone (PQQ): PQQ is another quinone that acts as a cofactor in bacterial dehydrogenases, enzymes that play a role in oxidation-reduction reactions involving substrates like alcohols and sugars. PQQ's redox capabilities enable these enzymes to facilitate electron transfer reactions essential for metabolic processes [30].

ENDOGENOUS QUINONES AND THEIR FUNCTIONS

Endogenous quinones, those produced within the body, have diverse functions that extend beyond cellular respiration and enzymatic activity.

Plastoquinone: Found in plants, plastoquinone (Fig. **19**) is involved in the photosynthetic electron transport chain. It functions similarly to ubiquinone in mitochondria, transporting electrons between photosystem II and the cytochrome b6f complex in the chloroplasts, playing a crucial role in the light-dependent reactions of photosynthesis.

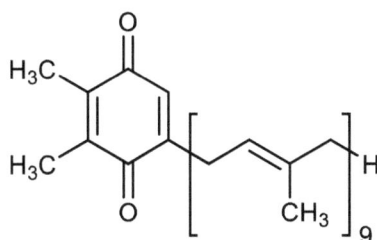

Fig. (19). Structure of Plastoquinone.

Menadione: Menadione (Vitamin K3) (Fig. **20**) is a synthetic precursor to vitamin K. In animals, it can be converted into active forms of vitamin K. It is involved in various cellular processes, including modulation of redox states and regulation of gene expression through redox-sensitive transcription factors.

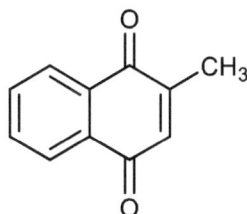

Fig. (20). Structure of Mendione (Vitamin K3).

Endogenous Antioxidants: Some quinones, like ubiquinone, also serve as endogenous antioxidants. They can neutralize reactive oxygen species (ROS), protecting cells from oxidative damage. This antioxidant property is vital for maintaining cellular health and preventing diseases associated with oxidative stress [31, 32].

THERAPEUTIC APPLICATIONS OF QUINONES

Quinones exhibit a range of therapeutic properties, including anti-cancer, antimicrobial, anti-inflammatory, and antioxidant effects. They also have applications in treating malaria and other parasitic diseases.

Anti-cancer Properties of Quinones

Quinones have demonstrated significant anti-cancer properties through various mechanisms of action.

Mechanisms of Action

Some quinones can intercalate into DNA, disrupting its structure and function. This can inhibit DNA replication and transcription, leading to cell death. Quinones can undergo redox cycling, leading to the production of ROS. These ROS can cause oxidative damage to cellular components, including DNA, proteins, and lipids, ultimately inducing apoptosis (programmed cell death) in cancer cells [33].

KEY QUINONE-BASED ANTI-CANCER DRUGS

Doxorubicin: Doxorubicin (Fig. **21**) intercalates into DNA, inhibiting the replication and transcription processes. It also generates ROS, contributing to its cytotoxic effects. It is widely used in the treatment of various cancers, including leukemia, breast cancer, and lymphomas.

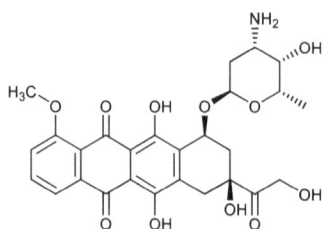

Biological Activity-anti-cancer

Targets- DNA topoisomerase 2-alpha, Telomerase reverse transcriptase, DNA, DNA topoisomerase 1, DNA topoisomerase 2-beta, Nucleolar and coiled-body phosphoprotein 1.

Fig. (21). Structure of Doxorubicin.

Mitomycin C: Mitomycin C (Fig. **22**) is a bio-reductive alkylating agent that, once activated, forms cross-links in DNA, inhibiting DNA synthesis and leading to cell death. It is used in treating stomach, pancreatic, and bladder cancers.

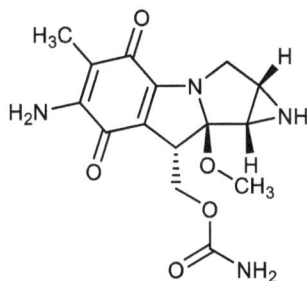

Biological Activity- Anti-cancer.

Target- DNA

Fig. (22). Structure of Mitomycin C.

Antimicrobial Properties

Quinones possess antimicrobial activities against a variety of pathogens, including bacteria, fungi, and viruses.

Mechanisms Against Bacteria, Fungi, and Viruses

Quinones can disrupt bacterial cell walls, inhibit bacterial enzymes, and interfere with DNA replication. Some quinones may inhibit the synthesis of essential cellular components, such as ergosterol, in fungal cell membranes, leading to fungal cell death. Quinones can interfere with viral replication and assembly, preventing the proliferation of viruses within host cells.

EXAMPLES OF QUINONE-BASED ANTIMICROBIAL AGENTS

Plumbagin: Found in the roots of Plumbago species, plumbagin (Fig. **23**) exhibits antimicrobial activity against a range of bacteria and fungi by generating ROS and inhibiting key enzymes.

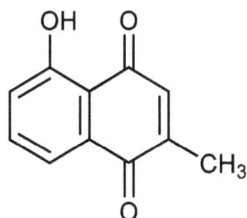

Biological Activity-Anti-microbial.

Target- Dihydroorotate dehydrogenase (quinone), mitochondrial.

Fig. (23). Structure of Plumbagin.

Lapachol: Derived from the bark of the Tabebuia tree, lapachol (Fig. **24**) has shown activity against various bacterial and fungal pathogens by disrupting cell membranes and inhibiting DNA synthesis.

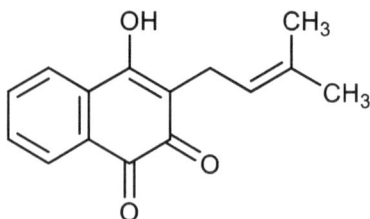

***Biological Activity*-**Anti-microbial
***Target*-** Disrupting cell membranes and inhibiting DNA synthesis.

Fig. (24). Structure of Lapachol.

ANTI-INFLAMMATORY AND ANTIOXIDANT EFFECTS

Quinones have been found to modulate redox balance and exhibit significant anti-inflammatory and antioxidant properties. Quinones can scavenge free radicals and reduce oxidative stress, protecting cells from damage. They can also regulate the expression of antioxidant enzymes and proteins.

KEY COMPOUNDS AND THEIR THERAPEUTIC POTENTIAL

Coenzyme Q10 (Ubiquinone): CoQ10 (Fig. **25**) is a powerful antioxidant that protects cells from oxidative damage. It has therapeutic potential in treating conditions associated with oxidative stress, such as cardiovascular diseases and neurodegenerative disorders.

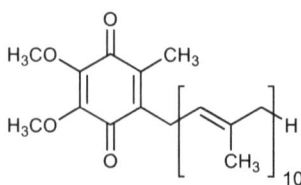

***Biological Activity*-**Anti-oxidant

***Targets*-**NADH dehydrogenase [ubiquinone] flavoprotein 3, mitochondrial, Succinate dehydrogenase [ubiquinone] flavoprotein subunit, mitochondrial

Fig. (25). Structure of Ubiquinone.

Tanshinone: Extracted from Salvia miltiorrhiza. Tanshinone (Fig. **26**) exhibits anti-inflammatory effects by inhibiting pro-inflammatory cytokines and signaling pathways, making it useful in treating inflammatory diseases [34, 35].

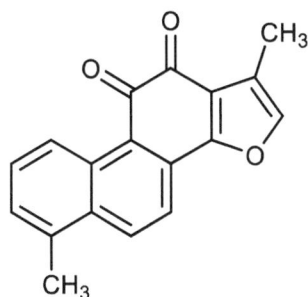

***Biological Activity*-** Anti-inflammatory, Anti-oxidant.

***Target*-** inhibiting pro-inflammatory cytokines and signaling pathways.

Fig. (26). Structure of Tanshinone.

OTHER MEDICAL APPLICATIONS

Quinones also have applications in treating malaria and other parasitic diseases.

Antimalarial: Quinones like **atovaquone** (Fig. **27**) inhibit the mitochondrial electron transport chain in Plasmodium species (the parasites responsible for malaria), leading to parasite death.

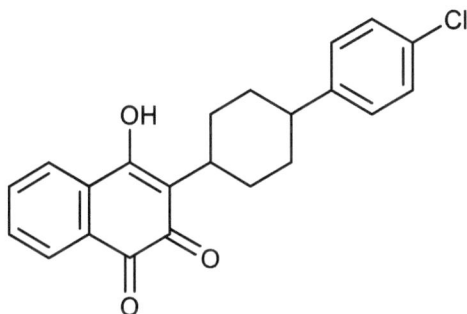

***Biological Activity*-** Anti-malarial, Anti-parasitic.

***Targets*-**Cytochrome b, Dihydroorotate dehydrogenase (quinone), mitochondrial

Fig. (27). Structure of Atovaquone.

Anti-parasitic: Quinones can also target other parasites by disrupting their metabolic processes and causing oxidative stress [36].

QUINONE COMPOUNDS IN DRUG DEVELOPMENT

Quinone compounds hold significant potential in drug development due to their diverse biological activities. However, developing quinone-based drugs involves strategic design, structure-activity relationship (SAR) studies, and overcoming various challenges such as toxicity and stability.

Strategies for Designing Quinone-Based Drugs

Designing quinone-based drugs involves several strategies aimed at maximizing therapeutic efficacy while minimizing adverse effects:

Target Specificity: Quinone-based drugs can be designed to target specific cellular components or pathways. This is achieved by modifying the quinone structure to enhance binding affinity to target proteins or DNA.

Prodrug Approaches: To improve selectivity and reduce toxicity, quinones can be developed as prodrugs. These are inactive compounds that are metabolized into active quinone species within the target cells.

Redox Cycling: Designing drugs that undergo controlled redox cycling can help in generating reactive oxygen species (ROS) selectively in cancer cells, leading to targeted cytotoxicity.

Conjugation with Targeting Moieties: Conjugating quinones with molecules that have high affinity for specific cell types or receptors can enhance drug delivery to the desired site of action [37].

STRUCTURE-ACTIVITY RELATIONSHIP (SAR) STUDIES

SAR studies are essential in understanding the relationship between the chemical structure of quinones and their biological activity. Key considerations in SAR studies include:

Substituent Effects: Modifying the quinone core with different substituents can significantly impact its reactivity, solubility, and ability to interact with biological targets. For example, the addition of alkyl groups can increase lipophilicity and cell membrane permeability.

Redox Potential: The redox potential of quinones affects their ability to undergo redox cycling and generate ROS. Optimizing the redox potential can enhance the therapeutic effects while minimizing damage to healthy cells.

Functional Groups: Incorporating specific functional groups can improve binding to target proteins or DNA. For instance, amino groups can enhance binding to DNA, while hydroxyl groups can increase solubility [38].

CHALLENGES IN DRUG DEVELOPMENT

Developing Quinone-Based Drugs Faces Several Challenges

Toxicity: Quinones can be highly toxic due to their ability to generate ROS and cause oxidative damage. Balancing therapeutic efficacy with minimizing toxicity to healthy cells is a significant challenge.

Stability: Quinones can be chemically unstable, undergoing rapid reduction or oxidation. Stabilizing quinone compounds to ensure they remain effective during storage and within the biological environment is crucial.

Selectivity: Achieving selectivity for target cells, such as cancer cells, without affecting normal cells is challenging. Strategies such as prodrug design and targeted delivery systems are employed to enhance selectivity.

CASE STUDIES OF SUCCESSFUL QUINONE-BASED DRUGS

Several quinone-based drugs have been successfully developed and are used in clinical practice:

Doxorubicin: This anthracycline antibiotic intercalates into DNA and inhibits topoisomerase II, preventing DNA replication and transcription. It also generates ROS, contributing to its cytotoxic effects. Doxorubicin is widely used in treating various cancers, including breast cancer, lymphoma, and leukemia.

Mitomycin C: This bioreductive alkylating agent cross-links DNA, inhibiting DNA synthesis and leading to cell death. It is effective against a range of cancers, including stomach, pancreatic, and bladder cancers.

Atovaquone: Used as an antimalarial, atovaquone inhibits the mitochondrial electron transport chain in Plasmodium species, leading to the collapse of mitochondrial membrane potential and parasite death. It is also used in treating Pneumocystis pneumonia in immunocompromised patients [39, 40].

TOXICOLOGICAL ASPECTS OF QUINONES

Quinones, despite their therapeutic potential, can exhibit significant toxicological effects. Understanding the mechanisms of quinone-induced toxicity, dose-response relationships, safety profiles, and strategies to mitigate toxicity is crucial for developing safe and effective quinone-based drugs.

Potential Toxic Effects of Quinones

Quinones can cause a range of toxic effects, which can impact various organs and systems in the body:

Oxidative Stress: Quinones can generate reactive oxygen species (ROS), leading to oxidative stress and damage to cellular components such as lipids, proteins, and DNA.

Cytotoxicity: Quinones can induce apoptosis or necrosis in cells, leading to tissue damage. This is particularly problematic for non-target cells, causing adverse effects in healthy tissues.

Cardiotoxicity: Some quinone-based drugs, such as doxorubicin, are known to cause cardiotoxicity, which can manifest as cardiomyopathy and heart failure.

Hepatotoxicity: Quinones can also induce liver damage, affecting liver function and potentially leading to liver failure in severe cases.

Neurotoxicity: Quinones can impact the nervous system, causing neurodegenerative effects and affecting cognitive and motor functions [41].

Mechanisms of Quinone-Induced Toxicity

The toxic effects of quinones are mediated through several mechanisms:

Redox Cycling and ROS Generation: Quinones can undergo redox cycling, repeatedly being reduced and oxidized. This process generates ROS, leading to oxidative stress and damage to cellular structures.

Alkylation of Biomolecules: Quinones can form covalent bonds with nucleophiles in proteins, DNA, and other biomolecules, disrupting their normal function.

Mitochondrial Dysfunction: Quinones can interfere with the mitochondrial electron transport chain, disrupting ATP production and leading to cell death.

Inflammatory Response: Quinones can induce the production of pro-inflammatory cytokines, contributing to tissue inflammation and damage [42, 43].

DOSE-RESPONSE RELATIONSHIPS AND SAFETY PROFILES

Understanding the dose-response relationship is critical in determining the safety profiles of quinone-based drugs:

Therapeutic Window: The therapeutic window is the range of doses at which a drug is effective without causing unacceptable side effects. For quinones, it is essential to identify the optimal dose that maximizes therapeutic effects while minimizing toxicity.

Toxicity Thresholds: Establishing toxicity thresholds helps in understanding the doses at which quinones start to exhibit toxic effects. This involves conducting preclinical studies in animal models and clinical trials in humans.

Cumulative Toxicity: Some quinones can cause cumulative toxicity with repeated doses, necessitating careful monitoring and dose adjustments during prolonged treatments [44].

STRATEGIES TO MITIGATE TOXICITY

Several strategies can be employed to mitigate the toxicity of quinone-based drugs:

Prodrug Design: Developing quinones as prodrugs can help in reducing toxicity. Prodrugs are inactive compounds that are metabolized into active quinone species within the target cells, minimizing exposure to non-target tissues.

Targeted Delivery: Conjugating quinones with targeting moieties, such as antibodies or peptides, can enhance selective delivery to target cells, reducing off-target effects.

Antioxidant Co-therapy: Co-administering antioxidants can help in neutralizing ROS generated by quinones, protecting healthy cells from oxidative damage.

Dose Optimization: Optimizing the dose and scheduling of quinone-based drugs can help in balancing therapeutic efficacy and toxicity. This involves careful monitoring of patient responses and adjusting doses as needed.

Chemical Modification: Modifying the chemical structure of quinones to enhance selectivity and reduce reactivity can help in mitigating toxicity. For example, introducing specific substituents can reduce the redox cycling potential and ROS generation [45].

QUINONES IN CLINICAL USE

Quinone-based drugs are used in various therapeutic applications, notably in cancer treatment, antimicrobial therapies, and other medical conditions. This section provides an overview of currently approved quinone-based drugs, clinical trial data and therapeutic outcomes, case studies in patient management, and future prospects for emerging therapies.

Current Clinically Approved Quinone-Based Drugs

Several quinone-based drugs have been approved for clinical use:

Doxorubicin (Adriamycin): An anthracycline antibiotic used primarily in chemotherapy for various cancers, including breast cancer, lymphomas, and leukemia.

Mitomycin C: An alkylating agent used to treat stomach, pancreatic, and bladder cancers. It is also used topically in ophthalmic surgery to prevent scarring.

Atovaquone: An antimalarial drug also used to treat Pneumocystis jirovecii pneumonia in immunocompromised patients.

Menaquinone (Vitamin K2): Used to treat and prevent vitamin K deficiency, which can lead to bleeding disorders.

CLINICAL TRIAL DATA AND THERAPEUTIC OUTCOMES

Doxorubicin

Efficacy: Doxorubicin has shown significant efficacy in treating various cancers. Clinical trials have demonstrated its effectiveness in reducing tumor size and improving survival rates in patients with breast cancer, lymphomas, and sarcomas.

Side Effects: Common side effects include myelosuppression, nausea, vomiting, alopecia, and cardiotoxicity. Long-term use is limited by cumulative dose-related cardiotoxicity.

Study Example: A study published in the Journal of Clinical Oncology reported that patients with metastatic breast cancer treated with doxorubicin had a response rate of approximately 50%, with improved overall survival compared to other chemotherapy agents.

Mitomycin C

Efficacy: Mitomycin C is effective in treating upper gastrointestinal and genitourinary cancers. It has been particularly useful in bladder cancer as an intravesical therapy to prevent recurrence after transurethral resection.

Side Effects: Potential side effects include myelosuppression, renal toxicity, and pulmonary toxicity. Topical use in ophthalmology can lead to complications such as delayed wound healing.

Study Example: A clinical trial published in The Lancet showed that intravesical mitomycin C significantly reduced the recurrence rate of non-muscle invasive bladder cancer compared to placebo.

Atovaquone

Efficacy: Atovaquone is highly effective in treating malaria and Pneumocystis pneumonia. It has been used successfully as an alternative to trimethoprim-sulfamethoxazole in patients with sulfa drug allergies.

Side Effects: Generally well-tolerated but can cause gastrointestinal disturbances, rash, and elevated liver enzymes.

Study Example: A study in the New England Journal of Medicine demonstrated that atovaquone was as effective as trimethoprim-sulfamethoxazole in treating Pneumocystis pneumonia, with fewer adverse effects [46].

CASE STUDIES AND PATIENT MANAGEMENT

Case Study 1: Doxorubicin in Breast Cancer

Patient: A 45-year-old female with HER2-positive breast cancer.

Treatment Plan: Administered doxorubicin in combination with cyclophosphamide, followed by paclitaxel and trastuzumab.

Outcome: Significant reduction in tumor size and no evidence of disease at the 6-month follow-up. The patient experienced manageable side effects, including temporary hair loss and mild cardiotoxicity, which were monitored and controlled with cardioprotective agents.

Case Study 2: Mitomycin C in Bladder Cancer

Patient: A 68-year-old male with non-muscle invasive bladder cancer.

Treatment Plan: Underwent transurethral resection of bladder tumor (TURBT) followed by intravesical mitomycin C therapy.

Outcome: No recurrence of cancer at the 12-month follow-up. The patient reported mild local irritation, which was resolved with symptomatic treatment.

FUTURE PROSPECTS AND EMERGING THERAPIES

The future of quinone-based therapies includes exploring new quinone compounds and improving existing ones for better efficacy and safety:

Novel Quinone Derivatives: Research is ongoing to develop new quinone derivatives with enhanced selectivity and reduced toxicity. These compounds are being designed to target specific cancer cells or pathogens more effectively.

Targeted Delivery Systems: Advances in nanotechnology and drug delivery systems are being explored to improve the targeting of quinone-based drugs to specific tissues or cells, minimizing systemic exposure and side effects.

Combination Therapies: Combining quinone-based drugs with other therapeutic agents, such as immunotherapy or other chemo-therapeutics, is being investigated to enhance overall treatment efficacy and overcome resistance.

Personalized Medicine: Tailoring quinone-based therapies based on individual patient profiles, including genetic and metabolic factors, can improve treatment outcomes and reduce adverse effects [47, 48].

FUTURE DIRECTIONS AND RESEARCH OPPORTUNITIES

The research and development of quinone-based compounds continue to evolve, offering promising directions for future therapies. Key areas of focus include emerging trends, novel derivatives, combination therapies, and advances in drug delivery systems.

Emerging Trends in Quinone Research

Redox Biology and Mechanisms: Understanding the redox biology of quinones is crucial. Studies focus on how quinones modulate redox balance within cells and how this impacts their therapeutic and toxicological profiles.

Biomarker Discovery: Identifying biomarkers that predict patient response to quinone-based therapies can enhance personalized medicine approaches.

Cancer Metabolism: Investigating the role of quinones in cancer metabolism, particularly how they affect cellular energy production and oxidative stress, is a growing area of research [49].

Novel Quinone Derivatives and Their Potential Applications

Improved Selectivity and Potency: Designing quinone derivatives with improved selectivity towards specific cellular targets can enhance their therapeutic efficacy. For example, modifying the quinone core to create derivatives that preferentially accumulate in cancer cells.

Multifunctional Quinones: Developing quinones that can target multiple pathways or cellular processes simultaneously. These multifunctional agents can have synergistic effects, enhancing their overall therapeutic potential.

Anti-inflammatory and Neuroprotective Agents: Novel quinone derivatives are being explored for their potential in treating inflammatory and neurodegenerative diseases, such as Alzheimer's and Parkinson's diseases, due to their antioxidant properties [50].

INTEGRATION OF QUINONE COMPOUNDS IN COMBINATION THERAPIES

Chemotherapy and Radiotherapy: Combining quinone-based drugs with traditional chemotherapy or radiotherapy can enhance treatment efficacy. Quinones can sensitize cancer cells to radiation or other chemotherapeutic agents, making them more susceptible to treatment.

Immunotherapy: Integrating quinone compounds with immunotherapeutic strategies, such as checkpoint inhibitors, can potentially boost the immune response against cancer cells.

Synergistic Drug Combinations: Identifying and developing drug combinations where quinones work synergistically with other agents to achieve greater therapeutic effects while minimizing toxicity.

ADVANCES IN DRUG DELIVERY SYSTEMS FOR QUINONE COMPOUNDS

Nanoparticle Delivery Systems: Nanotechnology offers innovative ways to deliver quinone compounds more effectively. Nanoparticles can encapsulate quinones, protecting them from premature degradation and enhancing their delivery to target tissues.

Liposomes and Micelles: These vesicular systems can improve the solubility and bioavailability of quinones. They can also provide sustained and controlled release of the drug, reducing the frequency of dosing.

Targeted Delivery Mechanisms: Conjugating quinones with targeting ligands (*e.g.*, antibodies, peptides) ensures that the drug is delivered specifically to diseased cells, minimizing off-target effects and improving safety profiles.

Responsive Delivery Systems: Developing delivery systems that respond to specific stimuli (*e.g.*, pH, temperature, enzymes) present in the tumor microenvironment or diseased tissues can enhance the precision and effectiveness of quinone-based therapies [51].

Research Opportunities

High-Throughput Screening: Utilizing high-throughput screening methods to identify new quinone derivatives with potent biological activities.

Preclinical Models: Developing advanced preclinical models, such as organoids and patient-derived xenografts, to better predict the clinical efficacy of quinone-based therapies.

Clinical Trials: Conducting well-designed clinical trials to evaluate the safety and efficacy of novel quinone compounds and combination therapies.

Mechanistic Studies: Deepening the understanding of the molecular mechanisms by which quinones exert their effects, which can inform the design of more effective and safer drugs [52].

CONCLUSION

Quinone compounds, with their distinctive redox properties and diverse chemical structures, play a crucial role in various biological systems and have significant therapeutic potential. This chapter has detailed the chemical nature and classification of quinones, elucidating their mechanisms of action through electron transfer, radical formation, and interactions with cellular components. The multifaceted roles of quinones in cellular respiration, enzymatic reactions, and as endogenous compounds underline their biological importance.

Therapeutically, quinones exhibit potent anti-cancer, antimicrobial, anti-inflammatory, and antioxidant properties, with clinically approved drugs like doxorubicin and mitomycin C demonstrating their efficacy. The development of quinone-based drugs involves strategic design, understanding structure-activity relationships, and overcoming challenges related to toxicity and stability. Successful case studies emphasize their potential, while ongoing research focuses on novel derivatives, combination therapies, and advanced drug delivery systems.

The future of quinone-based therapies looks promising, with emerging trends highlighting new applications and personalized medicine approaches. The integration of quinones in combination therapies and advancements in delivery technologies are expected to enhance their therapeutic outcomes. As research progresses, quinones are likely to contribute significantly to innovative treatments and improved patient care, solidifying their importance in modern medicine.

REFERENCES

[1]   Smith JP, Brown LM. Quinones and Their Reactions. J Org Chem 2010; 75(10): 3493-503.

[2]   Green DR, Reed JC. Mitochondria and Apoptosis. Science 1998; 281(5381): 1309-12.
[http://dx.doi.org/10.1126/science.281.5381.1309] [PMID: 9721092]

[3]   Roberts DV. Physical Properties of Quinones. J Chem Educ 2003; 80(12): 1420-3.

[4]   Mitchell P. Possible molecular mechanisms of the protonmotive function of cytochrome systems. J Theor Biol 1976; 62(2): 327-67.
[http://dx.doi.org/10.1016/0022-5193(76)90124-7] [PMID: 186667]

[5]   McCord JM, Fridovich I. Superoxide Dismutase. J Biol Chem 1969; 244(22): 6049-55.
[http://dx.doi.org/10.1016/S0021-9258(18)63504-5] [PMID: 5389100]

[6]   Trumpower BL. The protonmotive Q cycle. Energy transduction by coupling of proton translocation to electron transfer by the cytochrome bc1 complex. J Biol Chem 1990; 265(20): 11409-12.
[http://dx.doi.org/10.1016/S0021-9258(19)38410-8] [PMID: 2164001]

[7]   Morton JF. Henna, Lawsonia inermis. Journal of Economic Botany 1975; 29(2): 139-45.

[8]   Siegel D, Ross D. Immunodetection of NAD(P)H:quinone oxidoreductase 1 (NQO1) in human tissues11This work is dedicated to the memory of Professor Lars Ernster, who provided us with enthusiastic support, scientific insight, and constant encouragement in our many interactions. Free Radic Biol Med 2000; 29(3-4): 246-53.
[http://dx.doi.org/10.1016/S0891-5849(00)00310-5] [PMID: 11035253]

[9]   Begleiter A, Leith MK. Role of quinones in cancer chemotherapy. Cancer Chemother Pharmacol 1997; 40(5): 343-9.

[10] Pelletier PJ, Caventou JB. Sur les quinones. Ann Chim Phys 1838; 68: 132-6.

[11] Wöhler F, Kekulé A. Ueber die Benzochinone. Annalen der Chemie und Pharmacie 1869; 150: 1-29.

[12] Ribaudo JM, Kletzien RF. Atovaquone: a new therapeutic agent for Pneumocystis carinii pneumonia. Antimicrob Agents Chemother 1990; 34(5): 793-7.

[13] Crane FL, Hatefi Y, Lester RL, Widmer C. Isolation of a quinone from beef heart mitochondria. Biochim Biophys Acta 1957; 25(1): 220-1.
[http://dx.doi.org/10.1016/0006-3002(57)90457-2] [PMID: 13445756]

[14] Minotti G, Menna P, Salvatorelli E, Cairo G, Gianni L. Anthracyclines: molecular advances and pharmacologic developments in antitumor activity and cardiotoxicity. Pharmacol Rev 2004; 56(2): 185-229.
[http://dx.doi.org/10.1124/pr.56.2.6] [PMID: 15169927]

[15] Ernster L, Dallner G. Biochemical, physiological and medical aspects of ubiquinone function. Biochim Biophys Acta Mol Basis Dis 1995; 1271(1): 195-204.
[http://dx.doi.org/10.1016/0925-4439(95)00028-3] [PMID: 7599208]

[16] Suttie JW. Vitamin K and human nutrition. J Am Diet Assoc 1993; 93(5): 599-605.
[PMID: 1573141]

[17] Dandawate PR, Vyas AC, Padhye SB, Singh MW, Baruah JB. Perspectives on medicinal properties of benzoquinone compounds. Mini Rev Med Chem 2010; 10(5): 436-54.
[http://dx.doi.org/10.2174/138955710791330909] [PMID: 20370705]

[18] Nematollahi A, Aminimoghadamfarouj N, Wiart C, Safavi M, Sharifzadeh M, Ajani Y. Reviews on 1,4-naphthoquinones from *Diospyros* L. J Asian Nat Prod Res 2012; 14(1): 80-8.

[http://dx.doi.org/10.1080/10286020.2011.633515] [PMID: 22263598]

[19]   Rahman MM, Islam MR, Akash S, *et al*. Naphthoquinones and derivatives as potential anticancer agents: An updated review. Chem Biol Interact 2022; 368: 110198.
[http://dx.doi.org/10.1016/j.cbi.2022.110198] [PMID: 36179774]

[20]   Zhao L, Zheng L. A review on bioactive anthraquinone and derivatives as the regulators for ROS. Molecules 2023; 28(24): 8139.
[http://dx.doi.org/10.3390/molecules28248139] [PMID: 38138627]

[21]   Mitchell P. Ubiquinone and other quinones in biological electron transfer. Biochim Biophys Acta 1976; 456(3): 89-105.

[22]   Bolton JL, Trush MA, Penning TM, Dryhurst G, Monks TJ. Mechanisms of quinone-induced toxicity. Chem Res Toxicol 2000; 13(3): 135-60.
[http://dx.doi.org/10.1021/tx9902082] [PMID: 10725110]

[23]   Monks TJ, Jones DC. Quinone-induced alkylation of DNA and proteins. J Biol Chem 2002; 277(7): 4895-903.

[24]   Thornburg LD, Britt BM. Enzyme inhibition by quinones: mechanistic aspects.Enzyme inhibition and drug design. Totowa, NJ: Humana Press 2001; pp. 259-76.

[25]   Arora A, Nair MG, Strasburg GM. Chemical properties of quinones and their impact on biological systems. Chem Rev 2012; 112(8): 5258-80.

[26]   Cores Á, Carmona-Zafra N, Clerigué J, Villacampa M, Menéndez JC. Quinones as Neuroprotective Agents. Antioxidants (Basel) 2023; 12(7): 1464.
[http://dx.doi.org/10.3390/antiox12071464]

[27]   Ji Q, Zhang L, Jones MB, *et al*. Molecular mechanism of quinone signaling mediated through S-quinonization of a YodB family repressor QsrR. Proc Natl Acad Sci USA 2013; 110(13): 5010-5.
[http://dx.doi.org/10.1073/pnas.1219446110] [PMID: 23479646]

[28]   Chesis PL, Levin DE, Smith MT, Ernster L, Ames BN. Mutagenicity of quinones: pathways of metabolic activation and detoxification. Proc Natl Acad Sci USA 1984; 81(6): 1696-700.
[http://dx.doi.org/10.1073/pnas.81.6.1696] [PMID: 6584903]

[29]   Bolton JL, Dunlap T. Formation and Biological Targets of Quinones: Cytotoxic *versus* Cytoprotective Effects. Chem Res Toxicol 2017; 30(1): 13-37.
[http://dx.doi.org/10.1021/acs.chemrestox.6b00256] [PMID: 27617882]

[30]   Dias GG, King A, de Moliner F, Vendrell M, da Silva Júnior EN. Quinone-based fluorophores for imaging biological processes. Chem Soc Rev 2018; 47(1): 12-27.
[http://dx.doi.org/10.1039/C7CS00553A] [PMID: 29099127]

[31]   Schulz CE, Dutta AK, Izsák R, Pantazis DA. Systematic High☐Accuracy Prediction of Electron Affinities for Biological Quinones. J Comput Chem 2018; 39(29): 2439-51.
[http://dx.doi.org/10.1002/jcc.25570] [PMID: 30281169]

[32]   Bittner S. When quinones meet amino acids: chemical, physical and biological consequences. Amino Acids 2006; 30(3): 205-24.
[http://dx.doi.org/10.1007/s00726-005-0298-2] [PMID: 16601927]

[33]   Begleiter A. Clinical applications of quinone-containing alkylating agents. Front Biosci 2000; 5(1): e153.
[http://dx.doi.org/10.2741/begleit] [PMID: 11056078]

[34]   Ferreira VF, de Carvalho AS, Ferreira PG, Lima CGS, da Silva FC. Quinone-Based Drugs: An Important Class of Molecules in Medicinal Chemistry. Curr Med Chem 2021; 17(10): 1073-85.

[35]   Madeo J, Zubair A, Marianne F. A review on the role of quinones in renal disorders. Springerplus 2013; 2(1): 139.
[http://dx.doi.org/10.1186/2193-1801-2-139] [PMID: 23577302]

[36]   Faizan S, Mohammed Abdo Mohsen M, Amarakanth C, *et al.* Quinone scaffolds as potential therapeutic anticancer agents: Chemistry, mechanism of Actions, Structure-Activity relationships and future perspectives. Results Chem 2024; 7: 101432.
[http://dx.doi.org/10.1016/j.rechem.2024.101432]

[37]   Dahlem MA Junior, Nguema Edzang RW, Catto AL, Raimundo JM. Quinones as an Efficient Molecular Scaffold in the Antibacterial/Antifungal or Antitumoral Arsenal. Int J Mol Sci 2022; 23(22): 14108.

[38]   Zhang L, Zhang G, Xu S, Song Y. Recent advances of quinones as a privileged structure in drug discovery. Eur J Med Chem 2021; 223: 113632.
[http://dx.doi.org/10.1016/j.ejmech.2021.113632] [PMID: 34153576]

[39]   Gordaliza M. Synthetic strategies to terpene quinones/hydroquinones. Mar Drugs 2012; 10(2): 358-402.
[http://dx.doi.org/10.3390/md10020358] [PMID: 22412807]

[40]   Chan-Zapata I, Borges-Argáez R, Ayora-Talavera G. Quinones as Promising Compounds against Respiratory Viruses: A Review. Molecules 2023; 28(4): 1981.
[http://dx.doi.org/10.3390/molecules28041981] [PMID: 36838969]

[41]   Bolton JL, Trush MA, Penning TM, Dryhurst G, Monks TJ. Role of quinones in toxicology. Chem Res Toxicol 2000; 13(3): 135-60.
[http://dx.doi.org/10.1021/tx9902082] [PMID: 10725110]

[42]   Monks T, Jones D. The metabolism and toxicity of quinones, quinonimines, quinone methides, and quinone-thioethers. Curr Drug Metab 2002; 3(4): 425-38.
[http://dx.doi.org/10.2174/1389200023337388] [PMID: 12093358]

[43]   Siraki AG, Chan TS, O'Brien PJ. Application of quantitative structure-toxicity relationships for the comparison of the cytotoxicity of 14 p-benzoquinone congeners in primary cultured rat hepatocytes *versus* PC12 cells. Toxicol Sci 2004; 81(1): 148-59.
[http://dx.doi.org/10.1093/toxsci/kfh182] [PMID: 15178806]

[44]   Irons RD. Quinones as toxic metabolites of benzene. J Toxicol Environ Health 1985; 16(5): 673-8.
[http://dx.doi.org/10.1080/15287398509530777] [PMID: 4093989]

[45]   Kumagai Y, Taguchi K. Toxicological Effects of Polycyclic Aromatic Hydrocarbon Quinones Contaminated in Diesel Exhaust Particles. Asian Journal of Atmospheric Environment 2007; 1(1): 28-35.
[http://dx.doi.org/10.1007/BF03654884]

[46]   Krayz GT, Bittner S, Dhiman A, Becker JY. Electrochemistry of Quinones with Respect to their Role in Biomedical Chemistry. Chem Rec 2021; 21(9): 2332-43.
[http://dx.doi.org/10.1002/tcr.202100069] [PMID: 34107155]

[47]   Bolton JL, Dunlap T. Formation and Biological Targets of Quinones: Cytotoxic versus Cytoprotective Effects. Chem Res Toxicol 2017; 30(1): 13-37.

[48]   Gong H, He Z, Peng A, *et al.* Effects of several quinones on insulin aggregation. Sci Rep 2014; 4(1): 5648.
[http://dx.doi.org/10.1038/srep05648] [PMID: 25008537]

[49]   Hasan F, Mahanta V, Abdelazeez AAA. Quinones for Aqueous Organic Redox Flow Battery: A Prospective on Redox Potential, Solubility, and Stability. Adv Mater Interfaces 2023; 10(24): 2300268.
[http://dx.doi.org/10.1002/admi.202300268]

[50]   Redal MA, Luis QS. Future directions: challenges, opportunities and limitations 2017.

[51]   Ega SP, Srinivasan P. Quinone materials for supercapacitor: Current status, approaches, and future directions. J Energy Storage 2022; 47: 103700.

[http://dx.doi.org/10.1016/j.est.2021.103700]

[52]　Zheng L, Jin J, Shi L, *et al.* Gamma tocopherol, its dimmers, and quinones: Past and future trends. Crit Rev Food Sci Nutr 2020; 60(22): 3916-30.
　　　[http://dx.doi.org/10.1080/10408398.2020.1711704] [PMID: 31957471]

CHAPTER 10

Recent Study on Quinone Derivatives and their Applications

Suryakant R. Rode[1] and **Ashutosh Kumar Dash**[2,*]

[1] *Jai Research Foundation Valvada, Valsad, Gujrat, India*

[2] *Senior Research Scientist (R&D), Drug Discovery Division, Macleods Pharmaceutical Ltd, Mumbai, India*

Abstract: Quinone and its derivatives have manifold applications in pharmaceutical industries. In this chapter, we look over the current practices of quinones and their derivatives in several fields. Recent studies have found that quinone-enhanced humification in food waste composting is a strategy for hazard mitigation and nitrogen retention. Quinone derivatives such as diazanthraquinone dimers have been demonstrated as high-capacity organic cathode materials for rechargeable lithium batteries. Their preparation and advantage over conventional batteries have been explained. Quinone-chlorophyll conjugation synthesized by the Diels-alder approach as conformers, called atropisomers, is a recent invention. Currently, in the field of pharmacological practices, quinone and its class of molecules have demonstrated a wide range of therapeutic properties, such as anticancer, anti-inflammatory, and antibiotic.

Keywords: Anticancer agents, Benzoquinone anthraquinone, Diel's alder reaction, Lithium-ion batteries, Naphthoquinone, Pictet Spengler annulation, Quinone.

INTRODUCTION

Quinones are electron carriers that play a role in photosynthesis. As vitamins, they represent a class of molecules preventing and treating several illnesses such as osteoporosis, cardiovascular diseases, cancer [1, 5], bacterial infection, *etc*. They are used in Li-ion batteries [3] and food waste composting [2]. Quinone and chlorin are conjugated *via* the Diels-Alder reaction; the resulting compound can exhibit unique electronic properties due to the new conjugated π-system [4]. One fascinating study observed the synthesis of bis(arylamino) pentiptycenes using pentiptycene quinone in a one-pot process [6]. Quinones exist in nature in many forms, such as benzoquinones, naphthoquinones, anthraquinones, and polycyclic

---

*Corresponding author Ashutosh Kumar Dash: Jai Research Foundation Valvada, Valsad, Gujrat, India; E-mail: ??

quinones [7 - 9]. For example, vitamin K (phylloquinone) include naphthoquinones, emodin, physcion, cascarin, catenarin, and rhein. Anthraquinones and benzoquinones are present in nature and are named carthamins. In this article, we have discussed about recent novelty of work on quinone and its derivative.

CLASSIFICATION OF QUINONES

Benzoquinones

Benzoquinones (Fig. **1**), such as lawsone, plumbagin, and 1,4-benzoquinone (menadione), exhibit various biological activities, including antioxidant, antibacterial, and anticancer effects. Pharmacological targets and pathways include NAD(P)H: quinone oxidoreductase 1 (NQO1), topoisomerases, and the proteasome. Key pathways involve reactive oxygen species (ROS) generation, DNA damage, and inhibition of the proteasome [9, 10].

Fig. (1). Structure of benzoquinone.

Naphthoquinones

Naphthoquinones (Fig. **2**) have two carbonyl groups within their naphthalene ring structure. Lawsone, a naphthoquinone, is derived from the henna plant and is a ideal example in this category. The cytotoxic and antitumor properties of naphthoquinones are well-documented, and their potential as anticancer agents has been extensively researched. Pharmacological targets and pathways for naphthoquinones include thioredoxin reductase, topoisomerases, and the mitochondrial electron transport chain. Key biological pathways involve redox regulation, DNA damage, and mitochondrial dysfunction [9, 10].

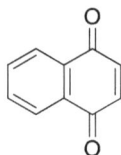

Fig. (2). Structure of naphthoquinones.

ANTHRAQUINONES

The nucleus consists of tricyclic anthracenes featuring two carbonyl groups, which can be readily sourced from plants and fungi. Notable examples include emodin, aloe-emodin, and rhein. Anthraquinones (Fig. **3**) are known for their diverse biological activities, including anti-inflammatory, anticancer, and antibacterial properties. Mode of action as targets includes protein kinase C (PKC), NF-κB, and topoisomerases in cancer and other illnesses. Associated biological pathways encompass the modulation of protein kinases, inflammatory processes, and responses to DNA damage [9 - 11].

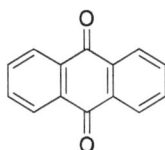

Fig. (3). Structure of anthraquinone.

Heteroquinones

Heteroquinones (Fig. **4**) comprise one or more heteroatoms, such as oxygen, sulfur, or nitrogen, within their ring structure. Examples include menadione bisulfite, a water-soluble form of menadione, and plumbagin, both of which are naturally occurring compounds featuring a quinone-oxygen bridge. These compounds often possess unique chemical and biological properties that make them promising candidates for drug development [9, 10, 12].

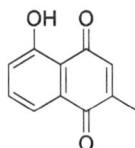

Fig. (4). Structure of heteroquinone.

Pharmacological targets include topoisomerases and DNA methyltransferases, along with reactive oxygen species (ROS) generation. The associated biological pathways involve DNA damage, epigenetic modulation, and oxidative stress responses.

These quinone derivatives have recently been used for emerging sustainable and highly efficient batteries, surpassing traditional lithium-ion battery technology. The development of diazaanthraquinone dimers has led to high-capacity organic cathode materials for rechargeable lithium batteries. 2,2′-bi(1,- -diazaanthraquinone) (Li8-BDAAQ) is a recent example. The unique structure of Li8-BDAAQ, with its multiple redox-active sites and the ability to coordinate with lithium ions, makes it a promising candidate for high-performance battery materials. The general process of formulating has been described as follows [3].

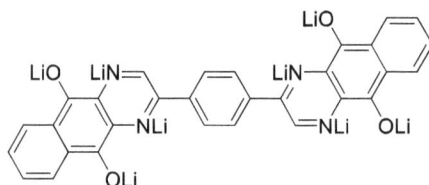

Fig. (5). Lithium-ion interacted molecule used in batteries.

GENERAL PROCEDURE FOR DIAZAANTHRAQUINONE PREPARATION IN THE USE OF LI-ION BATTERIES

Compounds **1** and **2**were heated at 80°C for 12 h to obtain **3**, followed by Wolff-Kishner reduction using hydrazine hydrate ($N_2H_4.H_2O$) at 65°C for 3 h to get compound **4**. In step 3, the condensation reaction between **4** and **5** provided**6,** followed by single ion reduction accompanied by Li-ion intercalation, which finally gave**7**, applied in Li-ion batteries [3].

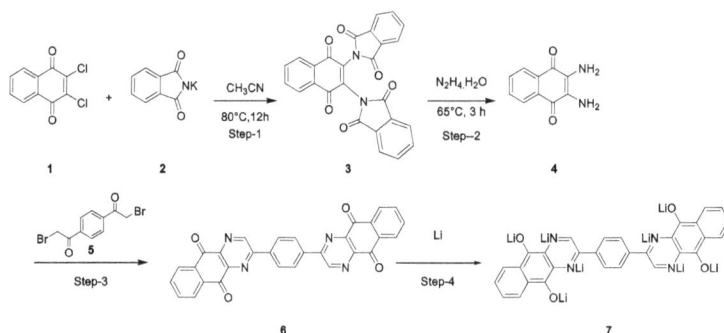

Fig. (6). Preparation of single-electron reduction accompanied by Li-ion intercalation molecule.

KEY FEATURES AND BENEFITS OF DIAZAANTHRAQUINONE DIMERS

Stability: The incorporation of nitrogen atoms within the quinone framework can enhance the stability of the molecule, making it more resistant to degradation during cycling [3].

Lithium coordination: The ability of the molecule to coordinate with lithium ions at multiple sites can improve the efficiency of lithium-ion insertion and extraction processes, enhancing the overall performance of the battery [3].

MECHANISM OF OPERATION

Lithiation and delithiation: During the charging process, lithium ions from the electrolyte are inserted into the Li8-BDAAQ structure, undergoing a reduction reaction. During discharging, the lithium ions are extracted from the Li8-BDAAQ structure, undergoing an oxidation reaction. This reversible process allows the battery to store and release energy efficiently [3].

Redox reactions: The quinone moieties within Li8-BDAAQ can undergo reversible redox reactions, contributing to the overall capacity of the battery. The presence of nitrogen atoms can further stabilize these redox reactions, improving the cycle life of the battery.

APPLICATION OF LI8-BDAAQ IN LITHIUM-ION BATTERIES

As cathode/anode material: Li8-BDAAQ can be utilized as a cathode material in lithium-ion batteries. Its elevated redox potential and various redox-active sites facilitate the effective storage and release of significant energy during charge and discharge cycles. The structure of Li8-BDAAQ can facilitate fast lithium-ion diffusion, leading to improved charge/discharge rates and better power density. While less common, Li8-BDAAQ can also be explored as an anode material. Its ability to undergo multiple electron transfers can be leveraged to enhance the capacity and performance of the anode [3].

ADVANTAGES OVER TRADITIONAL MATERIALS

Enhanced capacity and stability: Compared to traditional cathode materials such as lithium cobalt oxide (LiCoO2), Li8-BDAAQ offers a higher theoretical capacity and improved stability due to its unique structure [3].

Environmental benefits: Organic materials like Li8-BDAAQ are generally more environmentally friendly compared to inorganic materials used in conventional batteries. They can be synthesized from renewable resources and are easier to recycle.

CHALLENGES AND RESEARCH DIRECTIONS OF QUINONES IN SOME OTHER RESPECTS

Conductivity: One of the challenges with using organic materials like Li8-BDAAQ is their lower electrical conductivity compared to inorganic materials. This can be addressed by combining Li8-BDAAQ with conductive additives or designing composite materials [3].

Optimization: Further research is needed to optimize the structure and formulation of Li8-BDAAQ-based electrodes to maximize their performance. This includes improving the synthesis methods, enhancing the electrode formulation, and optimizing the battery assembly process.

QUINONES ENHANCE HUMIFICATION IN FOOD WASTE COMPOSTING

Studies reveal that adding p-benzoquinone (PBQ) can effortlessly promote humification and nitrogen retention in organic waste. The process of reducing the toxicity of quinone-containing waste through co-composting involves quinones converting into amino-quinone structures *via* biochemical reactions, which fosters the early production of stable humic acid (HA) in significant amounts [2]. The addition of external quinones speeds up the humification process and enhances nitrogen incorporation into the HA while minimizing the loss of carbon and nitrogen during composting. This results in a final product that is less toxic.

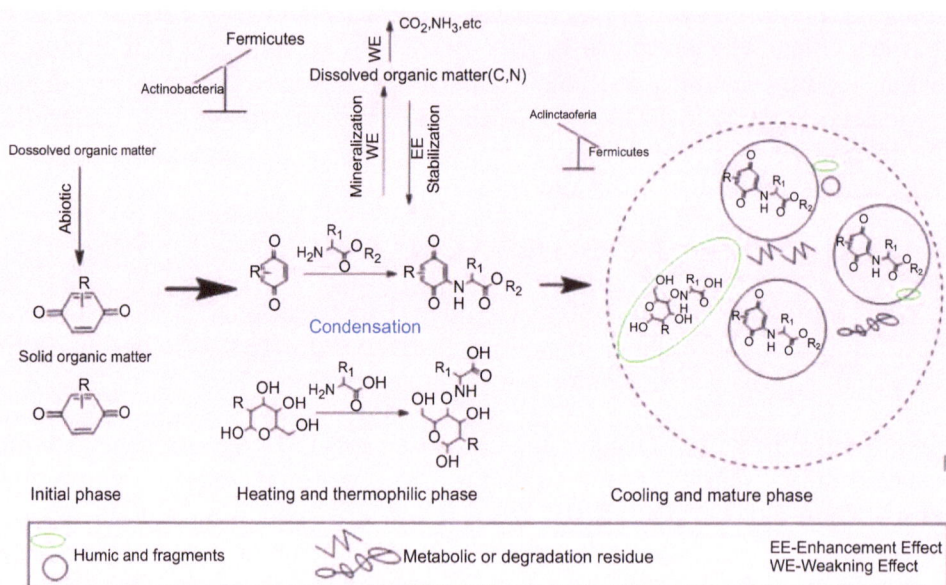

Fig. (7). Graphical representation of humification.

Fig. (7) shows that in the initial phase, the mixing of plant residues, animal remains, and other organic waste materials takes place. In the heating and thermophilic phase, microbial activity generates heat, leading to a rise in temperature (40-70°C) as microbes break down easily degradable organic compounds. Thermophilic microorganisms take over, further breaking down complex organic compounds. Quinones are introduced to the system, enhancing microbial activity. They act as electron acceptors and hasten microbial processes, breaking down lignin and other resistant molecules. Polymerization (smaller molecules combine to form larger, stable structures) and condensation reactions (*e.g.*, amino acids, peptides, and sugars undergo condensation reactions, forming complex macromolecules) lead to the formation of humic substances.

Conclusively, cooling and mature phase formation of stable humic substance rallies soil fertility and structure.

CONJUGATION OF CHLORO-QUINONE FORMING ADVANCED MOLECULE [4]

The conjugation of chlorin-quinone *via* the Diels-Alder reaction and its effect on fluorescence through intramolecular electron transfer are fascinating topics. Its synthetic protocol is elucidated as follows.

A solution of 3-(1,3-butadienyl) chlorin in chlorobenzene degassed under reduced pressure with a continuous flow of argon was prepared initially. To this solution, p-benzoquinone was added, and the mixture refluxed in the dark for one day (synthesis in Fig. **8**). After the reaction was complete, the solvent was removed under reduced pressure, and the product was isolated using flash chromatography. The resulting mixture of compounds **15** and **16** was further purified by reversed-phase HPLC to isolate compound **15**. This compound was then treated with 1,4-benzoquinone for three days, resulting in the formation of compound **16** as a 1:1 mixture of atropisomers. Stereoisomers so formed were successfully separated using HPLC. A similar reaction was performed with 1,4-naphthoquinone to obtain anthraquinone derivatives. The significant fluorescence quenching observed in compound **16** was attributed to intramolecular electron transfer from the photoexcited chlorin to the quinone. The quenching efficiencies exceeded 99% and were unaffected by the rotational stereochemistry. Additionally, the naphthoquinone conjugate exhibited slightly greater quenching compared to the anthraquinone conjugate, which was likely due to the more favorable electrochemical reduction of naphthoquinone [4, 19].

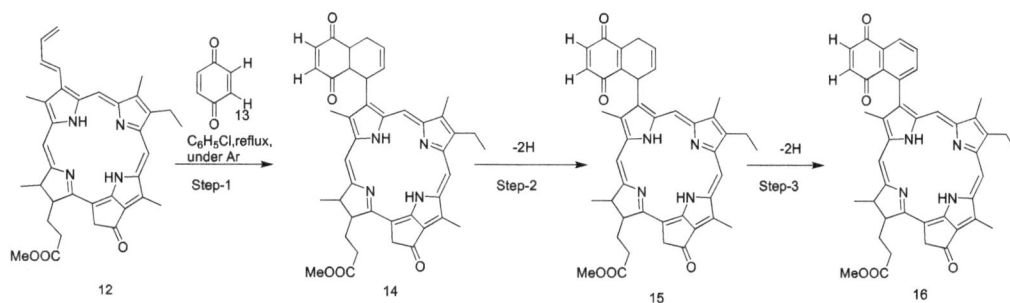

Fig. (8). Synthesis of chloro-quinone conjugate.

IDENTIFICATION OF ATROPISOMERS OF NAPHTHOQUINONE DERIVATIVE

^{1}H NMR spectra of two atropisomers of naphthoquinone derivative after HPLC separation are given below [4].

Chromatogram of 2nd Isomer

With superficial observation, we cannot distinguish between these two atropisomers (Fig. **9** and **10**). However, by examining their ¹H NMR spectra, we can observe slight variations in chemical shifts, small differences in coupling constants, and relative peak areas. Additionally, High-Performance Liquid Chromatography (HPLC) can separate these two isomers, showing them as distinct peaks.

Isomer 1st

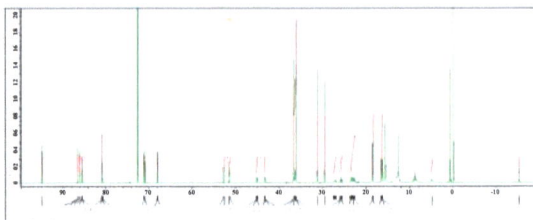

Fig. (9). ¹HNMR isomer Ist isomer of atropisomers.

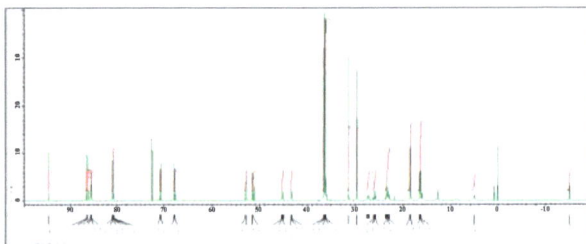

Fig. (10). ¹HNMR isomer IInd.

APPLICATIONS OF CHLORIN-QUINONE CONJUGATES

As Fluorescent Probes and Sensors

The unique fluorescence properties of chlorin-quinone conjugates can be harnessed to develop highly sensitive fluorescent probes and sensors. These can be used in several processes.

Biological imaging: For tracking and imaging biological processes.

Chemical sensing: Detecting the presence of specific ions or molecules in a solution.

Photodynamic Therapy (PDT)

PDT is a recent application in the mitigation of various diseases. In this direction, chlorine conjugates have been used in PDT for cancer treatment. The introduction of quinone can potentially modify the photophysical properties, leading to more efficient or targeted therapy options [18].

QUINONE AND ITS DERIVATIVES HAVING CANCER-TREATING POTENTIAL

Quinones possess a strong capability to engage in redox processes, and this unique reversible reduction and oxidation property makes them valuable in cancer therapy, as well as promising candidates for anti-inflammatory agents [5]. Quinones quickly convert to hydroquinone, which can then revert to quinones, creating a redox system. During this redox cycling, hydroxyl radicals can transform glutathione (GSH) into its oxidized form (GSSG) in the presence of hydrogen peroxide (Fig. **11**). This conversion occurs without the involvement of enzymes such as glutathione S-transferase (GST). A variety of medications, environmental toxins, and both organic and inorganic compounds can lead to the formation of quinone-glutathione (GSH) conjugates and/or result in the depletion of GSH [13, 14].

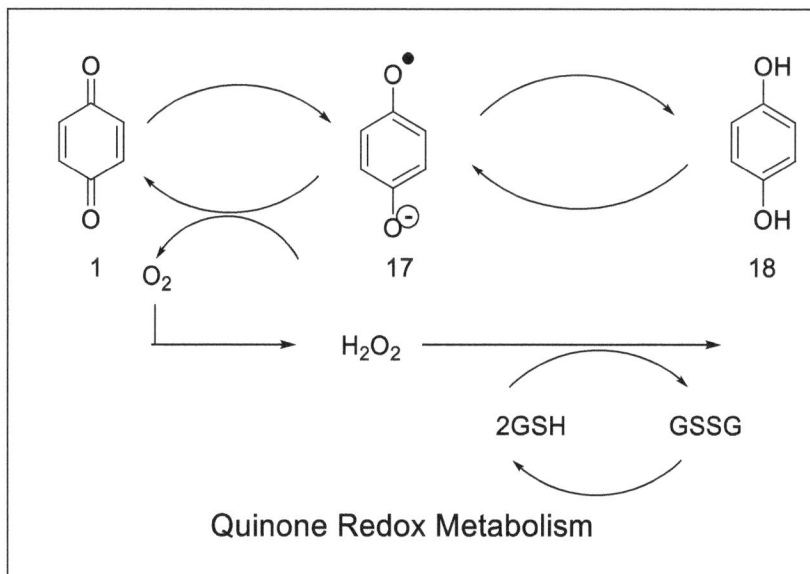

Fig. (11). Conversion of GSH to GSSG in the presence of hydrogen peroxide.

The redox potential, influenced by structural changes, determines the efficiency of electron transfer and the generation of reactive oxygen species (ROS). These ROS can induce oxidative stress, potentially leading to the death of cancer cells.

QUINONES AS ANTICANCER AGENTS DUE TO THEIR UNIQUE MECHANISMS OF ACTION IN ROS [5]

Quinones play a significant role as anticancer agents due to their ability to undergo redox cycling and generate reactive oxygen species (ROS). Here is an overview of the mechanisms through which quinones exert their anticancer effects:

Redox cycling and ros generation: Quinones can undergo redox cycling, where they are reduced to semiquinones and then deoxidized back to quinones. This redox cycling process generates reactive oxygen species (ROS) such as superoxide anions, hydrogen peroxide, and hydroxyl radicals. Elevated levels of ROS can induce oxidative stress, leading to:

Dna damage: ROS can cause single and double-strand breaks in DNA, leading to mutations and apoptosis.

Lipid peroxidation: ROS can oxidize lipids in cell membranes, resulting in membrane damage and cell death.

Protein oxidation: ROS can oxidize critical cellular proteins, disrupting their function and leading to cell death.

ALKYLATION AND CROSS-LINKING OF DNA

Some quinones can directly alkylate DNA, forming covalent bonds with DNA bases. This alkylation can result in other ways as follows.

Quinones interact with DNA by forming adducts, disrupting the processes of replication and transcription, and inhibiting cell growth. They can cause both inter- and intra-strand DNA cross-links, leading to stalled replication forks and cell cycle arrest. Additionally, quinones inhibit topoisomerases, enzymes essential for DNA replication, transcription, and recombination, resulting in the accumulation of DNA breaks and promoting cell death. By inhibiting topoisomerases, quinones also impair the cell's ability to repair damaged DNA, amplifying their cytotoxic effects.

MODULATION OF SIGNAL TRANSDUCTION PATHWAYS

Quinones can modulate various cellular signaling pathways [5], such as:

Activation of apoptotic pathways: Quinones can activate pro-apoptotic proteins such as p53, Bax, and caspases, leading to programmed cell death.

Inhibition of cell survival pathways: Quinones can inhibit survival pathways such as PI3K/Akt and NF-κB, reducing cell proliferation and inducing apoptosis.

Epigenetic modulation: Some quinones can influence epigenetic modifications, such as:

Histone modification: Quinones can alter histone acetylation and methylation, affecting gene expression and promoting apoptosis.

Dna methylation: Quinones can influence DNA methylation patterns, leading to the activation of tumor suppressor genes and the inhibition of oncogenes.

EXAMPLES OF QUINONES AS ANTICANCER AGENTS AS MARKETED PRODUCTS

  i. **Doxorubicin:** An anthracycline quinone that intercalates into DNA, inhibits topoisomerase II, and generates ROS, leading to DNA damage and apoptosis [20, 21].
 ii. **Mitomycin c:** A quinone that undergoes bioreductive activation to form DNA cross-links, inhibiting DNA synthesis and inducing apoptosis.
iii. **Menadione (vitamin k3):** A quinone that generates ROS and induces oxidative stress, leading to cancer cell death.

Structure-activity relationships (SAR): play a key role in understanding how the structural characteristics of quinones influence their anticancer properties. Here are the critical factors in the SAR of quinones to understand the quinone core [5].

Quinone Core Structure: The type of quinone core, such as naphthoquinones (*e.g.*, plumbagin) or anthraquinones (*e.g.*, doxorubicin), strongly influences anticancer activity. These quinones demonstrate potent effects through DNA intercalation and reactive oxygen species (ROS) generation. Electron-withdrawing groups (*e.g.*, nitro, cyano) on the quinone ring enhance anticancer activity by increasing electrophilicity, facilitating redox cycling and ROS production. Substituents like hydroxyl or methoxy groups affect redox potential, solubility, and cellular uptake.

Substituent Position and Nature: The location of substituents on the quinone ring (*e.g.*, ortho, meta, or para) influences how the molecule interacts with biological targets. Ortho-quinones generally show higher reactivity, forming covalent bonds with biomolecules and exhibiting stronger anticancer effects.

Ring Size and Fused Ring Systems: The addition of rings to the quinone core, such as a fused benzo ring, can enhance anticancer activity. Variations in ring size, such as those in naphthoquinones and anthraquinones, affect potency, with larger ring systems often showing increased efficacy [17].

Oxidation State and Redox Properties: The redox potential of quinones is crucial for their anticancer effects. Quinones with suitable redox potentials participate effectively in redox cycling, generating ROS that induce oxidative stress and promote cancer cell death [13, 14].

Linker and Conjugation: The addition of linkers or conjugation with specific functional groups can modify quinone stability, solubility, and cellular absorption. Changes in the linker can affect quinone stability, reactivity, and interaction with biological targets. Conjugation with peptides or targeting ligands may improve selectivity and enhance delivery to cancer cells [15, 16].

In summary, the anticancer efficacy of quinones is strongly linked to factors such as their core structure, substituents, redox potential, lipophilicity, and capacity to generate reactive oxygen species (ROS) (Fig. **12**). A thorough understanding of these structure-activity relationship (SAR) aspects is essential for developing more effective quinone-derived anticancer agents.

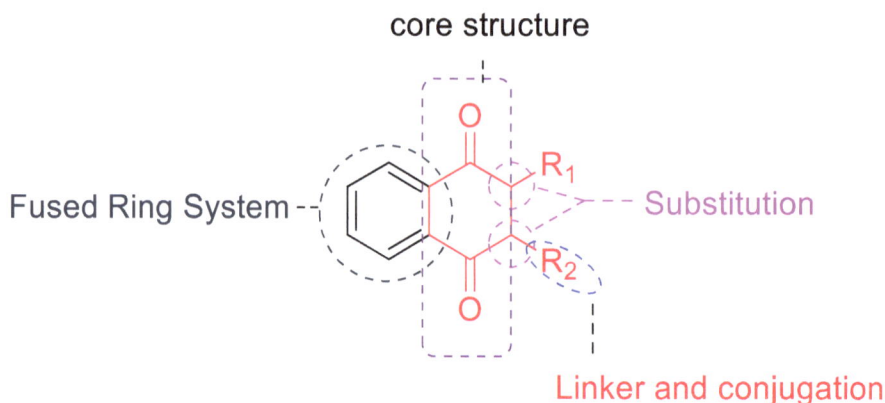

Fig. (12). SAR of quinone.

QUINONES IN SUPRAMOLECULAR CHEMISTRY AND POLYMER CHEMISTRY

Pentiptycene is useful for supramolecular chemistry and polymer chemistry. One of the research studies proclaimed the synthesis of Bis (aryl amino) pentiptycenes in an 8-step process, but the researchers optimized it in a single pot by using pentiptycene. Quinone is a key starting material and reagent like Ar-NH2, TiCl$_4$, and DABCO [6].

By using the same procedure, they conjugated 20 different amines with pentiptycene quinone, for example R=Cl, Br, I, F, CN, NO$_2$, Ph, OH. OCH$_3$, COOCH$_3$, CH$_3$, some amino pyridines, *etc*.

Among the many examples present in the literature, one is mentioned to discuss this conversion [6].

ONE-POT SYNTHESIS PROCEDURE OF BIS (ARYL AMINO) PENTIPTYCENES USING ANILINE [6]

Step 1: To a two-neck bottle equipped with a stirring bar containing pentiptycene quinone 1 (460 mg, 1 mmol, 1 equiv), aniline (931 mg, 10 mmol, 10 equiv), and DABCO (673 mg, 6 mmol, 6 equiv), PhCl was added (20 mL) under nitrogen atmosphere. The two-neck bottle was heated to 60°C with an oil bath, followed by a slow addition of TiCl4 (0.67ml, 6 mmol, 6 equiv) at 60°C. The reaction mixture was stirred under 140°C for 2 days (synthesis in Fig. **13**). After the reaction mixture was cooled to rt, the reaction mixture was poured into 100 mL of DCM, quenched by NaHCO$_3$(aq), and extracted with DCM (3 × 50 mL). If undissolved solid residues remained, the solid residue was filtered and washed with DCM/MeOH cosolvent (DCM/M eOH = 10/1) or THF, and the organic solution was combined with the DCM layer. The combined organic solution was dried over MgSO$_4$ and then concentrated. The resulting crude product was purified by recrystallization or column chromatography (the solvent system for each case is shown independently in section 2.2) using silica gel to afford the isolated yield as the yield of one-pot synthesis. By using this process, we can isolate 18- 90% yield within a single pot [6].

ANALYTICAL DATA

The analytical data for the compound Bis (aryl amino) pentiptycene is given in Figs. (**14** and **15**).

^{1}H NMR (400 MHz, CDCl$_3$) δ 7.25 – 7.17 (m, 4H), 7.17 – 7.06 (m, 8H), 6.92 – 6.83 (m, 10H), 6.59 – 6.52 (m, 4H), 5.54 (s, 4H).

^{13}C NMR (126 MHz, CDCl$_3$) δ 147.4, 145.1, 141.9, 129.5 (2C), 125.0, 123.7, 118.6, 114.2, 77.2, 49.6. **HRMS (ESI) m/z**: [M-H]- Calcd for C$_{46}$H$_{33}$N$_2$ 613.2638; found 613.2611.

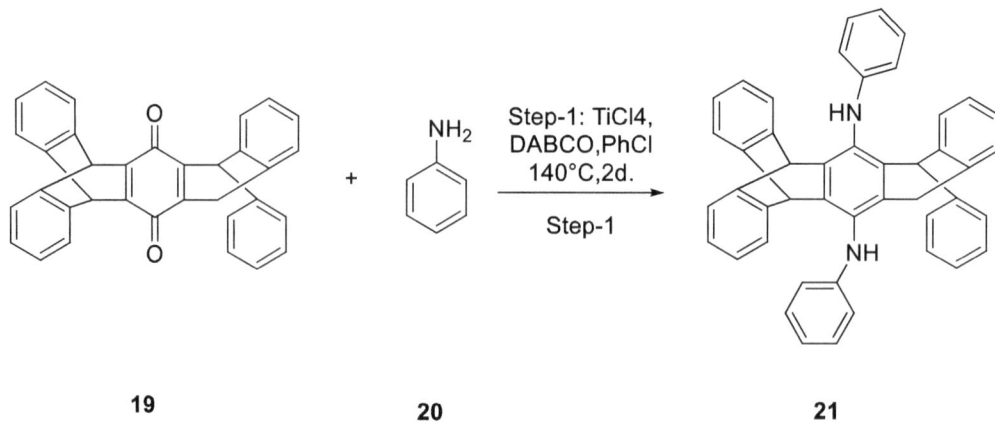

Fig. (13). Synthesis of Bis (aryl amino) pentiptycenes.

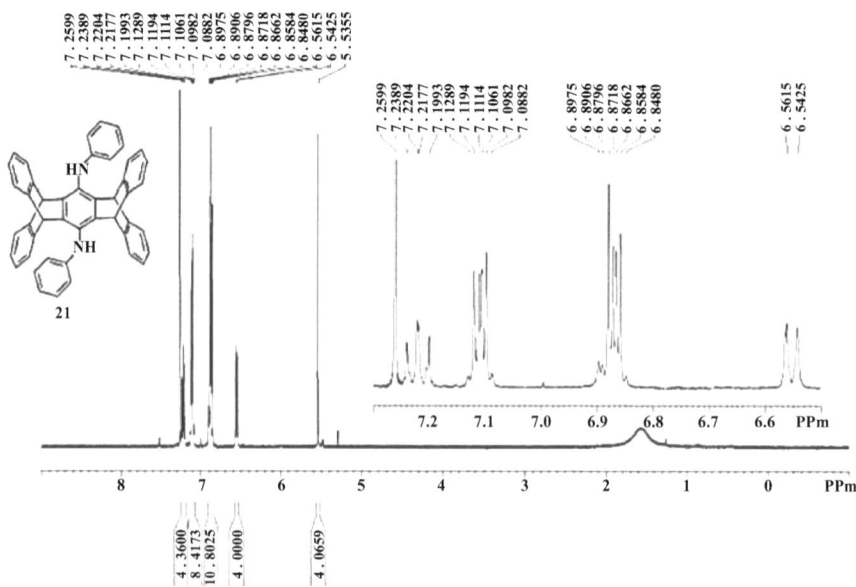

Fig. (14). ^{1}H NMR of Bis (aryl amino) pentiptycenes.

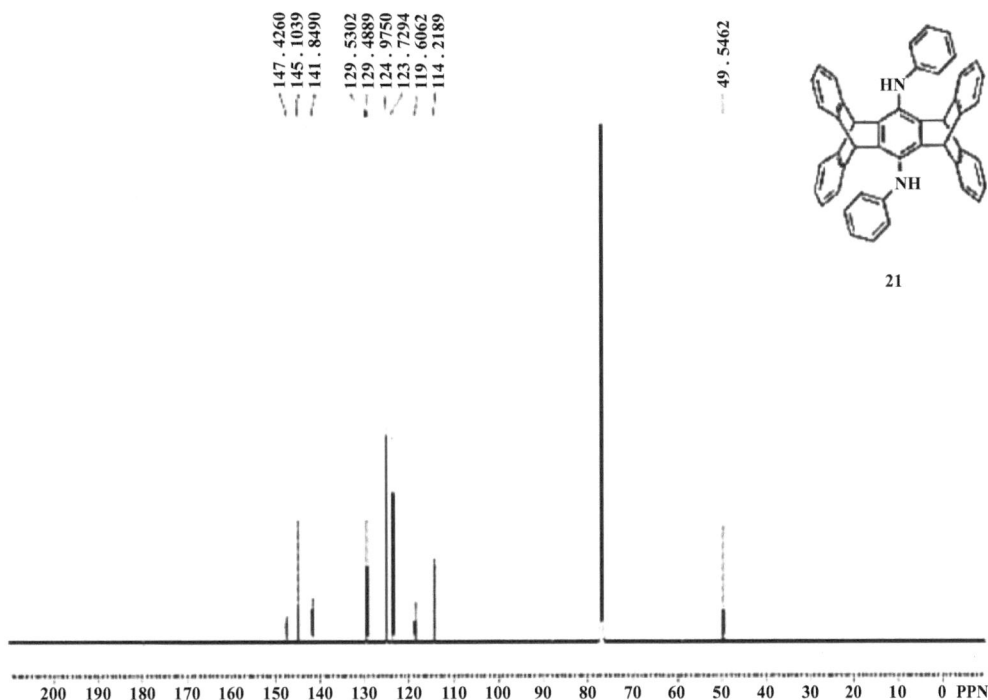

Fig. (15). ^{13}C NMR of Bis (aryl amino) pentiptycenes.

APPLICATION OF BIS (ARYL AMINO) PENTIPTYCENES

Bis (aryl amino) pentiptycenes are a fascinating class of compounds with unique structural features and potential applications in various fields due to their distinct properties. Here are some key applications and potential uses of bis (aryl amino) pentiptycenes.

Organic electronics: The rigid and extended π-conjugated system of pentiptycenes can be advantageous in organic semiconductor applications, including organic light-emitting diodes (OLEDs), organic photovoltaics (OPVs), and organic field-effect transistors (OFETs)

Molecular recognition and sensing: Bis(aryl amino) pentiptycenes can be designed to recognize specific molecules or ions, making them useful in chemical sensing applications. Their large surface area and functional groups can interact selectively with target analytes.

Catalysis: Functionalized bis (aryl amino) pentiptycenes can act as ligands for metal catalysts, enhancing the efficiency and selectivity of catalytic processes.

PENTIPTYCENES USED IN MEDICINAL CHEMISTRY AS NDDS:

The unique structure of pentiptycenes can be exploited to develop novel drug delivery systems that improve the solubility, stability, and targeting of therapeutic agents.

One more issue is discussed in the Journal of Synthesis where they claimed that Cu(OAc)$_2$-catalyzed [4+2] annulation of N-substituted pyrrole-2-carbonitriles with quinones leads to the formation of quinone-8-aminoindolizine hybrids (Fig. **16**). This is achieved through a cascade reaction involving intermolecular Michael addition, thorpe–Ziegler type cyclization, and aromatization. These quinone amino indolizine derivatives revealed significant anticancer effects [7].

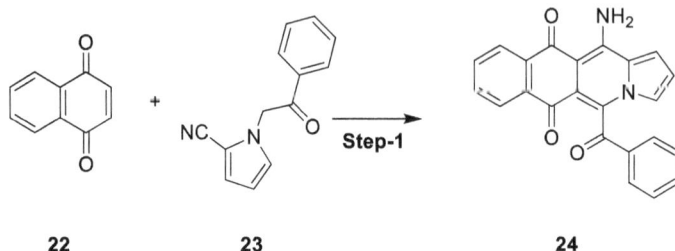

22   **23**   **24**

Fig. (16). Synthesis of quinone-8-aminoindolizine hybrids.

The synthesis can be attributed to naphthoquinone, 3-(1-Benzyl-1H-imidaol-4-yl)-2-phenylacrylonitrile, in equimolar amounts. Copper (II) acetate (5-10 mol%) and the Lewis acid are added to the flask. Acetonitrile is added to the flask to dissolve the reagents, and the reaction vessel is purged with nitrogen to create an inert atmosphere. The reaction mixture is heated to a reflux temperature and stirred continuously. The reaction progress is monitored by TLC.

SOME OTHER APPLICATIONS OF QUINONES

Anticancer agents: Compounds with quinoline and indole structures are known for their anticancer properties. The structure, with its multiple carbonyl groups and aromatic rings, could interact with various biological targets, potentially inhibiting the growth of cancer cells [20, 21, 23].

Antimicrobial agents: Quinoline derivatives are often used in antimicrobial applications. The presence of additional functional groups like carbonyls and the indole moiety could enhance antimicrobial activity against a range of bacterial and fungal pathogens [22].

USED IN ORGANIC CHEMISTRY SYNTHESIS

Regioselective synthesis of 5-substituted-1,4-benzodiazepine scaffolds takes place by using p-quinone through Pictet–Spengler type cycloannulation as a high-yielding robust method for the synthesis of 5-substituted-1,4-benzodiazepine scaffolds, which represent a new molecular hybrid. In this article, the author utilized the Pictet-Spengler cycloannulation approach, so let`s discuss that first. The Pictet-Spengler reaction is a well-known chemical transformation used to synthesize tetrahydroisoquinolines and related heterocyclic compounds. It involves the cycloannulation of a β-arylethylamine with an aldehyde or ketone, followed by acid-catalyzed cyclization. Here is a detailed mechanism of the Pictet-Spengler reaction [8]:

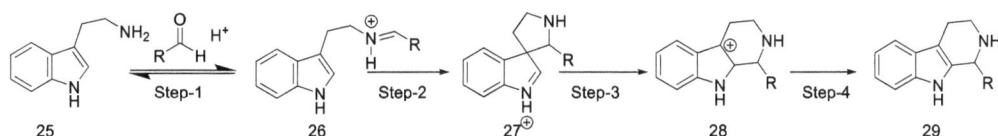

Fig. (17). Mechanism of Pictet-Spengler reaction.

MECHANISM OF THE SYNTHESIS

The mechanism of the synthesis includes [8]:

Imine formation: β-arylethylamine reacts with an aldehyde or ketone to form an imine (Schiff base). This is typically an equilibrium process.

Protonation of the imine: The imine nitrogen is protonated under acidic conditions, making it more electrophilic.

Cyclization: The aryl ring undergoes an electrophilic aromatic substitution (EAS) with the iminium ion. The electron-rich aromatic ring attacks the iminium carbon, forming a new C-C bond and resulting in a tetrahydroisoquinoline intermediate.

Deprotonation: The intermediate loses a proton, resulting in the formation of the final tetrahydroisoquinoline product.

The conversion starts from a bromo-p-quinone conjugate reacting with aniline to form 2-azide-3-arylamino-p-quinone. This intermediate is then reduced by sodium borohydride to yield 2-amino-3-arylamino-p-quinone. Subsequently, this compound is treated with an aldehyde and $InCl_3$ through a Pictet-Spengler type cycloannulation to obtain the final product (synthesis in Fig. **18**).

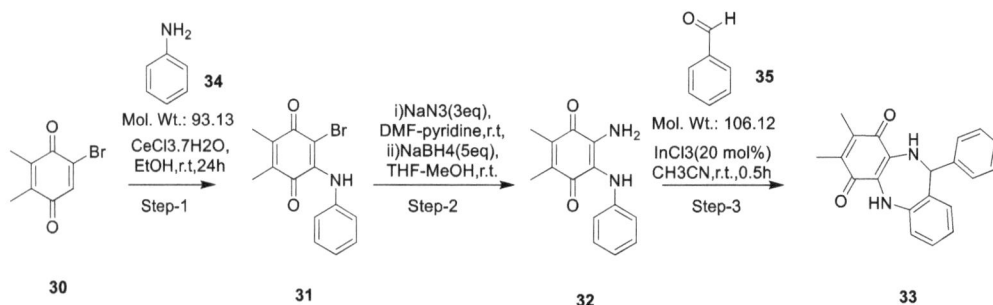

Fig. (18). Synthesis of 5-substituted-1,4-benzodiazepine scaffolds using p-quinone.

CONCLUSION

Quinones' unique redox activity, due to the ability to reversibly accept and donate electrons, makes them valuable in various applications across different fields.

In this chapter, we covered all the fields where quinones exhibit their unique role: Energy storage and conversion, biological systems, medicinal chemistry (as anticancer agent and antibiotic), organic synthesis (use as catalysts and reagents), and environmental applications (pollutant degradation).

Quinones exhibit their anticancer activity through multiple mechanisms, including redox cycling and ROS generation, DNA alkylation and cross-linking, inhibition of topoisomerases, modulation of signal transduction pathways, and epigenetic modifications. These diverse mechanisms make quinones potent and versatile agents in cancer therapy. However, their use is also associated with potential toxicity, particularly due to their ability to generate ROS, which can affect normal cells. Therefore, the therapeutic application of quinones requires careful consideration of their dosing and delivery to minimize side effects. These recent studies illustrate the versatility and potential of quinone derivatives in addressing critical challenges in energy, environment, and health. The ongoing research and development of these compounds are likely to yield even more innovative applications in the future.

REFERENCES

[1]   Quinone derivatives, pharmaceutical compositions, and use there off. WO2009042544A1.

[2]   Quinones-enhanced humification in food waste composting: A novel strategy for hazard mitigation and nitro genretention. Environmental 2024; 349
[http://dx.doi.org/10.1016/j.envpol.2024.123953]

[3]   Zhang P, Gan X, Huang L, *et al.* Facile Synthesis of Diazaanthraquinone Dimers as High-Capacity Organic Cathode Materials for Rechargeable Lithium Batteries. ACS Appl Mater Interfaces 2024; 16(12): 14929-39.
[http://dx.doi.org/10.1021/acsami.4c00586] [PMID: 38483071]

[4]   Kichishima S, Funayama N, Tamiaki H. Synthesis of chlorophyll–quinone conjugates by Diels–Alder

reaction and their fluorescence quenching by intramolecular electron transfer. Dyes Pigments 2024; 227(August): 112193.
[http://dx.doi.org/10.1016/j.dyepig.2024.112193]

[5]   Quinone scaffolds as potential therapeutic anticancer agents: Chemistry, mechanism of Actions, Structure-Activity relationships and future perspectives. Result in Chemistry 2024; 101432.
[http://dx.doi.org/10.1016/j.rechem.2024.101432]

[6]   One-Pot Synthesis of Bis (aryl amino) pentiptycenes by TiCl4-DABCO Assisted Reductive Amination of Pentiptycene Quinone. Organic Letter 2024; 26(17, 3): 3547-51.
[http://dx.doi.org/10.1021/acs.orglett.4c00939]

[7]   Lee S, Lee Y, Namkung W, Kim I. Access to 8-Aminoindolizine Fused with Quinone *via* Cu(OAc)2-Catalyzed Domino [4+2] Annulation. Synthesis 2024; 56(11): 1799-806.
[http://dx.doi.org/10.1055/a-2259-3283]

[8]   High-yielding regioselective synthesis of p-quinone fused 5-substituted-1,4-benzodiazepine scaffolds via Pictet–Spengler type cycloannulation New J Chem 2024. Advance Article. HTTPs.

[9]   Naturally Occurring Anthraquinones: Chemistry and Therapeutic Potential in AutoimmuneDiabetes. 2015.
[http://dx.doi.org/10.1155/2015/357357]

[10]   Perspectives on Medicinal Properties of Benzoquinone Compounds 2010; 10(5): 436-54.
[http://dx.doi.org/10.2174/138955710791330909]

[11]   El-Najjar N, Gali-Muhtasib H, Ketola RA, Vuorela P, Urtti A, Vuorela H. The chemical and biological activities of quinones: overview and implications in analytical detection. Phytochem Rev 2011; 10(3): 353-70.
[http://dx.doi.org/10.1007/s11101-011-9209-1]

[12]   Anthraquinone derivative C10 inhibits proliferation and cell cycle progression in colon cancer cells *via* the Jak2/Stat3 signalling pathway. Toxicol Appl Pharmacol 2021; 418: 1.115481.doi. org/10.1016/j.taap.2021.115481

[13]   Zhao B, Yang Y, Wang X, *et al.* Redox-active quinones induces genome-wide DNA methylation changes by an iron-mediated and Tet-dependent mechanism. Nucleic Acids Res 2014; 42(3): 1593-605.
[http://dx.doi.org/10.1093/nar/gkt1090] [PMID: 24214992]

[14]   NAD(P)H quinone oxidoreductase (NQO1): an enzyme which needs just enough mobility, in just the right places Biosci Rep 2019; 31(39(1))
[http://dx.doi.org/10.1042/BSR20180459]

[15]   Cenas N, Nivinskas H, Anusevicius Z, Sarlauskas J, Lederer F, Arnér ESJ. Interactions of quinones with thioredoxin reductase: a challenge to the antioxidant role of the mammalian selenoprotein. J Biol Chem 2004; 279(4): 2583-92.
[http://dx.doi.org/10.1074/jbc.M310292200] [PMID: 14604985]

[16]   Li J, Lu D, Wang J, Liu G. Synthesis and characterization of a chlorin–quinone conjugate as a potential probe for mitochondrial imaging. Tetrahedron Lett 2019; 60(23): 1567-70.
[http://dx.doi.org/10.1016/j.tetlet.2019.04.036]

[17]   Liu G, Li J, Lu D, Zhang H. Synthesis, characterization and photophysical properties of a chlorin–quinone conjugate. Dyes Pigments 2017; 144: 412-7.
[http://dx.doi.org/10.1016/j.dyepig.2017.05.030]

[18]   Sakaguchi S, Takahashi K, Okada T. Synthesis and photophysical properties of boron-dipyrromethene-flavin and chlorin-quinone dyads. Org Biomol Chem 2018; 16(38): 7012-8.
[http://dx.doi.org/10.1039/c8ob01956j] [PMID: 30232498]

[19]   Albers L, Hudhomme P, Barsu C, Ruppert R, Weiss J. Impact of the Nature of the Diene on the Formation of Chlorin-Quinone Adducts from Cycloadditions of Chlorins with Quinones. Eur J Org

Chem 2009; 2009(21): 3629-38.
[http://dx.doi.org/10.1002/ejoc.200900274]

[20]   Park SJ, Yoon SH, Kim SB. Quinone-based anticancer agents: an update. Arch Pharm Res 2014; 37(8): 893-903.
[http://dx.doi.org/10.1007/s12272-014-0408-9]

[21]   Kim YJ, Lim HS, Lee JW. Quinone-Based Anticancer Agents: 1,4-Benzoquinone as a Prominent Core Scaffold in Anticancer Drug Discovery. Molecules 2019; 24(13): 2475.
[http://dx.doi.org/10.3390/molecules24132475] [PMID: 31284478]

[22]   Pezzani R, Salehi B, Vitalini S, Iriti M, Zuniga FA, Sharifi-Rad J. Anti-inflammatory and Antioxidant Potential of Plants in Cancer Prevention and Treatment. Int J Mol Sci 2019; 20(20): 4981.
[http://dx.doi.org/10.3390/ijms20204981] [PMID: 31600949]

[23]   Sudhakar K, Nazeer N, Al-Dhabi NA. Quinone-based chemotherapeutic agents: A comprehensive review from benzoquinones to quinone hybrids. Eur J Med Chem 2020; 207: 112798.
[http://dx.doi.org/10.1016/j.ejmech.2020.112798]

SUBJECT INDEX

www.ingramcontent.com/pod-product-compliance
Lightning Source LLC
Chambersburg PA
CBHW050820220326
41598CB00006B/273